D0026749

Richard E. Miller, EdD

Epidemiology
for Health Promotion
and Disease Prevention
Professionals

Pre-publication
REVIEWS,
COMMENTARIES,
EVALUATIONS . . .

"For the field of health promotion to advance, practitioners will have to better integrate themselves within the medical care system. Epidemiology represents the science of this system and thus the gateway into understanding how it functions. *Epidemiology for Health Promotion and Disease Prevention Professionals* represents, perhaps, the only text that presents this information from the perspective of the health promotion field. It is an ideal forum for both professionals and students to understand the concepts important to the underpinnings of medicine and the medical care system. There are many useful sections, but the chapter 'Epidemiology and Programs' may be most relevant because of how it positions health promotion appropriately into the disease management process. From an instructor's perspective, the glossary of terms, list of Web sites, test questions, and references to Healthy People 2010 objectives are valuable complements to the material presented. Richard Miller should be commended for developing a much-needed resource for the profession."

Thomas Golaszewski, EdD
Associate Professor,
Department of Health Science,
State University of New York
College at Brockport

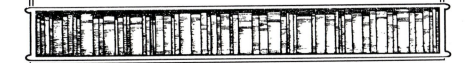

The Haworth Press®
New York • London • Oxford

Epidemiology for Health Promotion and Disease Prevention Professionals

Epidemiology for Health Promotion and Disease Prevention Professionals

Richard E. Miller, EdD

The Haworth Press®
New York • London • Oxford

The Haworth Press, Inc., 10 Alice Street, Binghamton, NY 13904-1580.

Cover design by Jennifer M. Gaska.

Library of Congress Cataloging-in-Publication Data

Miller, Richard E., EdD.
  Epidemiology for health promotion and disease prevention professionals / Richard E. Miller.
    p. cm.
  Includes bibliographical references and index.
  ISBN 0-7890-1598-6 (hard : alk. paper)—ISBN 0-7890-1599-4 (soft : alk. paper)
  1. Epidemiology. 2. Health promotion. I. Title.
  [DNLM: 1. Epidemiology. 2. Primary Prevention. WA 105 M649e 2002]
RA652 .M554 2002
614.4—dc21
                                                                                      2002068631

CONTENTS

ABOUT THE AUTHOR

Richard Miller, EdD, is an associate professor of health education in the Health, Fitness, and Recreation Resources Department at George Mason University in Fairfax, Virginia. Dr. Miller instructs undergraduate courses in the Health, Fitness, and Recreation Resources and BSEd Physical Education programs as well as graduate courses in the Master of Exercise, Fitness, and Health Promotion program. Prior to coming to GMU in 1989, he held corporate and occupational health management positions at Xerox and the University of Rochester Medical Center in Rochester, New York.

Preface

Epidemiology for Health Promotion and Disease Prevention Professionals is aimed at present and future health promotion and disease prevention professionals, and seeks to encourage them to incorporate epidemiology into their health care practices. Epidemiology is a science customarily studied by professionals in public health, medicine, nursing, health science, environmental health, and allied health fields. Emerging from these professions are epidemiologists who investigate the occurrence of diseases and other morbid conditions, which oftentimes results in improved health promotion and disease prevention practices. Therefore, in an effort to better understand its role in health promotion and disease prevention, professionals in health education and communication, fitness and sports medicine, health counseling, and assistance should also study epidemiology.

Health promotion and disease prevention professionals play collaborative roles in epidemiological activity. They participate on health care teams recruited during investigations or research studies. These professionals are consumers of epidemiological findings, meaning they are expected to be familiar with current developments established through epidemiological activity, as well as be able to provide information and research findings. During client services, they deliver sound advice and instruction based on epidemiological surveillance, investigations, and studies.

This textbook's goal is to be used by health promotion and disease prevention professionals. Whereas epidemiology can be presented in technical form for aspiring "disease detectives," it should also be applicable to those who practice everyday health promotion and disease prevention. Although the content is in-depth, numerous examples have health promotion and disease prevention implications. Chapter activities consist of knowledge tests on Healthy People 2010 (2000) focus areas. As a national health policy, Healthy People 2010 has organized its agenda into twenty-eight focus areas. Web site resources connect readers to relevant developments in the field. All said, readers are invited to learn more about epidemiology, the underlying science of their professional practice.

Acknowledgments

This text began as a good idea that evolved into a massive undertaking. Many persons helped along the way. My family tolerated my professional obsession; my colleagues offered their encouragement; and my students assessed the material for relevance and readability. I am grateful to the academic and marketing reviewers, especially Thomas J. Golaszewski, EdD, SUNY College at Brockport. He provided valuable input regarding the content of this book. I appreciate the many undergraduate and graduate students in several of my courses at George Mason University from whom I learned so much as I instructed epidemiology's application to health promotion and disease prevention.

Chapter 1

Introduction to Epidemiology

Epidemiology is an applied science and is fundamental to health promotion and disease prevention activity. Its concepts, theories, and methodologies are derived from other disciplines and put to use during epidemiological investigations and studies (Stone et al., 1996). Customarily, professionals in public health, medicine, nursing, health science, environmental health, and the allied health fields study epidemiology. They emerge as epidemiologists who investigate and control the occurrence of diseases and other health-affecting conditions. Many have earned master's degrees in public health and received additional training in epidemic intelligence services. They have been assigned the moniker "disease detectives" and are dramatically portrayed in the media. Realistically, many epidemiologists are community health nurses responding to local disease outbreaks, infection control specialists maintaining health care standards, environmental health managers monitoring the quality of living conditions, etc. Epidemiologists can be investigators, researchers, clinicians, and even public policymakers. They wrest diseases, protect the public, and promote the health of communities.

All professionals who promote health and prevent disease should study and incorporate epidemiology into their work. This includes professionals not commonly associated with epidemiological practice such as health and patient educators, fitness and exercise science specialists, athletic and personal trainers, and other specializations. Operating at all levels of prevention, these professionals respond to health promotion and disease prevention needs through instruction, training, advice, care, and programming. During service delivery, it is likely that health promotion and disease prevention professionals will interact with epidemiologists. More so, health promotion and disease prevention professionals will communicate and collaborate with health care professionals who rely on a common body of knowledge established through epidemiological investigations and studies. Therefore, it behooves health promotion and disease prevention professionals to know and to be able to apply epidemiological concepts in their activities.

WHAT IS EPIDEMIOLOGY?

What is **epidemiology**? The term is derived from Greek words *epi* and *demos,* which literally mean "on or upon the people." The definition of epidemiology can vary based on one's branch of knowledge or teaching. For example, a biological definition might be "the study of the distribution of a disease or physiological condition in human populations and of the factors that influence this distribution" (Lilienfeld and Stolley, 1994, p. 4). A nursing care professional might define it as "the study of how various states of health are distributed in the population and what environmental conditions, life-styles, or other circumstances are associated with the presence or absence of disease" (Valanis, 1999, p. 3). A more pragmatic definition has been offered by professionals in the allied health fields: "Epidemiology is the study of how and why diseases are distributed in the population . . . why some get sick and some don't" (Austin and Werner, 1974, p. 4).

The International Epidemiological Association (IEA) has compiled a dictionary of epidemiological terms. Within this publication, epidemiology has been defined using a public health approach: "the study of the distribution and determinants of health related states or events in specified populations, and the application of this study to the control of health problems" (Last, 1988, p. 42). It should be noted that throughout this text, **bolded** epidemiological terminology is consistent with IEA definitions whenever possible. Related to this, terms more challenging to pronounce can be located in various online encyclopedias and dictionaries (see Web Site Resources at the end of each chapter).

For professionals in health promotion and disease prevention, epidemiology can be considered the study of the occurrence and distribution, cause and control, and prevention and treatment of diseases as well as other morbid conditions. Note that in this definition the term **diseases** refers to pathological conditions of an organism resulting from various causes and characterized by clinical signs and/or symptoms of illness. **Signs** are objective indicators of disease based on professional observation; **symptoms** are subjective interpretations of feeling ill. Later in this text, diseases will be categorized according to cause as well as signs and symptoms. Also contained in this definition of epidemiology is the term **morbid conditions,** which are any departures, subjective or objective, from physical or mental well-being. Similar to disease, morbid conditions can negatively affect a person's health status and possibly lead to death. Examples include unintentional or intentional injuries, behavioral health disorders (e.g., distress, anxiety disorders, addiction, etc.), nutritional deficiencies, and congenital conditions. For the purpose of this text, **health status** is a person's standing in terms of physical functioning, emotional well-being, daily life activity performance, and feelings of fulfillment, productivity, and social responsibility. Through health risk appraisals and other measurements, health status is considered the appraised age of an individual compared to his or her actual age. Determining personal health status is one of this chapter's activities.

WHAT IS HEALTH PROMOTION AND DISEASE PREVENTION?

During the latter part of the twentieth century, personal and public health focus shifted from treating and curing diseases to preventing them. The expression **health promotion and disease prevention** (HP/DP) can be defined as the aggregate of all purposeful activities designed to improve personal and public health (Joint Committee on Health Education Terminology, 1991, p. 103). With the acronym HP/DP (pronounced *hip-dip*) and the new goal of promotion and prevention, professionals in epidemiology, public health, health care, allied health services, health education, fitness, and so forth now had a common agenda. Contributing to the systematic body of knowledge on health promotion and disease prevention has been the effort of epidemiologists. A primary example of this is **Healthy People 2010,** a national health promotion and disease prevention initiative that brings together national, state, and local government agencies; non-profit, voluntary, and professional organizations; businesses; communities; and individuals to improve the health of all Americans, eliminate disparities in health, and improve years and quality of healthy life (Healthy People 2010, 2000). The initiative has twenty-eight focus areas:

1. Access to Quality Health Services
2. Arthritis, Osteoporosis, and Chronic Back Conditions
3. Cancer
4. Chronic Kidney Disease
5. Diabetes
6. Disability and Secondary Conditions
7. Educational and Community-Based Programs
8. Environmental Health
9. Family Planning
10. Food Safety
11. Health Communication
12. Heart Disease and Stroke
13. HIV
14. Immunization and Infectious Diseases
15. Injury and Violence Prevention
16. Maternal, Infant, and Child Health
17. Medical Product Safety
18. Mental Health and Mental Disorders
19. Nutrition and Weight Management
20. Occupational Safety and Health
21. Oral Health
22. Physical Activity and Fitness
23. Public Health Infrastructure
24. Respiratory Diseases
25. Sexually Transmitted Diseases
26. Substance Abuse
27. Tobacco Use
28. Vision and Hearing

Healthy People 2010 knowledge tests, found at the end of each chapter, address important material related to each of the twenty-eight focus areas. These tests not only acquaint the reader with Healthy People 2010 targets for improvement, but also present examples of how epidemiology is the underlying science to health promotion and disease prevention. Each test is comprised of items relevant to each objective within each focus area. For instance, focus area 1, *Access to Quality Health Services,* and focus area 2, *Arthritis, Osteoporosis, and Chronic Back Conditions,* are covered at the end of this chapter.

Health Promotion and Disease Prevention Professionals

Applying epidemiology to the work of HP/DP professionals makes sense for three reasons. First, these professionals can play collaborative roles in how epidemiology is conducted, for example, they can participate on teams recruited during epidemiological investigations or research studies. Another reason this makes sense is because HP/DP professionals rely on knowledge generated from epidemiological inquiry, meaning they are expected to be familiar with and understand current epidemiological findings. Third, HP/DP professionals are the logical conveyors of epidemiological findings. During client services, these professionals deliver sound instruction, training, and advice based on epidemiological reasoning.

Who are HP/DP professionals? They represent a range of specialists and practitioners involved in **health promotion programming,** and can provide any planned combination of educational, political, regulatory, and organizational supports for actions and living conditions conducive to the health of individuals, groups, or communities (Green and Krueter, 1999). Examples of these supports include implementing a smoke-free workplace policy, developing community walking trails, or teaching the skills of healthy meal preparation. These professionals are involved in **disease prevention programming** which centers on the continuum of care, an array of health services and settings for the prevention, diagnosis, treatment, management, and rehabilitation of disease, injury, and disability. Included are clinical preventive services (e.g., screening tests, immunizations, risk assessments, and counseling about health) as well as primary care and specialized clinical services provided by community organizations, hospitals, trauma centers, and rehabilitation and long-term care facilities (Lohr, 1998).

Who are the people promoting health and preventing disease? They are health educators, promoters, and counselors. They are exercise specialists, managers, and physiologists. They are primary, allied, and ancillary health care professionals. They work in schools and off-campus facilities, clinical and nonclinical settings, and public or private sectors. They teach, treat, and administrate. They provide services to clients, family members, and significant others. They work side by side at all levels of prevention. To get a better idea of these professionals, the reader is encouraged to visit the Web sites of professional associations listed at the end of this chapter.

HP/DP professionals are active in professional associations such as the American Public Health Association and the Society for Public Health Education. Beyond this, there are still more professional associations for those who specialize in epidemiological practice and research specifically, such as the Association for Professionals in Infection Control and Epidemiology, The Society for Epidemiologic Research, the American College of Epidemiology, and the aforementioned International Epidemiological Association. These professional associations are also listed in Web Site Resources at the end of this chapter.

Physicians and Personal Trainers Collaborate

Representatives from health and fitness professional associations and medical care institutions have recognized the increasing collaboration between physicians and personal trainers. Commenting on this was Michael Pratt, a medical epidemiologist at the U.S. Centers for Disease Control and Prevention, explaining that both parties benefit from the collaboration. Medical doctors do not always feel confident in prescribing exercise to their patients, and personal trainers want referrals from MDs as well as insurance coverage for their client services (Krucoff, 2000). It can be inferred that health promotion and disease prevention professionals must understand the same language and approach to disease as medical doctors, meaning that health and fitness professionals need to know and understand the applied science of epidemiology.

This relates to Healthy People 2010 Objective 1-7: *(Developmental) Increase the proportion of schools of medicine, schools of nursing, and other health professional training schools whose basic curriculum for health care providers includes the core competencies in health promotion and disease prevention* (Healthy People 2010, 2000, 1-24).* (See Chapter 1 activities for more information.)

---

*Page numbers formatted as in original. First number represents section, second represents page within section. This standard will continue throughout this book.

HOW IS EPIDEMIOLOGY CONDUCTED?

With the objectives of inquiring, explaining, and controlling disease and other morbid conditions, epidemiology undertakes several specific tasks. These tasks can range from characterizing populations and determining the needs of public health programs to responding to disease cases and providing direct services to individuals. Epidemiology facilitates disease prevention and health promotion. To do so, epidemiology is conducted in three basic ways: (1) surveillance, (2) investigations, and (3) studies.

Epidemiological **surveillance** is the ongoing scrutiny of a population's disease experience to detect changes in occurrence and distribution through data collection, analysis, interpretation, and reporting. Essentially, surveillance helps epidemiologists understand the occurrence and distribution of disease and other morbid conditions. An example of surveillance would be a local public health department's reporting of infectious disease cases to the state health department. Another example would be a community's vital statistics system of reporting births, deaths, marriages, and divorces. Besides examining the occurrence and distribution of morbid events in a population, epidemiological surveillance data can be used in the first effort of determining the cause or **etiology** of the disease. Surveillance is used to alert professionals to the need for investigations and subsequent studies. Surveillance is further studied in Chapter 7.

Investigations are professional responses to disease occurrence, especially greater than expected or sudden appearances known as outbreaks or epidemics. An investigation has a twofold purpose of controlling the event and preventing any further occurrences. During an investigation, the actual cause of the outbreak or epidemic is determined. Problem-solving steps to investigating disease occurrences are covered in Chapter 8.

An epidemiological **study** is research designed to determine the distribution and cause of disease and other morbid conditions. Epidemiological studies are especially useful if the disease or condition has more than one risk factor or cause. A risk factor increases the possibility of morbidity—disease or other conditions that cause illness—or mortality—death—in exposed persons. The opposite of this is a protective factor, which is any factor (e.g., healthy life practice) that decreases the possibility of morbidity or death. Studies are also used to determine the effectiveness of interventions that are meant to prevent and treat disease and other morbid conditions. Kinds of studies are covered in Chapters 9 through 12.

HOW ARE EPIDEMIOLOGICAL FINDINGS USED?

Findings from epidemiological surveillance, investigations, and studies are the bases of a systematic body of knowledge on health promotion and disease prevention. Individuals, professionals, and communities utilize this knowledge, resulting in more informed consumers, better-defined professionals, and further health-enhanced communities (see Figure 1.1).

Concerned about personal health, individuals utilize disease prevention and health promotion knowledge, and are active consumers of health information, services, and resources. An example would be a person's concern about influenza, a viral infection of the respiratory tract. Heeding epidemiological surveillance alerts during the "flu season," the individual wonders about personal susceptibility to the disease. He or she takes an interest in media reports about the effectiveness and side effects of the flu vaccine. The individual may make an appointment with his or her personal health care provider (Barrett, 2000). As another example, an individual contemplates what he or she has read recently about hepatitis C, a blood/body fluid-borne viral infection of the liver. Being a member of a private fitness center, he or she might ask the professional staff about the nature of the disease and what can be done to prevent exposure. The professional responds with sound advice based on disease prevention and health promotion knowledge and then refers the member to his or her personal health care provider.

Epidemiology ⟶ Health Promotion and Disease Prevention

• Surveillance   • Activities to improve personal and public health

• Investigations

• Studies

FIGURE 1.1. Epidemiology relationship to health promotion and disease prevention

Professionals also utilize disease prevention and health promotion knowledge. Whether an epidemiologist or another health care specialist, this knowledge helps to define which services the professional is able to provide. One way an epidemiologist self-defines is through his or her research. Epidemiological research is distinguishable from research performed in other disciplines in that the dependent variable is either a disease or morbid condition affecting health status, whereas the independent variable is a suspected, or probable, cause. For example, an epidemiologist would rely on existing evidence of physical inactivity's relationship to health. Then, he or she would devise a study to determine whether regular walking in women decreased the incidence of cardiovascular disease, a category of chronic disease involving the pathology of the heart organ and its network of blood vessels. On the other hand, an exercise physiologist would be more intent upon studying the effects of regular walking on specific indicators of physical fitness such as oxygen uptake and recovery heart rate. In yet another example, the certified health education specialist is expected to undertake health needs assessments. Data for such assessments are provided by epidemiologists and are available from public health agencies. The needs assessment is a starting point from which a health educator plans, implements, and evaluates programs (National Commission for Health Education Credentialing, 2000). None of this could take place unless epidemiological activity fueled the ever-increasing body of disease prevention and health promotion knowledge.

The community also utilizes health promotion and disease prevention information. As a whole, the efforts of epidemiologists, health promotion and disease prevention professionals and other related specialists will ultimately improve the population's health status and quality of living. A primary example is the Healthy People 2010 initiative (Healthy People 2010, 2000). As previously noted, advocates from public and private sectors, representatives from all levels of government, and professionals in school and nonschool settings have come together to address twenty-eight focus areas of health concern and interest. Each focus area is linked to measurable and achievable objectives that have been composed from epidemiological findings derived from surveillance, investigations, and studies. This chapter highlights the first two focus areas in the chapter activities section. The goal of focus area 1, *Access to Quality Health Services,* is improvement of access to appropriate preventive care while addressing patient, provider, and system of care barriers. The goal of *Arthritis, Osteoporosis, and Chronic Back Conditions* is the prevention of these diseases and morbid conditions.

Osteoporosis and Physical Activity

Epidemiologists and other researchers have studied osteoporosis, a skeletal disease characterized by a reduction of bone mass and a deterioration of the microarchitecture of the bone leading to bone fragility, and how it can be prevented. Although osteoporosis occurs in both genders, females are at greater risk of developing this disease. Physical activity can increase bone mineral density and reduce bone loss in females throughout their lifecycle. In particular, weight-bearing exercises (e.g., walking, tennis, dance) and resistance training (weight lifting or calisthenics for muscle strength and endurance) act as key strategies along with adequate daily calcium and vitamin D intake for preventing and treating osteoporosis. In addition, perimenopausal and menopausal women might be prescribed therapy with estrogen, alendronate, or calcitonin. Safety precautions to prevent falls will also be urged. Physical activity along with the other strategies are important because women's bone mass decreases about 1 percent annually after age forty and throughout menopause. After menopause, however, estrogen declines and bone integrity is compromised markedly for about ten years before leveling off. On the average, most women lose about 15 percent of bone mass within five years after menopause. Nevertheless, women can lose as much as 40 percent of bone mass if they become significantly inactive such as during extended periods of bed rest. Whereas physicians and other clinical health care providers are prepared to screen, diagnose, and treat osteoporosis, health promotion and disease prevention professionals can play a crucial prevention role through instructional and activity programming (Katz and Sherman, 1998).

This relates to Healthy People 2010 Objective 2-9: *Reduction in the proportion of adults with osteoporosis* (Healthy People 2010, 2000, 2-3). (See Chapter 1 activities for more information.)

SUMMARY

Epidemiology can be applied by professionals in health promotion and disease prevention. These professionals rely on findings generated from epidemiological surveillance, investigations, and studies. Although epidemiology has varying definitions, for the purpose of this text it is defined as the study of the occurrence and distribution, cause and control, treatment and prevention of diseases and other morbid conditions. A primary example of health promotion and disease prevention is Healthy People 2010, which is composed of focus areas and objectives. Health promotion and disease prevention (HP/DP) professionals include health educators and promoters, fitness leaders, exercise scientists, sports medicine specialists, athletic and personal trainers, and specialists in health science. Health promotion and disease prevention professionals as well as epidemiologists have their respective professional associations. Epidemiological activity includes surveillance of the occurrence and distribution of diseases and other morbid conditions; investigations to determine etiology and to control diseases and other conditions; and studies to ascertain treatments and prevention strategies. Epidemiological activity yields health promotion and disease prevention knowledge that individuals, professionals, and the community can utilize.

REVIEW QUESTIONS

1. How is epidemiology an applied science? Who studies epidemiology and how does one become an epidemiologist?
2. Who are health promotion and disease prevention professionals and why should they study epidemiology?
3. What is the relationship between epidemiology and health promotion and disease prevention activity?
4. Do you know the various definitions of epidemiology, especially the one most relevant to health promotion and disease prevention professionals?
5. Do you know the definitions of the important terms in bold print throughout this chapter?
6. What is health promotion and disease prevention? Healthy People 2010? Can you identify the twenty-eight focus areas of Healthy People 2010?
7. Epidemiology should be applied by health promotion and disease prevention professionals for three reasons. What are they? Do you know the respective professional associations for health promotion and disease prevention professionals? For epidemiologists?
8. What are the objectives and tasks of epidemiology? How is epidemiology conducted through surveillance, investigations,

and studies? The ways epidemiology is conducted correspond well with the definition of epidemiology—please explain.

9. How do individuals, professionals, and communities use epidemiological findings? How would a health and fitness professional direct health promotion and disease prevention activity toward clients? How is epidemiological research distinctive from research in the health and fitness area such as exercise physiology? How does the community rely on Healthy People 2010 as a way to improve its health status and quality of living?

10. Do you know the answers to the following chapter activity questions based on objectives from Healthy People 2010 focus areas 1 and 2?

WEB SITE RESOURCES

Professional Associations

Aerobics and Fitness Association of America
15250 Ventura Blvd, Suite 200
Sherman Oaks, CA 91403
<http://www.afaa.com>

American Association for Health Education
1900 Association Drive
Reston, VA 22091
<http://www.aahperd.org/aahe/template.cfm>

American College of Epidemiology
1500 Sunday Drive, Suite 102
Raleigh, NC 27607
<http://www.acepidemiology.org/>

American College of Sports Medicine
401 W. Michigan St
Indianapolis, IN 46202-3233
<http://www.acsm.org>

American Council on Exercise
4851 Paramount Drive
San Diego, CA 92123
<http://www.acefitness.org>

American Public Health Association
800 I Street Northwest
Washington, DC 20001-3710
<http://www.apha.org/>

American School Health Association
P.O. Box 708
Kent, Ohio 44240
<http://www.ashaweb.org/>

Association of Professionals in Infection Control and Epidemiology
1275 K Street Northwest Suite 1000
Washington, DC 20005-4006
<http://www.apic.org/>

National Athletic Training Association
2952 Stemmons Freeway
Dallas TX, 75247-6196
<http://www.nata.org/>

National Strength and Conditioning Association
1955 North Union Blvd.
Colorado Springs, CO 80909
<http://www.nsca-lift.org>

National Strength Professionals Association
110 West Timonium Road
Timonium, MD 21113
<http://www.nspainc.com>

National Wellness Institute
1300 College Ct.
PO Box 827
Stevens Point, WI 54481-0827
<http://www.nationalwellness.org/>

Society for Epidemiological Research
P. O. Box 64655
Baltimore, MD 21264-4655
<http://www.jhsph.edu/Publications/JEPI/ser.htm>

Society for Public Health Education
750 First St Northeast #910
Washington, DC 20002-4242
<http://www.sophe.org>

Terminology

Encyclopedia Britannica
<http://www.britannica.com/>

Encyclopedia Smithsonian
<http://www.si.edu/resource/faq/start.htm>

Free Internet Encyclopedia
<http://www.cam-info.net/enc.html>

Healthy People 2010
Healthy People 2010: Objectives for improving health
<http://www.health.gov/healthypeople/>

REFERENCES

Austin, D.F. and Werner, S.B. (1974). *Epidemiology for the health sciences.* Springfield, IL: Charles C Thomas Publisher.

Barrett, E. (Ed.) (2000). Prevention and control of influenza: Recommendations of the Advisory Committee on Immunization Practices. *Epidemiology Bulletin* 100(8): 1-9.

Green, L.W. and Kreuter, M.W. (1999). *Health promotion planning: An educational and ecological approach* (Third edition). Mountain View, CA: Mayfield Publishing Company.

Healthy People 2010 (2000). Healthy People 2010: Objectives for improving health. Washington, DC: Office of Disease Prevention and Health Promotion, U.S. Department of Health and Human Services.

Joint Commission on Health Education Terminology (1991). Report of the 1990 Joint Commission on Health Education Terminology. *Journal of Health Education* 22(2): 103.

Katz, W.A. and Sherman, C. (1998). Osteoporosis. *The Physician and Sports-medicine* 26(2): 33-42.

Krucoff, C. (2000). Rx: Consult a personal trainer, new breed of exercise specialists aids people with medical conditions. *Washington Post,* October 31.

Last, J.M. (1988). *A dictionary of epidemiology.* New York: Oxford University Press.

Lilienfeld, D.E. and Stolley, P.D. (1994). *Foundations of epidemiology* (Second edition). New York: Oxford Press.

Lohr, K.N. (Ed.) (1998). *Medicare: A strategy for quality assurance.* Institute of Medicine, Washington, DC: National Academy Press.

National Commission for Health Education Credentialing (2000). Certified Health Education Specialists' Responsibilities and Competencies. Allentown, PA. Accessed online: <http://www.nchec.org/>.

Stone, D.B., Armstrong, W.R., Macrina, D.M., and Pankau, J.W. (1996). *Introduction to epidemiology.* Madison, WI: Brown & Benchmark.

Valanis, B. (1999). *Epidemiology in nursing and health care* (Third edition). Norwalk, CT: Appleton & Lange.

Purpose: (1) to acquaint the reader with Healthy People 2010 targets for improvement and (2) present examples of epidemiology as the underlying science to health promotion and disease prevention.

Directions: Check out your knowledge of these Healthy People 2010 focus areas by taking the following tests (answers follow in a separate section).

FOCUS AREA 1:
ACCESS TO QUALITY HEALTH SERVICES

The goal of this focus area is to improve access to appropriate preventive care, which requires addressing many barriers, including those involving the patient, provider, and system of care.

Clinical Preventive Care

1-1.   *Increase in the proportion of persons with health insurance.* Presently, about 83 percent of persons under age sixty-five are covered by health insurance. The 2010 target would be what percent of the under-sixty-five age group?
a. 83
b. 88
c. 93
d. 100

1-2.   *Increase the proportion of insured persons with coverage for clinical preventive services (developmental objective).* If this is so, what are these services?
a. Adult physical examinations
b. Well-child care (including immunizations)
c. Preventive screening tests such as mammograms
d. All of the above

1-3.   *Increase in the proportion of persons (adults aged eighteen years and older) appropriately counseled about health behaviors.* An example of such a health behavior would be:
a. Physical activity or exercise
b. Diet and nutrition
c. Smoking cessation
d. All of the above

Primary Care

1-4.   *Increase in the proportion of persons who have a specific source of ongoing care.* As of 1998, what proportion of persons in the Unites States did not have a usual heath care source?
a. 5 percent
b. 15 percent
c. 25 percent
d. 35 percent

1-5.   *Increase in the proportion of persons with a usual primary care provider.* As of 1996, what proportion of persons had a usual primary care provider?
a. 75 percent
b. 80 percent
c. 85 percent
d. 90 percent

1-6.   *Reduction of the proportion of families that experience difficulties or delays in obtaining health care or do not receive needed care for one or more family members.* As of 1996, about 12 percent of families experienced difficulties or delays in obtaining health care or did not receive needed care. This number is intended to be reduced to
a. 1 percent
b. 4 percent
c. 7 percent
d. 10 percent

1-7.   *Increase in the proportion of schools of medicine, schools of nursing, and other health professional training schools whose basic curriculum for health care providers includes the core competencies in health promotion and disease pre-*

vention (developmental objective). Which is an example of a
HP/DP competency to be addressed in the curriculum?
a. Environmental health hazards
b. Asthma management
c. Responding to natural and man-made disasters
d. All of the above

1-8.   *Increase in the proportion of all degrees awarded to members
of underrepresented racial and ethnic groups in the health
professions, in allied and associated health profession fields,
and in the nursing field.* If members of underrepresented racial or ethnic groups make up about 25 percent of the U.S.
population, their representation among health professionals
is in the range of:
a. 5 percent
b. 10 percent
c. 15 percent
d. 20 percent

1-9.   *Reduction in hospitalization rates for three ambulatory-care-
sensitive conditions—pediatric asthma, uncontrolled diabetes, and immunization-preventable pneumonia and influenza.*
Why have these three diseases been targeted for a 25 percent
reduction in hospitalization rates?
a. The three diseases are common problems encountered in
primary care and allow for monitoring of hospitalization
rates.
b. For each of these conditions, interventions can reduce hospitalization rates as well as long-term morbidity and possible mortality.
c. These three conditions have been chosen because coordination of community preventive services, public health interventions, clinical preventive services, and primary care
can reduce levels of these illnesses.
d. All of the above are true.

Emergency Services

1-10.   *Reduction in the proportion of persons who delay or have difficulty in getting emergency medical care (developmental ob-*

jective). To accomplish this objective, all of the following barriers have to be overcome except:
a. Lack of legislation guaranteeing access to emergency medical care
b. Psychocultural factors might keep some persons, even if insured, from seeking prompt care
c. Financial considerations might inhibit some persons, even if insured, from seeking prompt care
d. Limitations in number, location, or capability of emergency department might be apparent in certain geographic places

1-11. *Increase in the proportion of persons who have access to rapidly responding prehospital emergency medical services (developmental objective)*. One indicator of accomplishing this objective would be an interval of less than:
a. five minutes from placing emergency call until arrival at an urban scene for at least 90 percent of first-responder EMS
b. eight minutes from placing emergency call until arrival at an urban scene for at least 90 percent of transporting EMS
c. ten minutes from placing emergency call until arrival at a rural scene for at least 80 percent of EMS responses
d. All of the above

1-12. *Establishment of a single toll-free telephone number for access to poison control centers on a twenty-four-hour basis throughout the United States.* As of 1999, what percent of poison control centers shared the same toll-free telephone number?
a. 10 percent
b. 15 percent
c. 20 percent
d. 25 percent

1-13. *Increase in the number of tribes, states, and the District of Columbia with trauma care systems that maximize survival and functional outcomes of trauma patients and help prevent injuries from occurring.* As of 1998, how many states had a trauma care system?
a. Five
b. Ten

    c. Fifteen
    d. Twenty

1-14. *Increase in the number of states and the District of Columbia that have implemented guidelines for prehospital and hospital pediatric care.* As of 1998, how many states had such guidelines?
    a. Nine
    b. Eighteen
    c. Twenty-seven
    d. Thirty-six

Long-Term Care and Rehabilitative Services

1-15. *Increase the proportion of persons with long-term care needs who have access to the continuum of long-term care services (developmental objective).* To better understand this objective, which represents a long-term care service?
    a. Nursing home care
    b. Home health care
    c. Adult day care
    d. All of the above

1-16. *Reduction in the proportion of nursing home residents with a current diagnosis of pressure ulcers.* All of the following would more likely contribute to reaching this objective except:
    a. Increasing residents' mobility
    b. Having residents' reduce their blood pressure
    c. Improving residents' nutrition
    d. Maintaining/increasing residents' muscle mass

FOCUS AREA 2: ARTHRITIS, OSTEOPOROSIS, AND CHRONIC BACK CONDITIONS

This focus area's goal is preventing illness and disability related to arthritis and other rheumatic conditions, osteoporosis, and chronic back conditions.

Arthritis and Other Rheumatic Conditions

2-1.   *Increase in the mean number of days without severe pain among adults who have chronic joint symptoms (developmental objective).* To determine this, researchers asked persons if, during the past thirty days, for about how many days did pain make it hard for them to do usual activities such as:
a. Self-care
b. Work
c. Recreation
d. All of the above

2-2.   *Reduction in the proportion of adults with chronic joint symptoms who experience a limitation in activity due to arthritis.* As of 1997, what was the proportion of adults who experienced this limitation?
a. 27 percent
b. 37 percent
c. 47 percent
d. 57 percent

2-3.   *Reduction in the proportion of all adults with chronic joint symptoms who have difficulty in performing two or more personal care activities, thereby preserving independence.* Keeping this in mind, all of the following are correct about arthritis except:
a. Arthritis is a leading cause of difficulty in performing personal care activities.
b. Arthritis's limitation on activity directly causes persons to increase physical activity, decrease weight, and decrease their health risk.
c. Arthritis is the number one cause of activity limitations.
d. Arthritis is a leading cause of loss of independence.

2.4.   *Increase in the proportion of adults aged eighteen years and older with arthritis who seek help in coping if they experience personal and emotional problems.* Besides coping difficulties, which is another major personal or emotional problem experienced by persons with arthritis?
a. Depression
b. Anxiety

    c. Low self-efficacy
    d. All of the above

2-5.   *Increase in the employment rate among adults with arthritis in the working-aged population.* If 67 percent of adults with arthritis are currently employed, what is the target?
    a. 68 percent
    b. 78 percent
    c. 88 percent
    d. 99 percent

2-6.   *Elimination of racial disparities in the rate of total knee replacements (developmental objective).* Related to this, which of the following is correct?
    a. African Americans have much lower rates of total knee replacement than whites.
    b. Many persons are not getting needed interventions to reduce pain and disability.
    c. There are racial differences in medical care that are difficult to explain by financial or access-to-care issues.
    d. All of the above are true.

2-7.   *Increase in the proportion of adults who have seen a health care provider for their chronic joint symptoms (developmental objective).* With this objective in mind, which of the following is correct?
    a. A majority of adults have not seen a doctor for their arthritis.
    b. Arthritis is part of normal aging.
    c. Arthritis pain and disability can be reduced if health care providers encourage appropriate medical self-care, education, and physical activity for patients.
    d. Once a person develops arthritis, nothing can be done for it.

2-8.   *Increase in the proportion of persons with arthritis who have had effective, evidence-based arthritis education as an integral part of the management of their condition (developmental objective).* Related to this objective, all of the following are correct except:
    a. Educational interventions for arthritis are reaching a majority of persons with this painful and disabling condition.

    b. Educational interventions such as the Arthritis Self-Help Course are effective in reducing pain in arthritis patients as well as reducing the number of physician visits they make.

    c. Educational interventions for arthritis include information about community and self-help resources.

    d. Educational interventions for arthritis should be provided in a culturally and linguistically appropriate way.

Osteoporosis

2-9.   *Reduction in the proportion of adults with osteoporosis.* As of 1994, what was the proportion of adults with osteoporosis?
    a. 10 percent
    b. 20 percent
    c. 30 percent
    d. 40 percent

2-10.   *Reduction in the proportion of adults who are hospitalized for vertebral fractures associated with osteoporosis.* How much of a reduction in hospitalizations is intended in this objective?
    a. 10 percent
    b. 20 percent
    c. 30 percent
    d. 40 percent

Chronic Back Conditions

2-11.   *Reduction in activity limitation due to chronic back conditions.* With this in mind, who is most likely to experience lower back injury?
    a. Persons who are overweight
    b. Persons who frequently bend over or lift heavy objects
    c. Persons whose job requires repetitive lifting—bending and twisting forward
    d. All of the above

TEST ANSWERS

Focus Area 1

1-1.   (d) 100. The percent in 1997 of health insurance covered persons was 97 percent and the target for 2010 is 100 percent.*

1-2.   (d) All of the above. Although a majority of employer-sponsored health insurance plans cover these clinical preventive services, there is noticeable variability and that warrants a greater coverage for the insured. Prepaid insurance groups usually offer greater coverage than indemnity plans.

1-3.   (d) All of the above. Besides these health behaviors, counseling is recommended regarding alcohol use, safety practices, and hormonal therapy decisions. Clinical counseling should be directed at behaviors considered to be risky. Granted primary care time is limited, but epidemiologists have determined that clinical counseling is effective in getting patients to stop smoking and reduce problem drinking, and to adopt safer automobile travel practices (e.g., seat belts, child safety seat use).

1-4.   (b) 15 percent. It is important to decrease this number because persons having a usual health care source are more likely to access a variety of preventive health care services.

1-5.   (c) 85 percent. The higher the percent, the more continuity there will be in the health care delivery system. By having a primary care provider, persons will be better directed to appropriate care and rely less on unnecessary emergency care attention.

1-6.   (c) 7 percent. There are a variety of reasons that families experience difficulty in obtaining care or do not receive the care they thought they needed including lack of insurance, incorrect referrals, travel distance, lack of transportation, and other reasons. Thus, efforts are under way to decrease the proportion of families experiencing this difficulty from 12 to 7 percent of the overall population.

1-7.   (d) All of the above. This is a developmental objective of which proposed HP/DP competencies are to be considered for incorporation into premedical and medical school curric-

*Ages adjusted to the year 2000 standard population.

ula. HP/DP-enhanced curricula are also being considered for nursing, physician assistance, and allied health fields.

1-8.   (b) 10 percent. It will be necessary to increase this representation by more than onefold in most minorities and ethnicities. There are several significant reasons for this needed increase, among which are that minority health professionals are more likely to serve areas with high proportions of underrepresented racial and ethnic groups and to practice in or near designated health care shortage areas.

1-9.   (d) All of the above are true. These three diseases are representative of major age groups: children (asthma), working-age adults (diabetes), and the elderly (pneumonia and influenza). Managing asthma can reduce its ill health effects. The acute and long-term problems of diabetes can be prevented through primary care. Morbidity and mortality from pneumonia and influenza are avoidable through vaccines. To be effective, coordinated community, public, and clinical preventive services will have to be culturally competent and linguistically appropriate.

1-10.   (a) Lack of legislation guaranteeing accesses to emergency care. Actually, the Emergency Medical Treatment and Active Labor Act of 1986 specifies medical screening examination and appropriate stabilizing treatment for an emergency medical condition presented by any person to the emergency department of a medical center. This means that other reasons are standing in the way of persons accessing emergency care services when needed.

1-11.   (d) All of the above. Successful response to emergency care incidents requires prompt availability of sufficiently prepared and equipped medical care providers. To make this happen, there must be public awareness of how to engage EMS, properly prepared first responders (providers of first aid until EMS arrival), 911 connection to EMS, uniform ways for EMS to locate persons requesting assistance, reliable transportation, proper medical direction, and destination hospitals readied for EMS arrivals.

1-12.   (b) 15 percent. With over 2 million callers to poison control centers each year, it only makes sense that a single, easy-to-remember toll-free phone number would expedite persons trying to access this emergency care service. Most incidents are handled through telephone advice, thus preempting the need for more costly care at a medical center emergency department.

1-13.   (a) Five. As of 1998, only five states had a trauma care system, defined as an organized and coordinated effort in a defined geographic area to deliver the full spectrum of care to injured patients. The system's goal is to match the available trauma care resources in a community, region, territory, or state with individual patients' needs. This would ensure the patient efficient access to acute care and rehabilitative services.

1-14.   (b) Eighteen states. It is necessary for more states to have these guidelines. Pediatric emergency care is a particular challenge because prehospital providers may not routinely treat children and therefore have limited pediatric emergency care experience.

1-15.   (d) All of the above. Besides these services, others include assisted living and hospice care. Accessing all long-term care services is a challenge due to financial matters and limited services available.

1-16.   (b) Having residents reduce their blood pressure. Although this might seem like a risk reduction practice (that is, if the residents had high blood pressure to begin with), it is not relevant to the prevention and quality of care for pressure ulcers.

Focus Area 2

2-1.   (d) All of the above. Pain is prevalent among persons with arthritis leading them to prescription and over-the-counter drug use, surgery, and alternative health care approaches. By measuring days relatively pain free, research can determine health-related quality of life.

2-2.   (a) 27 percent. The objective is to reduce this to 21 percent of adults aged eighteen years and older with chronic joint symptoms that experienced activity limitation related to arthritis.

2-3.   (b) Arthritis's limitation on activity directly causes persons to increase physical activity, decrease weight, and decrease risk factors to other diseases. Actually, the activity limitations of arthritis indirectly affect a person's health and independence by decreasing physical activity, increasing weight, and placing him or her at higher health risk.

2-4.   (d) All of the above. This is a developmental objective. All are recognized as major personal and emotional problems experienced by persons with arthritis—especially among persons with physical pain. Since arthritis is a leading cause of physical pain, monitoring these mental health conditions can help to determine if physical pain interventions are working.

2-5.   (b) 78 percent. For adults with arthritis aged eighteen to twenty-four years, the target is a 10 percent increase in proportion that are employed.

2-6.   (d) All of the above. It is hard to determine why there are racial disparities in receiving this corrective surgical procedure. What it amounts to is that many persons are not receiving needed medical care intervention for pain and disability reduction.

2-7.   (c) Arthritis pain and disability can be reduced if health care providers encourage appropriate medical self-care, education, and physical activity for patients. About 16 percent of adults have not seen a doctor regarding their arthritis. One myth is that arthritis is part of normal aging and another myth is that nothing can be done for it.

2-8.   (a) Educational interventions for arthritis are reaching a majority of persons with this painful and disabling condition. Unfortunately, these interventions are reaching only about 1 percent of the intended target group. The existing evidence-based interventions represent opportunities for improving the health of persons with arthritis as well as reducing the impact of this problem nationwide.

2-9.   (a) 10 percent. About one in ten adults aged fifty years and older have osteoporosis as measured by low total femur bone mineral density. This objective has targeted a reduction to 8 percent of adults.

2-10.   (b) 20 percent. To achieve this objective, there would have to be a reduction from 15.5 to 14.0 hospitalizations per 10,000 adults aged sixty-five years and older who were hospitalized for vertebral fractures associated with osteoporosis.

2-11.   (d) All of the above. Besides these risks for lower back injury, other factors are vibration from vehicles or machinery, extended vehicular driving, certain sports activities, having osteoporosis, and age. Persons with past back problems are more likely to develop subsequent ones.

Chapter 2

Historical Perspectives

HISTORY AND EPIDEMIOLOGY

To appreciate the current practice of epidemiology, it is necessary to trace a selected review of history. It begins with a depiction of three major notions or beliefs about disease. Just as important, the roles of outstanding persons in the evolution of epidemiology are recognized and the work of twentieth-century contemporaries is honored citing landmark legislation along the way. All of this is presented according to its significance to the ever-increasing body of knowledge in health promotion and disease prevention.

Early Notions (and Potions)

Early notions or beliefs about disease took a variety of forms. Originating before recorded history, the **mystical notion** of disease refers to spiritual or mystical explanations of morbidity and mortality. Today, this belief is still held by various societies. Essentially, demons and evil spirits enter the body through spells, incantations, and devil possessions, sicken the person, and are then expelled through prayer, ritualistic practices, and potions. Someone of religious training or respect usually conducts the healing process. Without knowledge or concept of the microorganism or other hard-to-detect explanations of disease, it is understandable why people of yesteryear as well as uninformed contemporaries attribute illness and death to spiritlike forces. There remains today existing beliefs and practices of witchcraft, voodooism, sorcery, and demonic exorcism.

Another aspect of the mystical notion is the retaliatory higher power. That is, disease is the consequence of disobeying a supreme being or source of power that is worshipped in an organized religion. In many formal religions, the followers place their health status in the hands of their God. Some faiths consider disease the punishment for sinful behavior. Likewise, spiritual growth is needed before the stricken person can heal. Much of the mystical or spiritual notions about disease have been described in depth by Winslow (1943, pp. 3-52).

The **natural notion** of disease refers to the influence of naturally concurring events as explanations of illness and death. Specifically, the occurrence of disease is associated with other happenings in a person's life, erroneously concluding that an accompanying event has a causal relationship with disease. This faulty idea is based on the unrealistic powers or qualities as well as the existence of cosmic phenomena.

One interesting and long-held belief through the Middle Ages was that **miasmas,** poisonous gases assumed to emanate from swamps and putrid matter, caused disease. In fact, the disease **malaria**—a protozoan infection of the circulatory system resulting in periodic attacks of chills and fever, anemia, and an enlarged spleen, often with fatal complications—was named after swampy "bad air" believed to be the source of this infectious condition. Of course, it is now known that the female aenophiles mosquito, which inhabits still water, carries the protozoan and infects human hosts. For this reason, today's environmental health specialists realize the necessity of draining pools of standing surface water. Even so, the natural notion of miasma has been contemporarily interpreted and applied to public health efforts. Thus it is necessary to dispose of solid waste which can house microorganisms, and widely accepted is the importance of good room ventilation.

Related to the natural notion of disease causation is a compelling but erroneous belief called **spontaneous generation**. This belief holds that unhealthy environmental conditions create germs and **vermin,** rodent carriers of disease. For example, untidy living conditions spawn rodents associated with disease. It is now known that environmental conditions can act as the context, but not usually as the direct cause of most diseases.

If someone believes in natural causes of disease, he or she is bound to mythical cures for ailments. For example, if a toothache occurs because of what they believe are outside influences, a cure might be to "spit under a stone." Therefore, the cause of the disease is mistakenly attributed to a randomly concurring event or influence, and the treatment is illogically assumed to be effective. Trial and error, chance associations of events and disease occurances as well as cures all comprise the natural notion.

Over the years, many societies have ascribed **astrology,** the study of celestial body activity, with an influence on natural events and human affairs. Although there is little empirical evidence supporting astrology, it remains a highly practiced example of the natural notion.

The **scientific notion** of disease refers to biologically attributed events in the physical and social environments as causes for morbidity and mortality. This notion represents the start of **epidemiological reasoning.** Rather than inferring cause from the coincidence of two events, the epidemiological reasoner observes closely and takes into account all possible factors in the physical, social, and biological environments that might influence the disease event. Dunglison (1835) in this regard recorded preliminary efforts in his work on the influence of atmosphere and locality—changes in air and climate, seasons and other changes in the physical environment—on a person's hygiene. For example, if a person dies, there are a number of possible explanations, not just the exact correspondence of a quirky incident such as a change in the weather, the phase of the moon, or a rooster's crow. Suspected factors have to be identified and examined for their relationship to the cause of the disease and/or death. For the past 150 years, a public system for protecting health has grown and depended on both scientific discovery and social action (Institute of Medicine, 1988).

PARENTS OF EPIDEMIOLOGY

Hippocrates

Hippocrates' work dates about 400 years before the Common Era. As a Greek physician, he was probably the first person to establish a natural notion of disease, which later evolved into the scientific. **Hippocrates** has been given the title *parent of medicine.* Through direct and intense observation, he established a rational approach to disease causation and treatment. He organized his work in a collection of aphorisms, "Airs, Waters, and Places." Hippocrates was the first to posit that atoms were comprised of four basic environmental properties: hot, cold, moist, and dry. These properties influenced the human state and affected the balance of the four **humours,** or fluids, of the body: blood, phlegm (mucous), yellow bile (secretions), and black bile (excretions). Hence, healthy persons adjusted well to environment properties and experienced good humoural balance. Sick persons had too much or too little of one or more humours due to the flux of hot, cold, moist, or dry environmental properties. Medical treatment involved correcting humoural balance by purging one or more humours. Hippocrates' aphorisms were later incorporated into medical school training to which remnants are still adhered today (Salerno Society, 1966).

Although this explanation of disease might seem crude, there was in fact a medical basis to many of Hippocrates' conjectures. For example, persons have adopted the practice of "feeding a cold," believing it is important to eat well to maintain proper body temperature during times of coldlike conditions. Although the practice still exists, it is erroneous to "starve a fever," since proper nourishment is required throughout a malady. Hippocrates deserves greatest credit for discounting the notion of disease being a random occurrence or process. Rather, he established an epidemiologically sound explanation of disease, in that humoural balance was influenced by internal factors such as age, heredity, general fitness level, and external factors such as weather, soil conditions, seasons. For that, he deserves the added distinction of being called the *parent of early epidemiology.*

Hippocrates Advocated Patient Counseling

Hippocrates of Cos is best known for his clinical observations and explanations for diseases. However, he should also be recognized for his emphasis on patient counseling. He advocated that physicians educate their patients about the importance of a good bodily constitution and which health practices contributed to a proper balance of body humours (Legator, Harper, and Scott, 1985, p. 3).

This relates to Healthy People 2010 Objective 3-10: *Increase in the proportion of physicians and dentists who counsel their at-risk patients about tobacco use cessation, physical activity, and cancer screening* (Healthy People 2010, 2000, 3-22). (See Chapter 2 activities for more information.)

Galen

Galen of Pergamum, Turkey, conducted his work during the first and second centuries of the Common Era. He was heavily influenced by Hippocrates' work. A Greek physician, his understanding of disease lived well into the seventeenth century. He learned his profession from two sources: the great medical center at Alexandria, Egypt; and the Roman battlefields. Galen is considered the *parent of anatomy* since he perfected the skills of bodily dissection and surgery. However, he also spent time studying how plague, tuberculosis, and eye and skin infections were not so much of an anatomical condition as they were warnings not to associate with others having these conditions (Markel, 1997, p. 3).

His investigative work on succumbed gladiators and victims of war was demonstrated in public as well as applied to invasive means of treating disease. He was chief physician to Roman emperors. He demonstrated that arteries and veins carried blood and not air, as was the prevailing belief. Galen deserves credit for defying public opposition to the dissection of human corpses. He also made some mistakes while inferring human structure and function based on the comparative anatomy of nonhuman primates. Similar to Hippocrates, Galen believed in humoural balance in the body but went further to specify particular organs responsible for humoural production. He wrote of physical causes of illness and death until his own death at the age of eighty-seven.

Fracastoro

Girolamo Fracastoro's contributions to the study of disease took place during the fifteenth and sixteenth centuries in Venice, Italy. A physician, Fracastoro is considered the *parent of germ theory* since he proposed a germ or microbial explanation of disease three centuries before its scientific demonstration (Wain, 1970).

Fracastoro is best known for his work on **syphilis,** a bacterial sexually transmitted disease. During the Middle Ages, syphilis was **pandemic,** occurring across a wide geographic area affecting a high proportion of the population. While in the service of the Roman Catholic pope, Fracastoro presented the concept of **contagion,** which is the spread of disease through direct or indirect contact. He posited that disease was caused by specific minute bodies spread from the sick to other persons within whom the disease grew. Fracastoro's theory was in heavy competition with long-standing spiritual and mystical explanations of disease. His adamant defense of germ theory earned him the distinction of an informal derivative of his last name, fracas, meaning a noisy, disorderly fight or quarrel.

Baillou

A contemporary of Fracastoro was **Guillaume de Baillou,** recognized as the *parent of traditional epidemiology.* Throughout the late sixteenth and early seventeenth centuries, this French physician applied Hippocratic principles, or the natural notion, to disease causation. He observed and recorded the start, duration, and end of major epidemics of whooping cough, plague, measles, and diphtheria. Whooping cough, or **pertussis,** is a severe bacterial infection of the upper respiratory tract. Likewise, **diphtheria** is also a bacterial infection of the respiratory tract. **Measles** is an acute viral disease that causes rash, fever, and general discomfort. It is also believed that his work influenced the British physician Sydenham.

van Leewenhoek

Antonie van Leewenhoek's claim to fame was the invention of the microscope during the seventeenth century. By trade, he was a draper and haberdasher, but his leisure pursuit was grinding glass lenses to inspect small objects. Given this accomplishment, van Leewenhoek is given the title, *parent of microbiology,* for his invention, coupled with an emerging germ theory of disease, that helped to discount the faulty notion of spontaneous generation.

Graunt

Another important seventeenth-century figure in the study of disease was the Englishman, **John Graunt.** Although he is considered the founder of **demography,** the statistical study of human populations, Graunt should also be recognized as the *parent of vital statistics.* A merchant, he studied death records kept by municipalities, noting patterns in death statistics. He counted death cases, calculated death rates, and categorized them according to cause. He created the first death certificate. In his observations, annual death rates were higher in urban populations than they were in rural populations. Accordingly, annual death rates were higher for males than for females despite higher male birth rates, resulting in an even gender split in the adult census. Graunt is credited with devising the **life table,** which depicts age-specific survivorship, meaning he could predict the percentage of persons likely to live to their next age group, as well as their overall life expectancy, and average age of death. Graunt's methods have long been recognized for their statistical importance to public health. Perhaps his greatest contribution from his vital statistics work was the realization that mathematical analyses are useful only if the quality of the data is not suspect (Stroup and Berkelman, 1998).

Ramazzini

Bernardino Ramazzini was a seventeenth-century Italian physician and is considered the *parent of occupational medicine.* He studied diseases such as tumors resulting from exposure to irritating chemicals, dusts, metals, and other abrasive agents in several kinds of occupations. He also studied the malaria pandemic and its control through quinine derived from the cinchona bark. In fact, he was one of the first professionals in the study of morbid conditions to be concerned about repetitive motion injuries in workers. Influenced by Hippocrates and Galen, he advocated the use of purgatives in treating disease.

Ramazzini First to Observe Kidney Disease in Workers

Ramazzini was the first epidemiologist to investigate work-related physical agents and their influence on occupational health diseases and other morbid conditions. He was concerned about varicose veins occurring in workers who stood at their job for most the day. He examined different cases of **sciatica,** a painful condition of the legs due to inflammation of the sciatic nerve from musculoskeletal stress, in occupations requiring continual twisting and bending. Just as important, he was the first to observe kidney damage occurring in workers exposed to jarring motions such as couriers and others who rode excessively on bumpy, uneven roads. He found that the damage was actually located in the microvasculature of the kidney—a matter of concern for workers today (Timmreck, 1998).

This relates to Healthy People 2010 Objective 4-1: *Reduction in the rate of new cases of end-stage renal disease* (Healthy People 2010, 2000, 4-10). (See Chapter 2 activities for more information.)

Sydenham

Another notable Englishman of the seventeenth century was the physician **Thomas Sydenham.** Sometimes called the *English Hippocrates,* he was an intense observer of illness by meticulously recording details of disease. While studying water samples as well as human saliva, he spotted "animacules," which are now known as bacteria and protozoa. He is best known for his diagnostics and classification of various illnesses such as fevers. For example, he was the first to distinguish **scarlet fever,** resulting from streptococcal infection, from **measles,** caused by the rubeola virus. He also studied outbreaks of **hysteria,** a mental health disorder in which symptoms appear without an organic cause, and **St. Vitus' dance,** which he believed was a form of mass hysteria or dancing mania associated with the social stress of surviving during the time of the Black Death plague. Present-day medical specialists diagnose St. Vitus' Dance as a form of chorea, a nervous disorder marked by a lack of coordination and spasmodic movement that develops after a staphylococcal bacterial infection. Other accomplishments were Sydenham's formulation of **laudanum,** an early anesthetic comprised of alcohol and opiates, treatment of anemia through iron supplements, and using quinine in the care of malaria patients. Throughout his work, his contemporaries would not accept his exacting of diseases and epidemics. He clinically described cholera, dysentery, gout, malaria, measles, smallpox, syphilis, and tuberculosis with a notable emphasis on bedside observation (Winslow, 1943).

Lind

James Lind was a naval surgeon during the eighteenth century and is considered the *parent of naval hygiene* in England. It was his research that helped to rid **scurvy,** the nutritional deficiency of citric acid (vitamin C), from the naval arena. He performed probably the first experimental study in epidemiology when he assigned small groups of seamen different treatments for scurvy, discovering that fresh citrus fruits and lemon juice were the best remedies. The results of his research were significant, considering the great number of sailors dying from scurvy rather than from combat.

Through his observations, Lind recommended that ships be rid of lice to prevent outbreaks of **typhus,** a severe rickettsial infection causing fever, malaise, and body aches. He also recommended distilling seawater for drinking, thus reducing the risk of **dysentery,** a bacterial or protozoan-caused disease of the intestines resulting in inflammation, painful and bloody diarrhea, and dehydration (McNeill, 1976).

Snow

The mid-nineteenth century brought a surge of epidemiological advances, and one of the chief contributors was **John Snow.** Known as the *parent of modern epidemiology,* Snow is best known for investigating a series of cholera outbreaks in England between 1831 and 1866. **Cholera** is a water- or foodborne bacterial disease causing severe diarrhea, dehydration, vomiting, and cramps. Most famous was Snow's insistence that a common water source was contributing to the spread of infectious disease in the Golden Square area of London. In a symbolic determination to prevent further cases of cholera, he marched up to the Broad Street pump and removed its handle. By doing so, he prevented Londeners' access to contaminated water. He also made a statement regarding the poor quality of public health maintenance in that city.

Snow was the first to use epidemiological techniques such as **spot mapping,** marking the location of disease cases in a geographic area, and testing public water for contamination. Even more fascinating was that Snow's investigation took place before the identification of cholera bacteria was confirmed by his contemporary, Robert Koch (Karlen, 1995).

Koch

One of the primary contributors to the understanding of disease causation was Nobel prizewinner, **Robert Koch.** During the mid- to late nineteenth century, this German physician isolated the bacteria responsible for tuberculosis, cholera, and anthrax, thus earning him the designation, *parent of bacteriology.* **Tuberculosis** is a severe bacterial infection of the respiratory tract that is generally fatal unless successfully treated. **Anthrax** is a bacterial infection characterized by boillike lesions and swelling of the lymph glands.

As a surgeon, Koch built a small laboratory to study pathogenic microorganisms. Inspired by the work of his contemporaries, Koch set out to isolate and photograph these bacteria on microscope slides. He noted the life cycle of anthrax and how dried spores could survive in inhospitable conditions for years before infecting grazing livestock. Koch discovered ways to stain the tubercle bacillus (tuberculosis or TB) for better observation. He even devised a means to determine if a person had been exposed to the TB bacteria, the predecessor of today's PPD skin test. Koch also traveled to Egypt and India to successfully identify and picture cholera and amoebic dysentery microbes. Koch came near to identifying the mosquito vector to malaria, although credit for that discovery goes to British bacteriologist Ronald Ross. Probably the most important product of Koch's efforts are his *Postulates of Disease* (studied in Chapter 3), which represent fundamental principles for locating disease-causing microorganisms (Karlen, 1995).

Pasteur

From the mid- to latter nineteenth century, there were major developments in public health involving advances in scientific knowledge about the cause and prevention of numerous diseases (Institute of Medicine, 1988). One of Koch's mid-nineteenth century contemporaries was **Louis Pasteur,** a French chemist and microbiologist who is most well known for his contributions to immunizations. Thus, Pasteur has been dubbed the *parent of vaccines.* An enterprising scientist, Pasteur demonstrated that microorganisms could cause fermentation and disease. He was the first to develop vaccines for such diseases as rabies, anthrax, and various strains of cholera. **Rabies, or** *Lyssavirus,* is a highly virulent viral disease that is usually transmitted from animal to human host. He was contracted by various commercial industries essentially to save beer and wine from spoilage and to protect silkworms from invading microorganisms. On top of all that, Pasteur successfully ridded milk products of unhealthy microorganisms through a process he developed known as **pasteurization.**

Nightingale

Through most of the nineteenth century, **Florence Nightingale,** an English nurse, valiantly undertook a mission of promoting nursing as a professional practice (Unwin, Carr, and Leeson, 1997). For that, Nightingale is considered the *parent of nursing*. However, during her time she was called the "Lady of the Lamp."

Nightingale dedicated herself to training those in the nursing profession. During various British military conquests, such as the Crimean War in the Middle East, she was in charge of nursing in military hospitals where she faced deplorable conditions. She cared for patients in crowded wards amid poor sanitation and other disgraceful arrangements. Nightingale committed herself to improving the health care of the sick and injured. Whereas the physicians of that time were hostile to her improvement efforts, she answered by eradicating rat- and flea-infested hospital wards and personally cleaning up filth accumulated through inadequate sanitation. Her first requisition was 200 scrub brushes for washing the soldiers' clothing. She spent countless hours around the clock personally attending to the sick and injured. At war's end she was literally the last staff member to close down the hospital. Nightingale returned to England a national hero; however, she refused official transport home as well as any kind of public reception. After being received by Queen Victoria, she established a school of nursing, consulted with the military regarding health care conditions in India, trained midwives, and advocated for the health reform of workhouses. She accomplished all of this as an invalid lying on her couch for years. Her vision gradually diminished until her death in 1910. She received the Order of Merit—the first female to do so—and was proffered a national funeral, which was declined by her wish.

Semmelweis

Ignaz Philipp Semmelweis stands out as a pioneer in health care standards. During the early to mid-nineteenth century, Semmelweis, a Hungarian physician, determined the cause of puerperal fever. **Puerperal fever,** or childbed fever, is a systematic bacterial infection of the body. Because of his work in **antisepsis,** which is destruction of disease-causing microorganisms to prevent infection, Semmelweis is known as the *parent of infection control*.

To appreciate his work, it should be known that puerperal infection was epidemic in maternity wards throughout Europe with roughly 25 to 30 percent of delivering mothers dying from this systematic body infection. Although suspected causes ranged from poverty to illegitimacy to home deliveries, Semmelweis concluded that physicians and interns with unwashed hands inadvertently introduced the bacterial disease to the patients, which are referred to as **nosocomial infections** these days. In light of this perceived affront to health care practice, Semmelweis faced strong objections from the medical community. Semmelweis further observed that midwives assisting in deliveries were less likely to transmit disease compared to medical students who were called from anatomical dissections to the maternity clinics. He directed the students to wash their hands with chlorinated lime before pelvic examinations of women. Consequently, mortality rates in patients dropped to about 1 percent. So revolutionary was his idea of infection control that his superiors responded by dropping him from his clinical position within the hospital. Humiliated, Semmelweis abandoned clinical practice for a couple of years until a resurgence of puerperal fever in other obstetric clinics drew him back into professional action. He was again successful at significantly reducing maternal mortality rates through his emphasis on handwashing and other infection control techniques. Despite his successes, many authorities in the medical community continued to reject the notion of communicable diseases being spread by health care professionals. Such strong adversity gradually diminished Semmelweis's spirit until he experienced a clinical case of depression necessitating admittance to a mental hospital. He died while a patient at the hospital; ironically, from a bacterial disease. He contracted the disease prior to coming to the mental hospital as a result of operating on an infected patient at another facility. Thereafter, the medical community finally accepted Semmelweis's conclusion about disease transmission to patients and techniques for infection (Unwin, Carr, and Leeson, 1997).

Shattuck

American **Lemuel Shattuck's** work spanned the late nineteenth and early twentieth century. Shattuck was a leader in community-based disease control and therefore deserving of the honor, *parent of U.S. public health*. He submitted governmental reports advocating the establishment of state and local boards of health as well as data collection systems, sanitary inspections, and professional preparation of disease control specialists. He consulted for the federal government on such matters as quarantine of yellow fever and other disease cases—**yellow fever** is a viral disease spread by mosquitos that causes fever, chills, muscle aches, and death. It is believed that Shattuck's scholarly work was the basis of important public health-related legislation such as the founding of the U.S. Public Health Service (1902), and the Pure Food and Drug Act (1906) (Rosen, 1993, pp. 217-219).

Stern

Elizabeth Stern was a Canadian-born American researcher who throughout the twentieth century received acclaim for her work on cancer. **Cancer** refers to diseases characterized by abnormal and out-of-control cell division that can invade surrounding tissue and spread through the circulatory system to other body parts. Another term for cancer is **malignant neoplasm,** or rapid multiplication of under-developed cells. Essentially, she was the first person to explain the stages of a cell's progression from normal to cancerous state. She is recognized as the *parent of cytopathology,* the study of diseased cells. Stern published the first case report demonstrating the link between herpes simplex virus and cervical cancer. She was also successful in drawing a significant correlation between prolonged use of oral contraceptives and cervical cancer. Her findings prompted the development of cervical cancer screening tests.

HONORABLE MENTIONS
OF THE TWENTIETH CENTURY

There are several persons who conducted their epidemiological activity throughout the twentieth century, and their work deserves recognition:

- Several researchers have identified diseases resulting from nutritional deficiencies. For instance, **Joseph Goldberger** conducted his work on pellagra, a disease resulting from a deficiency of niacin, which causes general weakness, lower appetite, skin and mucous membrane inflammation, gastrointestinal problems, and emotional discomfort.

- We cannot overlook the important work of the research team, **Richard Doll** and **Austin Hill,** who conducted studies during the mid-1900s that established the causal relationship between cigarette smoking and lung cancer (Fox, Hall, and Elveback, 1970).
- In the latter portion of the twentieth century considerable attention was focused on breast cancer and other cancer research. A pioneer in this area was **Ruth Sager,** an American geneticist.
- One of the more important epidemiological findings during the twentieth century was the identification of risk factors to cardiovascular disease. Members of the team who started the Framingham Heart Study in 1948 were **William Kannel, Thomas Dawber,** and others. The study continues today.
- Vaccines for the crippling disease polio were developed mid-century by both **Albert Sabin** (oral vaccine) and **Jonas Salk** (injected vaccine).
- The human immunodeficiency virus (HIV) emerged in the 1980s with several research teams, funded by the U.S. Centers for Disease Prevention and Control, establishing an understanding of the disease process and effective treatments.
- Another noteworthy contributor to the epidemiology movement is **Bernadette Healey.** During the 1980s and 1990s she became the first female director of the National Institute of Health. It was through her leadership that female representation in analytical research, both as investigators and as subjects, was promoted.
- Another contemporary is **Ivor Lensworth Livingston,** an epidemiologist at Howard University. He is the first to compile a comprehensive review of epidemiological research on health problems, issues, and policies pertaining to African Americans (Livingston, 1994).

RECENT HISTORY OF PUBLIC AND ENVIRONMENTAL HEALTH

Recent and current epidemiologists share credit for their accomplishments in the nation's public health system. At the start of the twentieth century, infectious diseases reigned as leading causes of death, and life expectancy barely reached fifty years of age. Other morbid conditions were prevalent such as nutritional deficiencies, prenatal health problems, toxic exposures, and injuries related to industrial working conditions. Urban areas swelled in population, and this burdened an underdeveloped public health system.

During the first half of the twentieth century an impressive surge of health care development took place. It was launched due to intense social reform at the time. Important legislation was passed:

- Pure Food and Drug Act of 1906, and subsequent amendments, ensures safe, effective, and pure drugs and food preparations
- Public Health Services Act of 1912, which approved the founding of U.S. Public Health Service
- Workers' compensation statutes were passed on a state-by-state basis to protect the health and financial status of employees injured in the course of work
- Social Security Act of 1935 and its Medicare and Medicaid amendments (1965)
- National Housing Act of 1937 and related legislation, which allowed the federal government to subsidize the costs of constructing and managing housing for low-income families
- National Hospital Survey and Construction Act of 1946, also known as the Hill-Burton Act, which funded extensive medical center and health care clinic development
- National Mental Health Act of 1946, which allowed federal funds to support development of state mental hospitals and local mental health care systems
- National School Lunch Act of 1946, which offered reduced-price lunch meals to children attending schools

Private and public hospitals were accompanied by the birth of nonprofit health organizations such as the National Society for the Study and Prevention of Tuberculosis (later renamed the American Lung Association), the American Cancer Society, and others. By midway through the twentieth century, health care facilities and public health departments were flourishing. Still, the emphasis was more curative than preventive. However, things change. In 1979 the surgeon general published the Healthy People report, which continues to act as the health promotion and disease prevention agenda for the nation (Mc-

Kenzie, Pinger, and Kotecki, 1999, pp. 9-22; Rosen, 1993, pp. 320-462).

Even with this public health reform and development, with its foci on controlling infectious diseases and treating other morbid conditions, it might be difficult for some of us to imagine the environmental living conditions in the United States prior to the establishment of the Environmental Protection Agency (EPA) in 1970. Many aspects of the physical environment were deteriorating. Littering was a fact of life. Leaded gasoline was the sole product at the pump. Tobacco smoking was allowed in hospital patient rooms. Raw sewage and phosphates were openly discharged in recreational waterways, which subsequently were closed to the public. Airline schedules were often delayed or canceled due to smog conditions. Leaves and lawn debris were openly incinerated in street corner gutters. Home and car repair byproducts (e.g., oil) were flung over the backyard fence. All garbage, and any toxic substance therein, was deposited in open landfills. Schoolchildren were exposed to asbestos-lined classrooms. Workers were offered little protection against toxic and other health-threatening working conditions. There were few federal regulations for the commercial disposal of toxic substances. Only recently has any consideration been given to handling radioactive waste from atomic fission and fusion energy production. And the list of environmental travesties still goes on.

One plus was the recycling efforts of the American public during World War II when needed resources were scarce. However, by the 1950s, U.S. society had resumed its "throwaway" mentality and solid waste was accumulating. The public had a growing concern about environmental degradation and its subsequent effect on public health. Accordingly, on April 22, 1970, a remarkable event occurred that changed the environmental health history of the nation. U.S. citizens finally said, "Enough is enough," and staged Earth Day, the largest organized demonstration in U.S. history until then, which was centralized in the Washington, DC, Mall but concurrently was observed in major metropolitan areas across the nation. Millions of people expressed dissatisfaction with the state of the environment and insufficient policies to protect it. Citizens were urged to assume more personal responsibility for "cleaning up," while U.S. Congress was lobbied to enact more effective environmental legislation. Earth Day is still observed annually on April 22.

Although environmental health related legislation existed prior to the establishment of the Environmental Protection Agency in 1970, many say the agency is successful in its role as the collective environmental regulatory effort of the nation. Its mission is to protect public health and to safeguard and improve the natural environment. It ensures that the following federal legislation is implemented and enforced fairly and effectively:

- The Clean Air Act (1963) and its subsequent amendments furnished regulations and restrictions on the release of criteria air pollutants: carbon dioxide, lead, nitrogen dioxide, ozone, particulate matter, and sulfur dioxide.
- Occupational Safety and Health Act (1970), which set standards for ensuring a safe and healthy working environment.
- Lead-Base Paint Poisoning Prevention Act (1971) initiated a national effort to identify children with lead poisoning and to abate sources in the environment.
- The Clean Water Act (1972) and its subsequent amendments aimed at ensuring water quality in such a way as to make all rivers and lakes swimmable and fishable, and reduce discharge of pollutants in U.S. waters.
- Noise Control Act (1972) and its subsequent amendments aimed at regulating noise emissions from new consumer products. Later, standards were set for quiet communities.
- Safe Drinking Water Act (1974) set maximum contaminant levels for specific pollutant levels in drinking water (e.g., coliform bacteria).
- The Resource Conservation and Recovery Act (1976) and its subsequent amendments provide for "cradle-to-grave" regulation and disposal of solid (i.e., garbage) and hazardous (i.e., chemicals, biohazardous) waste.
- Comprehensive Environmental Response, Compensation, and Liability Act (1980) which responded to the public's demand to clean up leaking dump sites. This legislation created the Superfund.
- Nuclear Waste Policy Act (1982) outlined the procedures for the disposal of wastes from nuclear power plants.

Of course, there is a good deal of legislation taking place at the state level. Much of this regulation is a statutory extension of federal mandates. For example, each state self-determines the monitoring and control of radon exposure, although the original guidelines are set forth in the Resource Conservation and Recovery Act (1976). Likewise, global-level attention has been directed at environmental health conditions. For example, there have been earth summits— international conferences throughout the 1990s to curb global warming. However, the United States government has argued that such control would negatively impact industry and the economy (McKenzie, Pinger, and Kotecki, 1999, pp. 487-530; Sellers, 1997).

SUMMARY

The history of epidemiological activity is traced through important accomplishments, recognized leaders in the field, and landmark legislation. It is necessary to understand early notions or beliefs about disease. Spiritual and mystical explanations for disease and death are of limited effect today; however, the natural notion has been and remains at the heart of epidemiological reasoning. Several accomplished figures, prior to and during the Common Era, contributed to the evolution of epidemiological reasoning and are therefore considered parents of epidemiology. This review also acknowledges the distinguished professionals of the twentieth century, as well as the recent history of the U.S. environmental health movement. Legislation relevant to disease prevention and health promotion, including major efforts to reduce and control air, land, water, and other pollutants in the past thirty years, has also helped shape today's epidemiological climate.

REVIEW QUESTIONS

1. Do you know the early notions about disease? Can you describe them? Can you provide examples of each notion?
2. Do you know the definitions of the important terms that are in bold print in this chapter?

3. Who are the parents of epidemiology? Can you identify and present them in chronological order? Can you describe their important accomplishments?
4. Who are some of the "honorable mentions" in epidemiology during the twentieth century?
5. Can you cite landmark legislation relevant to disease prevention and health promotion?
6. Can you describe the recent history of public and environmental health in our country? What are important legislative acts during the twentieth century?
7. Do you know the answers to the chapter activity questions based on objectives from Healthy People 2010 focus areas 3 and 4?

WEB SITE RESOURCES

Centers for Disease Control and Prevention
<http://www.cdc.gov/>

Emory University School of Public Health
<http://www.sph.emory.edu/PHIL>

Environmental Protection Agency
<http://www.epa.gov/>

The Internet Classics Archive by Daniel C. Stevenson, Web Atomics
<http://classics.mit.edu/>

National Institute of Health
<http://www.nih.gov>

National Library of Medicine, Images from the History of Medicine
<http://www.nlm.nih.gov/hmd/hmd.htm>

University of California San Francisco, Epidemiological Links and Information
<http://www.epibiostat.ucsf.edu/epidem/epidem.html>

World Health Organization
<http://www.who.int/home-page>

Yale University Biomedicine: History of Science, Technology, and Medicine
<http://info.med.yale.edu/hismed/>

REFERENCES

Dunglison, R. (1835). *On the influence of atmosphere and locality.* Reprinted by Cellinie, J. (1977). *Human health: Elements of hygiene.* New York: Arno Press.

Fox, J.P., Hall, C.E., and Elveback, L.R. (1970). *Epidemiology: Man and disease.* London: The MacMillan Company, Collier-MacMillan Limited.

Healthy People 2010 (2000). *Healthy People 2010: Objectives for improving health.* Washington, DC: Office of Disease Prevention and Health Promotion, U.S. Department of Health and Human Services.

Institute of Medicine (1988). *The future of public health.* Washington, DC: National Academy Press.

Karlen, A. (1995). *Man and microbes.* New York: G.P. Putnam's Sons.

Legator, M.S., Harper, B.L., and Scott, M.J. (Eds.) (1985). *The health detective's handbook.* Baltimore, MD: The Johns Hopkins University Press.

Livingston, I.L. (1994). *Handbook of black American health.* Westport, CT: Greenwood Press.

Markel, H. (1997). *Quarantine!* Baltimore, MD: The Johns Hopkins University Press.

McKenzie, J.F., Pinger, R.R., and Kotecki, J.E. (1999). *An introduction to community health* (Third edition). Boston, MA: Jones and Bartlett Publishers.

McNeill, W.H. (1976). *Plagues and peoples.* New York: Doubleday.

Rosen, G. (1993). *A history of public health.* Baltimore, MD: The Johns Hopkins University Press.

Salerno Society (1966). *The school of Salernum.* Translated by J. Harrington (1607). *Regimen Sanitatis Salerni.* London: John Holme and John Press.

Sellars, C.C. (1997). *Hazards on the job.* Chapel Hill, NC: The University of North Carolina Press.

Stroup, D.F. and Berkelman, R.L. (1998). *History of statistical methods in public health.* In D.F. Stroup and S.M. Teutsch (Eds.), *Statistics in public health: Quantitative approaches to public health problems.* New York: Oxford University Press, pp. 3-4.

Timmreck, T.C. (1998). *An introduction to epidemiology* (Second edition). Boston, MA: Jones and Bartlett Publishers.

Unwin, N., Carr, S., and Leeson, J. (1997). *An introductory study guide to public health and epidemiology.* Philadelphia, PA: Open University Press.

Wain, H. (1970). *A history of preventive medicine.* Springfield, IL: Charles C. Thomas Publishers.

Winslow, C.-E.A. (1943). *The conquest of epidemic disease.* Madison, WI: The University of Wisconsin Press.

Purpose: (1) To acquaint the reader with Healthy People 2010 targets for improvement and (2) present examples of epidemiology as the underlying science to health promotion and disease prevention.

Directions: Check out your knowledge of these Healthy People 2010 focus areas by taking the following tests (answers follow in a separate section).

FOCUS AREA 3: CANCER

This focus area's goal is reducing the number of new cancer cases as well as the illness, disability, and death caused by cancer.

3-1. *Reduction in the overall cancer death rate.* How much of a reduction is targeted?
a. 11 percent
b. 21 percent
c. 31 percent
d. 41 percent

3-2. *Reduction in the lung cancer death rate.* How much of a reduction is targeted?
a. 12 percent
b. 22 percent
c. 32 percent
d. 42 percent

3-3. *Reduction in the breast cancer death rate.* Related to this objective, what percent of breast cancer deaths in fifty- to seventy-four-year-old females can be reduced through proper mammography screening?
a. 10-29 percent
b. 20-39 percent

c. 30-49 percent

d. 40-59 percent

3-4.   *Reduction in the death rate from cancer of the uterine cervix.*
Related to this objective, if cervical cancer is detected early
through a Pap test, the likelihood of survival is almost:

a. 70 percent

b. 80 percent

c. 90 percent

d. 100 percent

3-5.   *Reduction in the colorectal cancer death rate.* How much of a
reduction is targeted?

a. 14 percent

b. 24 percent

c. 34 percent

d. 44 percent

3-6.   *Reduction in the oropharyngeal cancer death rate.* Related to
this, which risk factor(s) explain oral cancer?

a. Alcohol consumption

b. Tobacco consumption

c. Combination of alcohol and tobacco consumption

d. Neither alcohol nor tobacco consumption

3-7.   *Reduction in the prostate cancer death rate.* Which of the following is correct about prostate cancer?

a. Other than skin cancer, prostate cancer is the most commonly diagnosed form of cancer in males.

b. Prostate cancer is the second leading cause of cancer death
among U.S. males.

c. Prostate cancer is most common in males aged sixty-five
years and older.

d. All of the above are correct.

3-8.   *Reduction in the rate of melanoma cancer deaths.* Which is a
risk factor to skin cancer?

a. Personal/family history of melanoma

b. Presence of atypical moles or a large number of moles

c. Intermittent sun exposure, sunburns early in life, freckles,
and sun-sensitive skin

d. All of the above

3-9. *Increase in the proportion of persons who use at least one of the following protective measures that may reduce the risk of skin cancer: avoid the sun between 10 a.m. and 4 p.m., wear sun-protective clothing when exposed to sunlight, use sunscreen with a sun-protective factor (SPF) of 15 or higher, and avoid artificial sources of ultraviolet light.* As of 1998, what percent of adults practiced at least one of these protective measures?
a. 37 percent
b. 47 percent
c. 57 percent
d. 67 percent

3-10. *Increase in the proportion of physicians and dentists who counsel their at-risk patients about tobacco use cessation, physical activity, and cancer screening.* What is the targeted proportion of providers who counsel their at-risk patients?
a. 65 percent
b. 75 percent
c. 85 percent
d. 95 percent

3-11. *Increase in the proportion of women who receive a Pap test.* As of 1998, about what percent of females eighteen years and older had a Pap test within the past three years?
a. 69 percent
b. 79 percent
c. 89 percent
d. 99 percent

3-12. *Increase in the proportion of adults who receive a colorectal cancer screening examination.* What is the targeted proportion of adults receiving a fecal blood occult test within the preceding two years?
a. 50 percent
b. 60 percent
c. 70 percent
d. 80 percent

3-13. *Increase the proportion of women aged forty years and older who have received a mammogram within the preceding two*

years. What is the targeted proportion of these adult females having a mammogram in the past 2 years?
a. 50 percent
b. 60 percent
c. 70 percent
d. 80 percent

3-14.   *Increase in the number of states that have a statewide population-based cancer registry that captures case information on at least 95 percent of the expected number of reportable cancers.* As of 1999, how many states had such a registry?
a. eleven
b. twenty-one
c. thirty-one
d. forty-one

3-15.   *Increase in the proportion of cancer survivors who are living five years or longer after diagnosis.* As of 1988-1995, what was the proportion of survivors?
a. 59 percent
b. 69 percent
c. 79 percent
d. 89 percent

FOCUS AREA 4: CHRONIC KIDNEY DISEASE

This focus area's goal: reducing new cases of chronic kidney disease and its complications, disability, death, and economic costs.

4-1.   *Reduction in the rate of new cases of end-stage renal disease.* How can end-stage renal disease be prevented?
a. Managing diabetes
b. Managing blood pressure
c. Detecting renal insufficiency
d. All of the above

4-2.   *Reduction in deaths from cardiovascular disease in persons with chronic kidney failure.* Related to this objective, which of the following is correct?

a. Cardiovascular disease is the major cause of death among patients with chronic renal failure and end-stage renal disease.
b. Reducing cardiovascular disease deaths will lead to a significant decrease in deaths for persons with chronic renal failure and end-stage renal disease.
c. Reducing cardiovascular disease risk factors can take place before the onset of terminal kidney failure.
d. All of the above are correct.

4-3. *Increase in the proportion of treated chronic kidney failure patients who have received counseling on nutrition, treatment choices, and cardiovascular care, twelve months before the start of renal replacement therapy.* As of 1996, what percent of patients received this counseling?
a. 45 percent
b. 55 percent
c. 65 percent
d. 75 percent

4-4. *Increase in the proportion of new hemodialysis patients who use arteriovenous fistulas as the primary mode of vascular access.* Related to this objective, what is arteriovenous fistula?
a. Joining a person's artery to a hemodialysis machine
b. Joining a person's own artery to a kidney transplant machine
c. Joining a person's own artery to the nearby vein
d. Joining a person's artery to his or her kidney

4-5. *Increase the proportion of dialysis patients registered on the waiting list for transplantation.* As of 1994-1996, what percent of patients were wait-listed for transplantation?
a. 10 percent
b. 20 percent
c. 30 percent
d. 40 percent

4-6. *Increase the proportion of patients with treated chronic kidney failure who receive a transplant within three years of registration on the waiting list.* Why do African Americans,

Native Americans, and Alaskan Americans "move up" the waiting list at a slower rate compared to other groups in the population?
a. Genetic and biological factors while matching kidney donor and recipient HLA tissue types
b. Patient registration procedures and locations of transplant centers
c. Cultural attitudes about organ donation
d. All of the above

4-7.   *Reduction in kidney failure due to diabetes.* Related to this objective, how does diabetes result in kidney failure?
a. Persons eat too much sugar in their diet
b. Persons have too much insulin in their blood
c. Persons experience long-standing effect of diabetes on the microvasculature of the kidney
d. Persons experience diabetic coma

4-8.   *Increase in the proportion of persons with type 1 or type 2 diabetes and proteinuria who receive recommended medical therapy to reduce progression to chronic renal insufficiency (developmental).* Related to this objective, what is the distinction between type 1 and type 2 diabetes?
a. Type 1 is more prevalent than type 2 diabetes.
b. Type 1 is also called adult-onset diabetes.
c. Type 2 represents 95 percent of all diagnosed cases of diabetes.
d. Type 2 is also called insulin-dependent diabetes.

TEST ANSWERS

Focus Area 3

3-1. (b) 21 percent. The present cancer death rate is 202.4 per 100,000 population, and the target is 159.9 per 100,000 population.*

3-2. (b) 22 percent. The present lung cancer death rate is 57.6 per 100,000 population, and the target is 44.9 per 100,000 population.*

3-3. (b) Epidemiological studies on the effectiveness of mammography screening have demonstrated a 20 to 39 percent decrease in breast cancer deaths in females aged fifty to seventy-four. Likewise, the same studies have demonstrated an approximate 17 percent decrease in females forty to forty-nine years old.

3-4. (d) 100 percent. Cervical cancer's preliminary signs are precancerous changes in cervical tissue detectable through a Pap test. Women complying with this routine screening and its recommended follow-up stand a survival ratio of almost 100 percent.

3-5. (c) 34 percent. The present colorectal cancer death rate is 21.2 per 100,000 population, and the target is 13.9 per 100,000 population.

3-6. (c) Combination of alcohol and tobacco consumption. Although each is an independent risk factor, when combined they explain about 90 percent of all oral cancers.

3-7. (d) All of the above. Prostate cancer accounts for about 29 percent of all cancers and about 11 percent of all cancer deaths in the United States. There are effective screening methods for this type of cancer.

3-8. (d) All of the above. It is important to know these risk factors since annual skin cancer rates have been increasing by about 2.5 percent over the past decade.

3-9. (b) 47 percent. The target is to increase this proportion to 75 percent. There is also a developmental subobjective for increasing the use of protective measures among adolescents.

---

*Ages adjusted to the year 2000 standard population.

3-10.   (c) 85 percent. Physicians, dentists and other primary care providers should be counseling at-risk patients in smoking cessation, healthy eating decisions, physical activity, and cancer screening in a linguistically and culturally appropriate manner.

3-11.   (b) 79 percent. The targeted improvement is 97 percent of all adult females having had a Pap test within the past three years.

3-12.   (a) 50 percent. The baseline proportion is 35 percent. Similar target and baseline percentages pertain to screening through sigmoidoscopy.

3-13.   (c) 70 percent. The baseline is 67 percent of females ages forty years and older having a mammogram in the past two years.

3-14.   (d) Forty one. The targeted increase is forty-five states having a population-based cancer registry capturing case information on 95 percent or more of the expected number of reportable cancers.

3-15.   (a) 59 percent. The target is 70 percent, which would represent a 19 percent increase.

Focus Area 4

4-1.   (d) All of the above. End-stage renal disease is also called treated renal failure and is cared for through dialysis and kidney transplantation. Unmanaged diabetes and blood pressure, plus other factors such as advancing age, proteinuria, genetics, and environmental exposures, contribute to chronic renal insufficiency, and over a span of 10 years, results in kidney failure. Earlier detection of chronic renal insufficiency is crucial, especially among some groups having higher rates of diabetes-driven chronic renal insufficiency such as African Americans, American Indians, or Alaskan Natives.

4-2.   (d) All of the above. Cardiovascular disease deaths are about three to four times greater in persons with end-stage renal disease compared to the general population. Any effort to reduce cardiovascular disease by managing its risk factors should reduce this kind of death in persons with end-stage renal disease. This is significant because cardiovascular disease risk factor management can take place before and during chronic renal insufficiency, which for ten years precedes end-stage renal disease. Cardiovascular disease risk factor management is crucial for persons who show elevated levels of proteinuria or creatinine, which are markers of declining kidney function.

4-3.   (a) The baseline is 45 percent of newly diagnosed patients with treated chronic kidney failure who receive counseling on nutrition, treatment choices, and cardiovascular care. The target is 60 percent.

4-4.   (c) Joining a person's own artery to the nearby vein. This increases blood flow in the vein leading to marked dilation of the blood vessel, thus allowing an easy needle insertion during dialysis.

4-5.   (b) 20 percent. Although there are a number of factors that explain whether a person receives a kidney transplant—the first step is registering on a waiting list. The target is 66 percent.

4-6.   (d) All of the above. Although the exact causes are unclear, all of these factors and more seem to play a role: the request/consent procedures of organ procurement organizations; organ acceptance practices at transplant centers; socioeconomic status of registrants; and availability of donated organs in local areas.

4-7.   (c) Persons experience long-standing effect of diabetes upon microvasculature of the kidneys. Diabetes complicates the kidney and other body organs causing blood vessel damage. There is also increased urine protein and decreased kidney function.

4-8.   (c) Compared to type 1 (insulin-dependent) diabetes, type 2 (adult-onset) diabetes is far more prevalent, especially in some racial and ethnic groups, and in older persons.

Chapter 3

Concepts and Principles

Recall the definition of epidemiology: the study of the occurrence and distribution, cause and control, prevention and treatment of disease and other morbid conditions. Each part of this definition will be addressed throughout this text, and so it will be necessary to cover important epidemiological concepts and principles that relate to each part of the definition. While doing so, it is important to know that a **concept** is a general idea obtained or deduced from specific phenomena or happenings. A **principle** is the relationship between two or more concepts that acts as a rule of understanding. In epidemiology, there are several concepts and principles to explore, along with their health promotion and disease prevention implications.

DISEASE OCCURRENCE AND DISTRIBUTION

Necessary and Sufficient Factors

When studying disease occurrence, a commonly accepted concept involves the agent. An **agent** is a necessary factor for the occurrence of disease or other morbid condition. As a **necessary factor,** the agent has to be present for morbidity, although its presence alone does not necessarily lead to disease. Disease occurrence requires the accompaniment of **sufficiency factors** that combine with the necessary factor. One of these sufficiency factors is the concept of host. A **host** is an organism on or within which another organism lives. For the purposes of this text, the human host will be studied. Another sufficiency factor to consider is the concept of **environment,** which includes the physical, biological, and psychosocial conditions surrounding an organism and affecting its growth, development, and survival.

What Is the Agent to Diabetes?

Diabetes is a chronic disease that usually manifests itself as one of two major types: type 1, mainly occurring in children and adolescents eighteen years and younger, in which the body does not produce insulin and thus insulin administration is required to sustain life; or type 2, occurring usually in adults over thirty years of age, in which the body's tissues become unable to use its own limited amount of insulin effectively. For years, it was believed that type 1 diabetes was due solely to a genetic factor and type 2 related more to lifestyle management. Medical science discoveries of the 1990s demonstrated that type 1 diabetes is partly the result of an autoimmune disorder developed in persons exposed to certain viruses such as coxsakie. Therefore, the medical understanding is that type 1 diabetes is an autoimmune disease that destroys insulin-producing cells of the pancreas and occurs in genetically susceptible individuals.

Type 2 diabetes, by contrast, is more of a lifestyle management consequence (e.g., excessive body weight, overnutrition) that studies have shown is more likely to manifest in genetically predisposed persons. So, diabetes is a disease that has more than one agent: biological, genetic, and behavioral. Given these developments in the study of diabetes, it is important that this information be provided to the public (Swinburn, 1996).

This relates to Healthy People 2010 Objective 5-1: *Increase in the proportion of persons with diabetes who receive formal diabetes education* (Healthy People 2010, 2000, 5-12). (See Chapter 3 activities for more information.)

Epidemiological Triad

All three concepts of agent, host, and environment interrelate in a principle known as the **epidemiological triad.** Within this principle, attention is given to the concept of **time,** which is a continuum of past, present, and future events comprising the disease occurrence.

There are two versions of the epidemiological triad (see Figure 3.1). The traditional version applies well to the occurrence of **infectious disease,** a pathological condition resulting from infection by a microorganism or its products. **Pathological** means there is an anatomical or functional manifestation of a disease. Hence, the agent could be a bacterium, virus, rickettsium, protozoan, or metazoan (to be discussed in Chapter 4). The host is an individual who becomes infected with an agent, and the environment is the surroundings that facilitate agent infestation in the host. The interaction of agent, host, and environment takes place within the context of time. As this description points out, the traditional triad applies well to disease occur-

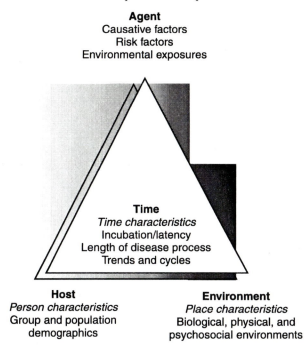

Agent
Causative factors
Risk factors
Environmental exposures

Time
Time characteristics
Incubation/latency
Length of disease process
Trends and cycles

Host
Person characteristics
Group and population
demographics

Environment
Place characteristics
Biological, physical, and
psychosocial environments

FIGURE 3.1. Epidemiological triad (*Source:* Adapted from Timmreck, 1998, p. 15.)

rence from a single causal agent that is environmentally supported to a make a person ill. That is why it is used to explain disease occur- rence in individual cases.

An application of the epidemiological triad is illustrated in a recent *E. coli* outbreak at the Washington County Fair in New York State in 1999. State health officials said the epidemic of 781 suspected cases could become the worst such contamination in U.S. history (CDC, 1999). One victim was believed to have become sick after drinking contaminated coffee at the fair, while another victim drank from a glass of contaminated water. Rain runoff is believed to have washed the potentially deadly *E. coli* bacteria from cow manure at a nearby cattle barn into the fair's underground water supply. *Escherichia coli,* or ***E. coli,*** is a naturally found bacteria and an integral part of the normal gastrointestinal inner environment. Sewage-contaminated water, milk, or food (e.g., undercooked beef) can transmit *E. coli.* Sometimes **vectors,** animate transmitters of an agent such as flies and other insects, carry the *E. coli* from a sewage source to a human food site. There are cases of *E. coli* in those who swim in sewage-contaminated water. Once the organism grows in greater numbers than can be tolerated in the digestive tract, it can cause severe, even bloody, diarrhea and abdominal cramps. Kidney failure, which can be fatal, occurs in about 2 to 7 percent of cases. However, these severe cases are more likely to occur in children under five years of age or in elderly adults. Therapy is largely that of replacing lost fluids, although specific antimicrobial agents can be effective in some cases. The outbreak at the county fair probably would have been prevented had the attendees accessed municipal water, or if they consumed commercially prepared packaged drinks (CDC, 1999).

To explain more complex disease occurrence, the contemporary epidemiological triad is preferred over the traditional just discussed. In fact, the contemporary triad can be used to better understand the distribution of disease cases. Typically, this version of the triad is applied to a **noninfectious disease,** a pathological condition resulting from exposure to risk factors or nonliving substances. Thus, the agent could be one or more unhealthy behaviors, unsafe practices, genetic predisposition, or unintended exposures to hazardous substances (more in Chapter 4). Rather than limiting the understanding of disease occurrence and distribution to a single person, the host is understood in terms of groups of people. This makes sense, because not every person exposed to agents or who practices unhealthy behaviors becomes sick—possibly due to varying influence of physical, biological, and psychosocial characteristics of the environment or place. Also, one person's pathology might differ from another's based on respective host characteristics. Time characteristics also play a role in the occurrence and distribution of disease (Timmreck, 1998, pp. 6-8). More will be studied about person, place, and time characteristics in Chapter 5.

Epidemic Curve

Another principle used in understanding the distribution of cases is the **epidemic curve,** a charting of case appearances during an epidemic along a time line (see Figure 3.2). During a **common source epidemic,** when each case is exposed to the same source host or envi-

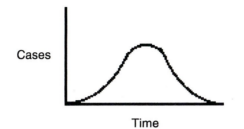

FIGURE 3.2. Epidemic curve (*Source:* Adapted from Lilienfeld and Stolley, 1994, p. 43.)

ronment, the distribution is likely to resemble a normal curve (time expressed logarithmically). During a **propagated epidemic,** when each case is exposed to a different source host, the time distribution of cases is uneven, extended, and skewed.

The epidemic curve is an important epidemiological principle because it depicts the time factor in disease occurrence and distribution. Without knowledge of the agent, epidemiologists can examine an epidemic curve and approximate the incubation period (explained later in this chapter) of the disease as well as identify the kind of epidemic. These two clues can also help the investigators narrow down the possible agents responsible for disease occurrence as well as better realize the spread or distribution of cases in an infected population (Lilienfeld and Stolley, 1994, pp. 269-276).

DISEASE CAUSE AND CONTROL

Two-by-Two Table

A good way to focus on suspected agents is by taking data from a number of cases and inserting them into a **two-by-two table.** As seen in Figure 3.3, the table is used to analyze the relationship between agent exposure and disease. It not only helps to determine a single cause to infectious diseases, it is useful in ascertaining multiple causes to noninfectious diseases. Epidemiologists can consider and control for various host and environmental variables. The underlying princi-

	Disease	No Disease
Exposed	# a	# b
Not exposed	# c	# d

FIGURE 3.3. Two-by-two table (*Source:* Adapted from Timmreck, 1998, p. 353.)

ple in this table is to compare exposed and nonexposed persons and whether they are disease cases or not. Once the counts of persons have been entered into the table, risk calculations can be performed (Stone et al., 1996).

A recent example of the two-by-two table's use documents an outbreak of illness among hikers in Roanoke, Virginia, during the summer of 1999. State and local health officials interviewed hikers who trekked the Appalachian Trail north of Roanoke, trying to determine the cause of an illness reported by thirty-six hikers. Complaints included nausea, vomiting, and diarrhea. Local epidemiologists interviewed the hikers who became ill, as well as an equal number of hikers who were not sick, to see what similarities and dissimilarities could be found. Only by comparing the experiences of well and sick hikers were they able to determine whether it was a common source or person-to-person epidemic. Both ill and nonill hikers were asked about their hygiene practices (e.g., hand washing); whether they filtered/boiled their drinking water (i.e., rather than drinking straight from streams); if they had consumed food or bottled water from a popular general store immediately off the trail; or if they had contact (e.g., handshaking) with another hiker who later became ill. Through this research, it was determined that the hikers had been exposed to the agent **Norwalk virus,** a highly contagious disease characterized by nausea, vomiting, and diarrhea. It is primarily spread by having direct contact with vomitus or feces from an infected person and then transferring the virus to the mouth from the hands (*VDH News,* 1999).

Risk

Another epidemiological concept is **risk,** the possibility of a group of persons experiencing morbidity or mortality. Risk calculation utilizes counts of cases that are entered into a two-by-two table. This calculation is usually performed during epidemiological investigations and studies (see Chapters 7 through 12). A risk calculation is usually expressed in a statement similar to: "The risk of developing 'such and such disease' is 'so many' times more likely in persons exposed to 'such and such factor.'" Although the factor is usually an agent, in a risk calculation the agent is called a **risk factor.** Accordingly, persons are considered **at risk** of developing a disease or morbid condition as a result of risk factor exposure.

Principle of Causality

During the nineteenth century Robert Koch set forth his postulates for infectious disease causation known as **Koch's Postulates of Disease.** These postulates are now considered integral to epidemiology:

- An agent occurs in every case of disease and under the circumstances that can account for the disease process.
- The agent cannot occur in other diseases.
- After being isolated, the agent can be grown in pure culture and, if allowed to infect, can initiate the disease process. (Lilienfeld and Stolley, 1994, p. 261)

Latter-day epidemiologists have modified these postulates to better explain causation of both infectious and noninfectious diseases:

- One or more risk factors are present in persons with the disease than are present in persons without the disease.
- Persons exposed to the risk develop the disease more frequently than those not exposed.
- The incidence of disease increases in relation to the duration and intensity of the risk factor.
- The removal of a risk factor lessens occurance of the disease. (Evans, 1976, pp. 175-195)

Perhaps an easier way to think about this is to rely on the **principle of causality,** a rule of understanding the causation of disease. Thinking in terms of "**P**" words:

- The agent/risk is always **p**resent when the disease/condition occurs.
- The agent/risk consistently **p**recedes the disease/condition.
- There is a **p**ropensity in the relationship—increase the agent/risk and there is a corresponding increase in the disease/condition.
- The agent/risk relationship to disease/condition appears in other **p**ersons. In other words, relationship is demonstrable in diverse populations of susceptible hosts.
- The agent/risk relationship to disease/condition appears to be consistent despite **p**lace.

This principle has been presented and described in terms of etiological hypotheses and categories of causes (Cassel, 1964), with respective variable relationships determined through mathematical equations (Susser, 1972). However, it all comes down to existence, time, strength of association, replication in others, and elimination of ecological fallacy.

Disease Process

Once the cause of a disease is known, the next logical step is to explore ways to control it. It would be a good idea to understand the disease process at the outset, sometimes referred to as the natural history of disease (Gordis, 1996), another important principle in epidemiology (see Figure 3.4). **Disease process** refers to a pathological progress starting with susceptibility, moving to exposure, through subclinical and clinical stages, and ultimately to a stage of full, partial, or no recovery. During each stage there are opportunities to control the disease. Within the disease process principle are related concepts. One is the **chain of infection,** the mechanism of an infectious agent leaving its source and entering and infecting a new host. Another concept is **infection control,** which is practiced at all disease process stages

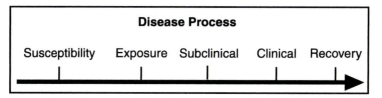

FIGURE 3.4. The disease process (*Source:* Adapted from Stone, Armstrong, Macrina, and Pankau, 1996, p. 36.)

during which standard precautions (i.e., cleanliness, protection, immunization, etc.) are performed for preventing the spread of infectious diseases.

The **susceptibility stage** is when agent, host, and environmental factors are conducive to disease occurrence. **Exposure** is when the host lays open to the agent. During the **subclinical stage** (or incubation or latency period), pathological changes are taking place in the host, although at best only subtle signs and symptoms are indicated. Recall that a sign is an objective indicator of disease based on professional observation whereas a symptom is a subjective indicator expressed by the infected host. Pathological changes will become clearly apparent and diagnosable during the **clinical stage.** The outcome of the disease will constitute no or some degree of **recovery**— that is, the host returning to a normal state of functioning.

Life Satisfaction for Persons with Disabilities

As persons progress through and survive the disease process, they will experience either full or some degree of recovery. This recovery might take the form of a **disability,** a general term used to represent the interactions between individuals with a health condition and barriers in their environment. Crucial to successful recovery is life satisfaction, that is, recovering persons feeling their physical, emotional, social, spiritual, and environmental support needs are being met. Monitoring the life satisfaction of people with disabilities, as well as the general population, provides the opportunity to evaluate society's efforts at accommodating the needs of people with disabilities (Patrick, 1997).

This relates to Healthy People 2010 Objective 6-6: *Increase in the proportion of adults with disabilities reporting satisfaction with life* (Healthy People 2010, 2000, 6-16). (See Chapter 3 activities for more information.)

The disease process principle is more often applied to infectious diseases, but is of value in understanding noninfectious diseases as well. Most diseases have a characteristic disease process; however, epidemiologists sometimes poorly understand the process of some diseases. The time line and expressed pathological changes can be specific to individual cases, and the process can be arrested at any point with correct preventive or therapeutic interventions. Hence, the disease will be controlled. More attention will be given to the disease process as it applies to both infectious and noninfectious diseases in Chapter 6.

Investigative Method

On a larger scale, epidemiologists control disease through investigations. During an epidemic or outbreak, epidemiologists rely on what is known as the **investigative method.** This principle involves determining the needs of a disease control program, designing appropriate interventive and preventive health services, and responding to the usual or unusual presence of disease in a population (Timmreck, 1998, p. 4). For example, serologic laboratory tests might be needed during an outbreak. These tests can include a range of measurements of blood and plasma-related protein molecules indicative of immune defense activity. Depending upon the particular test, investigators could detect the presence of both the agent and the host's immune efforts to eradicate it. A serologic test is more often employed after the investigators have narrowed down the possible suspected agents.

The investigative method is personified in the concept of the "disease detective." Relying on a balance of inductive and deductive reasoning, the disease detective uncovers the cause, confirms its presence, studies the spread, examines the transmission, identifies those who are susceptible, and institutes measure for control. A more detailed explanation of the investigative method can be found in the five-step problem-solving protocol presented in the next section.

DISEASE PREVENTION AND TREATMENT

Problem Solving

A primary means of determining causes and risk factors, as well as preventing and treating diseases and morbid conditions, is through epidemiological studies. During the study, epidemiologists can apply a **five-step problem-solving protocol:**

1. Determine the problem
2. Study the problem
3. Suggest a solution
4. Test the solution
5. Evaluate the solution

These steps are also used during epidemiological investigations (see Chapter 8). Problem solving during epidemiological studies will be presented in greater detail later in this book (see Chapters 9 through 12).

In actuality, an epidemiological study into the prevention and treatment of disease is more complex than the five steps of problem solving. The five-step protocol is being presented because it acts as a practical approach to conducting an epidemiological inquiry. In fact, epidemiologists in the field have encouraged health-related professionals to conduct modest studies of their own in hopes of answering one or more interesting problems, especially if they are in a position to collect and analyze appropriate data. To someone lacking previous experience in research, the task might appear formidable. However, following a basic problem-solving procedure assists the beginning researcher in addressing frequently encountered difficulties during a study (Freidman, 1987).

Levels of Prevention

It should be explained that epidemiological studies are conducted not only to determine the effectiveness of prevention and treatment interventions, but also to determine the distribution and cause of disease and other conditions. One way to categorize an epidemiological study is according to **levels of prevention**—gradient stages of risk for disease. If **primary prevention** is the focus, then the study targets subjects at low health risk. **Secondary prevention** focuses on persons at high health risk. During **tertiary prevention,** the researchers are concerned about persons who already are disease cases.

Levels of prevention are also used to categorize health promotion and disease prevention activity. Examples of primary prevention would include educating persons about the agents and risks of disease and other conditions, e.g., learning how overnutrition contributes to the risk of hypertension. Other primary prevention activities would include health care services, medical tests, counseling, health education, and other actions designed to prevent the onset of a targeted condition. Routine immunization of healthy individuals is another example of primary prevention (U.S. Preventive Services Task Force, 1995).

Secondary prevention activity includes screenings to detect risk factors to disease, e.g., blood pressure screening for hypertension, and other measures such as health care services designed to identify or treat individuals who have a disease or risk factors for a disease, but who are not yet experiencing symptoms of the disease. Pap tests and high blood pressure screening are further examples of secondary prevention (U.S. Preventive Services Task Force, 1995).

Once a disease case has been diagnosed, tertiary prevention is applied through health care, i.e., possible medication and lifestyle management counseling. Tertiary prevention can include preventive health care measures or services that are part of the treatment and management of persons with clinical illnesses. Examples of tertiary prevention include cholesterol reduction in patients with coronary heart disease and insulin therapy to prevent complications of diabetes (U.S. Preventive Services Task Force, 1995).

Whereas health promotion and disease prevention professionals might emphasize primary and secondary level prevention activity, other health professionals might be more inclined to administer tertiary level prevention. For example, the practice of modern (allopathic) medicine rests on three concepts: 1) the body can be reduced to parts (cells, tissues, organs, and systems) without much regard to how change in a part might affect the whole body; 2) if the disease is bad, the health professional can combat it, even if there are costs to pay such as side effects and consequential limitations; and 3) the disease or body condition cannot only be treated but prevented through chemicals such as medications (Neustaeder, 1996). This is not meant as a harsh statement about medical doctors and other health care team members. Rather, it is a reminder that professionals whose philosophy centers more on primary and secondary prevention will need to cooperate and collaborate with other professionals who practice tertiary level prevention.

An example of applying levels of prevention can be seen in the professional work of emergency medical technicians (EMTs). Every time an EMT or paramedic responds to a call for help, he or she is at risk of exposure to diseases and other morbid conditions such as injuries. All along, public health officials have been warning the community and its helping professionals about the hazard of **bloodborne pathogens.** These would be disease agents requiring blood or body fluid for transmission from an infected host (e.g., emergency care patient) to a new host (e.g., unsuspecting EMT). During the 1980s, primary prevention efforts were undertaken to train all EMTs in universal precautions for infection control. Now called standard precautions, EMTs and other health-related professionals prevent the unintentional exposure to HIV disease, hepatitis strains, and other infectious agents through immunization, personal protective equipment, and proper handling of biomedical hazards. To secondarily prevent disease, postexposure vaccines and other prophylaxis (e.g., cleansing) are practiced. All exposures are brought to the attention of primary care professionals; if disease ensues, tertiary prevention is administered through treatment, medication, and rehabilitation (Nixon, 2000).

Clinical Decision Making

Clinical decision making is the guiding principle in the treatment of disease and other morbid conditions. The clinician orders screenings, diagnostic tests, and procedures, ascertains a diagnosis, and then recommends appropriate clinical care. The decision making is based on necessary and essential choices. To implement this principle, clinicians are encouraged to frame a question and to create a decision tree (see Figure 3.5). The decision tree is a valuable concept that involves assigning probabilities and utilities to the possible outcomes as well as performing a follow-up sensitivity analysis. Clinical decision making and the decision tree are further explained in Chapter 12.

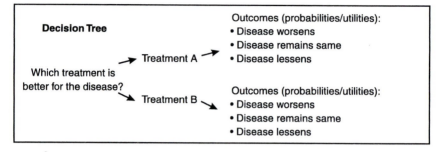

FIGURE 3.5. Decision tree in clinical decision making (*Source:* Adapted from Lilienfeld and Stolley, 1994, pp. 269-270.)

SUMMARY

Disease occurrence and distribution can be better understood through necessary and sufficient factors, the traditional and contemporary epidemiological triads, and the epidemic curve. Such principles and concepts help examine each part of the definition of epidemiology. Disease cause and control are addressed through the two-by-two table, risk, principle of causality, the disease process, and the investigative method. Disease treatment and prevention are explained through the problem-solving protocol, levels of prevention, and clinical decision making. These concepts and principles will be addressed further in subsequent chapters.

REVIEW QUESTIONS

1. What is a concept? Principle?
2. Do you know the definitions of the terms in bold print throughout this chapter?
3. Regarding disease occurrence and distribution, can you explain necessary and sufficient factors? Can you describe the epidemiological triad principle? Can you distinguish between the traditional and contemporary versions of the triad? How is it used to explain disease occurrence and distribution? How can the epidemiological triad be applied to an infectious disease such as *E. coli?*

4. Can you describe the epidemic curve and how it is used to explain disease distribution?

5. Regarding disease cause and control, can you describe the principle of the two-by two-table? How is the table utilized regarding disease causation? If given an example such as the Appalachian Trail hikers' illnesses, could you construct a table that depicts cases and noncases of this disease outbreak?

6. What is the concept of risk? What is a risk factor? What does it mean to be at risk? What is a risk statement?

7. Can you present Koch's Postulates of Disease for infectious disease causation? What is the principle of causation?

8. Can you describe the disease process principle? To which kind of disease is this principle more likely to be applied? Within this principle are the concepts of chain of infection and infection control. What are they?

9. Can you explain the investigative method as well as the concept of the "disease detective"?

10. Regarding disease treatment and prevention, what are the five steps of problem solving that can be used to understand how epidemiological investigations and studies are conducted?

11. What are the three levels of prevention? How can they be applied to health promotion and disease prevention activities such as emergency care response? If given examples of epidemiological studies, could you identify which level of prevention is being addressed?

12. If clinical decision making is the guiding principle to treating disease and other morbid conditions, how do clinicians use the concept of the decision tree?

13. Do you know the answers to the following chapter activity questions based on objectives from Healthy People 2010 focus areas 5 and 6?

WEB SITE RESOURCES

InteliHealth—John Hopkins Health Information
<http://www.intelihealth.com/>

International Institute for Health Promotion, American University
<http://www.healthy.american.edu/iihp.html>

John Hopkins Infectious Diseases
<http://www.Hopkins-id.edu/>

Medical Information on Diseases
<http://galaxy.einet.net/galaxy/Medicine.html>

Online Dictionary of Epidemiology
<http://www.ceid.ox.ac.uk/course/course-glossary.htm>

REFERENCES

Cassel, J. (1964). Social science theory as a source of hypothesis. *American Journal of Public Health* 54: 1482-1488.

CDC (1999). Summary of outbreaks of Escherichia coli 0157 and other Siga toxin-producing *E. coli* reported to the CDC in 1999. Atlanta, GA: Centers for Disease Control and Prevention, pp. 1-17.

Evans, A.S. (1976). Causation and disease: The Henle-Koch postulates revisited. *The Yale Journal of Biology and Medicine,* 49(2): 175-195.

Freidman, G.D. (1987). *Primer of epidemiology* (Third edition). New York: McGraw-Hill Book Company.

Gordis, L. (1996). *Epidemiology.* Philadelphia, PA: W.B. Saunders Company.

Healthy People 2010 (2000). *Healthy People 2010: Objectives for improving health.* Washington, DC: Office of Disease Prevention and Health Promotion, U.S. Department of Health and Human Services.

Lilienfeld, D.E. and Stolley, P.D. (1994). *Foundations of epidemiology* (Third edition). New York: Oxford Press.

Neustaeder, R. (1996). *The vaccine guide: Making an informed choice.* Berkeley, CA: North Atlantic Books.

Nixon, R.G. (2000). *Communicable disease and infection control for EMS.* Upper Saddle River, NJ: Brady/Prentice-Hall Health.

Patrick, D. (1997). Rethinking prevention for people with disabilities part 1: A conceptual model for promoting health. *American Journal of Health Promotion,* 11(4): 25-26.

Stone, D.B., Armstrong, W.R., Macrina, D.M., and Pankau, J.W. (1996). *Introduction to epidemiology.* Madison, WI: Brown and Benchmark.

Susser, M. (1972). Procedures for establishing causal associations. In G.T. Stewart. (Ed.), *Trends in epidemiology: Applications to health service, research and training* (pp. 23-101). Springfield, IL: Charles C Thomas.

7e

Swinburn, B. (1996). The thirty genotype hypothesis: How does it look after 30 years? *Diabetes Medicine,*13(5): 695-699.

Timmreck, T.C. (1998). *An introduction to epidemiology* (Second edition). Boston, MA: Jones and Bartlett Publishers.

U.S. Preventive Services Task Force (1995). *Guide to clinical preventive services* (Second edition). Washington, DC: U.S. Department of Health and Human Services.

VDH News (June 1999). Health Department launches investigation of hikers' illness. *VDH News,* Richmond, VA: Virginia Department of Health.

Purpose: (1) to acquaint the reader with Healthy People 2010 targets for improvement and (2) present examples of epidemiology as the underlying science to health promotion and disease prevention.

Directions: Check out your knowledge of these Healthy People 2010 focus areas by taking the following tests (answers follow in a separate section).

FOCUS AREA 5: DIABETES

This focus area's goal is, through prevention programs, to reduce the disease and economic burden of diabetes and improve the quality of life for all persons who have or are at risk for diabetes.

5-1. *Increase in the proportion of persons with diabetes who receive formal diabetes education.* As of 1998, what proportion received this formal education?
a. 25 percent
b. 35 percent
c. 45 percent
d. 55 percent

5-2. *Prevention of diabetes.* Related to this objective, what is prevention?
a. Primary prevention is the stopping or delaying onset of diabetes.
b. Secondary prevention is the early identification and stopping or delaying onset of complications.
c. Tertiary prevention is the stopping of disability from disease and its complications.
d. All of the above are true.

5-3.   *Reduction in the overall rate of diabetes that is clinically diagnosed.* Related to this objective, which is correct about diabetes?

a. It's a chronic disease due to either or both insulin deficiency and resistance to insulin action, and is associated with hyperglycemia (elevated blood glucose levels).

b. Over time, without proper preventive treatment, organ complications related to diabetes develop, including heart, nerve, foot, eye, and kidney damage; problems with pregnancy also occur.

c. Diabetes is classified into four major categories: type 1, type 2, gestational, and other types.

d. All of the above are correct.

5-4.   *Increase in the proportion of adults with diabetes whose condition has been diagnosed.* As of 1994, what proportion of adults with diabetes had been diagnosed?

a. 58 percent
b. 68 percent
c. 78 percent
d. 88 percent

5-5.   *Reduction in the diabetes death rate.* How much of an improvement is targeted in reducing this death rate?

a. 43 percent
b. 53 percent
c. 63 percent
d. 73 percent

5-6.   *Reduction in diabetes-related deaths among persons with diabetes.* How much of an improvement is targeted in reducing diabetes-related deaths?

a. 1 percent
b. 11 percent
c. 21 percent
d. 31 percent

5-7.   *Reduction in deaths from cardiovascular disease in persons with diabetes.* How much of an improvement is targeted in reducing these kinds of deaths?

a. 10 percent

b. 20 percent
c. 30 percent
d. 40 percent

5-8. *Decrease in the proportion of pregnant women with gestational diabetes (developmental).* Related to this objective, which is associated with reduced complications and deaths from gestational diabetes in the unborn and in newborns?
a. Proper prepregnancy and pregnancy glycemia control
b. Careful perinatal obstetrical monitoring of indications of diabetes in pregnant women
c. Good nutrition in pregnant women as well as for newborns
d. All of the above

5-9. *Reduction in the frequency of foot ulcers in persons with diabetes (developmental).* Related to this objective, besides foot ulcers, what is another complication of diabetes?
a. Hypoglycemia
b. Hypertension
c. Heart disease
d. All of the above

5-10. *Reduction in the rate of lower extremity amputations in persons with diabetes.* How much of a reduction in lower extremity amputations is targeted?
a. 35 percent
b. 45 percent
c. 55 percent
d. 65 percent

5-11. *Increase in the proportion of persons with diabetes who obtain an annual urinary microalbumin measurement (developmental).* Related to this objective, what is microalbumin measurement? A laboratory procedure to detect:
a. Very small quantities of protein in the urine, indicating early kidney damage
b. The need for lower extremity amputations
c. Diabetes-induced hypertension
d. Diabetes-related foot ulcers

5-12. *Increase in the proportion of adults with diabetes who have a glycosylated hemoglobin measurement at least once a year.*

As of 1998, what proportion of persons with diabetes had this blood glucose screening test on an annual basis?

a. 12 percent
b. 24 percent
c. 36 percent
d. 48 percent

5-13.   *Increase in the proportion of adults with diabetes who have an annual dilated eye examination.* What is the targeted proportion of adults with diabetes to have this examination annually?

a. 55 percent
b. 65 percent
c. 75 percent
d. 85 percent

5-14   *Increase in the proportion of adults with diabetes who have at least one annual foot examination.* What is the targeted proportion of adults with diabetes to have this examination annually?

a. 55 percent
b. 65 percent
c. 75 percent
d. 85 percent

5-15.   *Increase in the proportion of persons with diabetes who have at least an annual dental examination.* As of 1997, what was the proportion of adults with diabetes who had this examination annually?

a. 58 percent
b. 68 percent
c. 78 percent
d. 88 percent

5-16.   *Increase in the proportion of adults with diabetes who take aspirin at least fifteen times per month.* As of 1994, what was the proportion of adults with diabetes who consumed aspirin at this monthly rate?

a. 5 percent
b. 10 percent
c. 15 percent
d. 20 percent

5-17. *Increase in the proportion of adults with diabetes who per-form self-blood-glucose-monitoring at least once daily.* What is the targeted proportion of adults with diabetes who perform this daily monitoring?
  a. 50 percent
  b. 60 percent
  c. 70 percent
  d. 80 percent

FOCUS AREA 6:
DISABILITY AND SECONDARY CONDITIONS

This focus area's goal is to promote the health of people with disabilities, prevent secondary conditions, and eliminate disparities between people with and without disabilities in the U.S. population.

6-1. *Inclusion in the core of all relevant Healthy People 2010 sur-veillance instruments a standardized set of questions that identify "people with disabilities."* What percentage of Healthy People 2000 surveillance instruments included questions identifying people with disabilities?
  a. 0 percent
  b. 25 percent
  c. 50 percent
  d. 75 percent

6-2. *Reduction in the proportion of children and adolescents with disabilities who are reported to be sad, unhappy, or de-pressed.* As of 1997, what proportion of this population with disabilities reported being sad, unhappy, or depressed?
  a. 11 percent
  b. 21 percent
  c. 31 percent
  d. 41 percent

6-3. *Reduction in the proportion of adults with disabilities who re-port feelings such as sadness, unhappiness, or depression that prevent them from being active.* Of 1997, what propor-

tion of this population with disabilities reported being sad, unhappy, or depressed to the point of limiting their activity?
a. 18 percent
b. 28 percent
c. 38 percent
d. 48 percent

6-4. *Increase in the proportion of adults with disabilities who participate in social activities.* What is the targeted proportion of adults with disabilities who participate in social activities?
a. 25 percent
b. 50 percent
c. 75 percent
d. 100 percent

6-5. *Increase in the proportion of adults with disabilities reporting sufficient emotional support.* As of 1997, what proportion of adults with disabilities reported having sufficient emotional support?
a. 31 percent
b. 51 percent
c. 71 percent
d. 81 percent

6-6. *Increase in the proportion of adults with disabilities reporting satisfaction with life.* What is the targeted proportion of adults with disabilities reporting life satisfaction?
a. 31 percent
b. 51 percent
c. 71 percent
d. 91 percent

6-7. *Reduction in the number of people with disabilities in congregate care facilities, consistent with permanency planning principles.* Related to this objective, what is a congregate care facility?
a. An out-of-home facility providing housing for people with disabilities in which rotating staff members provide care (sixteen or more beds for adults, any number of beds for persons under twenty-one years of age)
b. A correctional facility

c. A long-term care nursing facility

d. A foster care home

6-8. *Elimination of disparities in employment rates between working-aged adults with and without disabilities.* As of 1995, what proportion of adults with disabilities between the ages of twenty-one and sixty-four years old were employed?

a. 32 percent

b. 52 percent

c. 72 percent

d. 92 percent

6-9. *Increase in the proportion of children and youth with disabilities who spend at least 80 percent of their time in regular education programs.* What is the targeted proportion of children and youth with disabilities spending 80 percent of their time in regular education programs?

a. 20 percent

b. 40 percent

c. 60 percent

d. 80 percent

6-10. *Increase in the proportion of health and wellness and treatment programs and facilities that provide full access for people with disabilities (developmental).* Related to this objective, which of the following represents health promotion for persons with disabilities?

a. Efforts to create healthy lifestyles and a healthy environment to prevent medical and other secondary conditions

b. Efforts at teaching people how to address their health care needs

c. Efforts at increasing opportunities for people to participate in usual life activities

d. All of above

6-11. *Reduction in the proportion of people with disabilities who report not having the assistive devices and technology needed (developmental).* Which of the following is correct about assistive technology for persons with disability?

a. The inability to pay is the main reason that persons with disabilities do not use assistive technology

b. Assistive technology can aid the independence and self-sufficiency of persons with disabilities

c. Assistive technology can enable persons with disabilities to work, attend school, and participate in community life.

d. All of the above are correct.

6-12.   *Reduction in the proportion of people with disabilities reporting environmental barriers to participation in home, school, work, or community activities (developmental).* Related to this objective, all of the following are correct except:

a. The most important outcome for all persons, including those with disabilities, is full participation as active, involved, and productive members of society.

b. A greater proportion of persons with disabilities report encountering problematic environmental barriers daily compared to persons without disabilities.

c. Full social participation for all persons cannot be achieved without eliminating environmental barriers found within architectural structures, technology, organizational policies and practices, and public attitudes.

d. Public health agencies should measure only the nature and extent of disability and not the extent to which environmental barriers impede social participation.

6-13.   *Increase the number of tribes, states, and the District of Columbia that have public health surveillance and health promotion programs for people with disabilities and caregivers.* How many states currently have such public health surveillance and health promotion programs?

a. Four states

b. Fourteen states

c. Twenty-four states

d. Thirty-four states

TEST ANSWERS

Focus Area 5

5-1.   (c) 45 percent. The target is 60 percent of persons with diabetes receiving formal diabetes education.* Formal diabetes education is self-management training that includes a process of initial individual patient assessment; instruction provided or supervised by a qualified health professional; evaluation of accumulation by the diabetic patient of appropriate knowledge, skills, and attitudes; and ongoing reassessment and training. An educated person can better manage the disease and its complications such as foot ulcers, hypoglycemia, and hypertension.

5-2.   (d) All of the above are true. Since there are three levels of prevention—before, during, and late-stage problem—all are correct answers.

5-3.   (d) All of the above are correct. It is important to know more about diabetes because it is one of the Healthy 2010 focus areas for which progress in achieving its 2000 objectives has not been in the desired direction, although increasing numbers of people are receiving formal education on diabetes.

5-4.   (b) 68 percent. The target is 80 percent. Diabetes's prevalence is growing, probably due to increases in new cases, decreases in deaths, and improvements in detection.

5-5.   (a) 43 percent. The baseline is 75 deaths per 100,000 population with the target at 45 deaths per 100,000 population.

5-6.   (b) 11 percent. The baseline is 8.8 deaths per 1,000 persons with diabetes and the target is 7.8 deaths per 1,000 persons with diabetes. Examples of diabetes-related deaths would be mortality from cardiovascular and/or kidney diseases for which diabetes is an underlying condition.

5-7.   (a) 10 percent. The baseline is 343 deaths from cardiovascular disease per 100,000 with diabetes. The target is 309 deaths per 100,000 persons with diabetes.

5-8.   (d) All of the above. All of these practices should be covered in formal diabetes education for persons with diabetes.

---

*Ages adjusted to the year 2000 standard population.

5-9.   (d) All of the above. In addition to these complications is the increased risk of end-stage renal disease.

5-10. (c) 55 percent. The baseline is 4.1 lower extremity amputations per 1,000 persons with diabetes and the target is 1.8 lower extremity amputations per 1,000 persons with diabetes per year.

5-11. (a) very small quantities of protein in the urine, indicating early kidney damage. Early intervention by detecting microalbumin in a person's urine can reduce the likelihood of microvascular complications of diabetes.

5-12. (b) 24 percent. The target for improvement is 50 percent of adults aged eighteen years and older with diabetes having a glycosylated hemoglobin measurement at least once a year.

5-13. (c) 75 percent. Presently about 47 percent of adults aged eighteen years and older with diabetes have a dilated eye examination annually. This is an example of tertiary prevention—screening for early diabetes complications in the eye.

5-14. (c) 75 percent. Presently about 55 percent of adults aged eighteen years and older with diabetes have an annual foot examination for ulcers. This is also an example of tertiary prevention.

5-15. (a) 58 percent. The targeted improvement is 75 percent of persons aged two years and older with diagnosed diabetes seeing a dentist at least once a year. Persons with diabetes are at increased risk for periodontal disease and tooth loss.

5-16. (d) 20 percent. The targeted improvement is 30 percent of adults aged forty years and older with diabetes taking aspirin at least fifteen times per month. This practice is associated with a reduced risk of microvascular and macrovascular complications, heart attack, and stroke.

5-17. (b) 60 percent. The baseline is 42 percent of adults aged eighteen years and older with diabetes performing self-blood-glucose-monitoring at least once daily. This is another practice that reduces the risks of microvascular and macrovascular complications from diabetes.

Focus Area 6

6-1.   (a) 0 percent. Since no Healthy People 2010 surveillance instruments include a standard set of questions that identify people with disabilities in 1999, a set of survey questions has been developed and tested through the Office of Health Promotion and Disease Prevention.

6-2.   (c) 31 percent. The target for improvement is a reduction to 17 percent. This would be equivalent to the proportion of children and adolescents without disabilities who reportedly experience these negative emotions.

6-3.   (b) 28 percent. The target for improvement is a reduction to 7 percent. This would be equivalent to the proportion of adults without disabilities who report feelings of sadness, unhappiness, or depression that prevent them from being active.

6-4.   (d) 100 percent. The baseline is 95.5 percent of adults aged eighteen years and older with disabilities participate in social activities. This would be equivalent to adults aged eighteen years and older without disabilities.

6-5.   (c) 71 percent. The target is 79 percent of adults aged eighteen years and older with disabilities report sufficient emotional support. This would be equivalent to adults eighteen years or older without disabilities.

6-6.   (d) 91 percent. The baseline is 87 percent of adults aged eighteen years and older with disabilities who report satisfaction with life.

6-7   (a) An out-of-home facility providing housing for people with disabilities in which rotating staff members provide care (sixteen or more beds for adults, any number of beds for persons under twenty-one years of age). The target for this objective is to reduce the number of adults in congregate care by 50 percent, and totally eliminate the number of persons under twenty-one years old in such care. The intended alternatives are community-based and in-home assistance services.

6-8.   (b) 52 percent. The target is 82 percent. This would represent a 58 percent improvement and make it equivalent to adults without disabilities.

6-9.   (c) 60 percent. The baseline is 45 percent of children and youth ages six to twenty-one years old with disabilities to spend at least 80 percent of their time in regular education programs. The improvement would be 33 percent.

6-10.   (d) All of the above. Persons with disabilities need to have access to programs and facilities that offer opportunities for physically and emotionally healthy lives. The Americans with Disabilities Act, with its enforcement section, can improve services and prevent secondary disabilities.

6-11.   (d) All of the above are correct. Assistive technology is any item, piece of equipment, or product system, whether acquired commercially, modified, or customized, that is used to increase, maintain, or improve the functional capabilities of individuals with disabilities.

6-12.   (d) Public health agencies should measure only the nature and extent of disability and not the extent to which environmental barriers impede social participation. It is important to study both disability as well as impedance to full social participation. This impedance can be in the forms of environmental barriers and universal design elements.

6-13.   (b) Fourteen states. The target is full coverage including all fifty states, the District of Columbia, and all Native American tribes.

Chapter 4

Agents

Recall that an agent is a necessary factor for the occurrence of disease and other morbid conditions. An agent can be a microorganism, chemical, energy form, individual/group behavior, or genetic message whose presence or, in some conditions, relative absence (e.g., nutritional deficiency) is needed for disease occurrence. A disease can have more than one agent. Accordingly, disease occurrence also requires the sufficiency factors of host and environment, all interacting within the context of time (Last, 1988).

Since there are two kinds of diseases, infectious and noninfectious, each has its respective agents. Sometimes called "communicable," infectious disease agents are biological in nature. With noninfectious diseases, a variety of agents such as chemical, physical, behavioral, social, and genetic can be necessary factors (Stone et al., 1996). Occurrence of a disease—be it infectious (e.g., common cold) or noninfectious (e.g., cancer)—rests on the likely exposure of a susceptible host to an infectious disease agent. Exposure can vary in duration and dose (amount of the agent present). Other sufficiency factors such as environmental conditions and host characteristics play important roles in disease occurrence (Timmreck, 1998).

BIOLOGICAL AGENTS

Biological agents are microorganisms, primary examples being bacteria, viruses, rickettsia, protozoa, and metazoa.

1. **Bacteria** are microscopic parasites that lack nuclear membranes but can live inside or outside the cells of their hosts. They are classified by shape: bacilli are rod-shaped like the foodborne disease pathogen *Clostridium perfringes.* Cocci are spherical

like streptococcus and staphylococcus. Spirochetes are spiral-shaped such as the agent to rat-bite fever.

2. **Viruses** are submicroscopic parasites that reproduce within the cells of their hosts, upon which they depend for vital life processes. The more common are cold virus strains.
3. **Rickettsia,** once considered a mix of viral and bacterial organisms, is actually a kind of bacteria.
4. **Protozoa** are microscopic unicellular parasites.
5. **Metazoa** are microscopic multicellular parasites. The more common are worms (e.g., hookworm, schistosomiasis, and onchocerciasis).

Other biological agents include fungi, which cause histoplasmosis and athlete's foot, and yeasts (e.g., candidiasis) (Moore, 2001).

It has been decided at a national level that the following diseases must be reported by health care providers to state health departments within seven days of occurrence (CDC, 1994):

Amebiasis	Malaria
Anthrax*	Meningitis*
Botulism*	Mumps
Brucellosis	Pertussis
Campylobacteriosis	Plague
Chicken pox	Poliomyelitis*
Chlamydia	Psittacosis*
Cholera*	Q fever
Diphtheria*	Rabies*
Encephalitis and arboviral	Rocky Mountain spotted fever
infections	Rubella and congenital syndrome
Escherichia coli 0157:H7 *(E. Coli)*	*Salmonellosis*
Giardiasis	Shigellosis
Gonorrhea	Syphilis
*Haemophilus influenzae**	Tetanus
Hepatitis A, B, or C*	Toxic shock syndrome
Histoplasmosis	Trichinosis
HIV/AIDS	Tuberculosis*
Legionellosis	Tularemia
Leprosy	Typhoid fever
Leptospirosis	Typhus
Listeriosis	Yellow fever*
Lyme disease	

*Must be rapidly reported to health department.

At the state level, health departments might require the reporting of additional infectious diseases such as influenza (the flu). The primary agent to most of these notifiable diseases is biological. Many of these infectious diseases are caused by bacteria: anthrax, botulism, brucellosis, campylobacteriosis, chlamydia, cholera, diphtheria, *E. coli,* gonorrhea, *Haemophilus influenzae,* legionellosis, leprosy, leptospirosis, listeriosis, Lyme disease, meningitis, pertussis, plague, psittacosis, salmonellosis, syphilis, tetanus, toxic shock syndrome, tuberculosis, tularemia, and typhoid fever. Viruses are responsible for the following diseases: chicken pox, encephalitis, hepatitis, HIV/AIDS, influenza, aseptic meningitis, mumps, poliomyelitis, rabies, rubella (measles), and yellow fever. Rickettsia are agents of Q fever, Rocky Mountain spotted fever, and typhus. Protozoa are responsible for amebiasis, giardiasis, and malaria. Metazoa, such as worms, are agents of trichinosis.

Even though it is important to report these diseases, the actual practice is not always the case. There are a few reasons for this, among which are decisions by patient and/or physician to conceal the case, and indifference by some physicians to the usefulness of reporting diseases such as hepatitis, influenza, and measles. Even so, notifiable disease reporting remains vital to the public's health, as data can act as a starting step for epidemiological investigations and studies which are the foundations to health promotion and disease prevention (Last, 1988).

The School Nurse and Notifiable Diseases

The practice of assigning a school health nurse to school systems began over 100 years ago. Since then, these professionals have played an important public health role with several key responsibilities, among which is identifying and reporting notifiable diseases. With the understanding that children's physical and mental health are linked to academic and social success, the school health nurse not only controls infectious diseases but provides supportive care to those infected. He or she also assesses children's development, screens for noninfectious diseases (e.g. hearing or vision impairment), provides health instruction, acts as a resource to special needs children, and serves as a liaison to the health care delivery system. With over 48 million youth in the nation's schools, it is imperative that the school population is able to avail itself of a licensed practical nurse or registered nurse. The desired ratio is one school nurse per every 750 students (Kann, Collins, and Pateman, 1995).

(continued)

(continued)
    This relates to Healthy People 2010 Objective 7-4: *Increase in the propor-tion of the nation's elementary, middle, junior high, and senior high schools that have a nurse-to-student ratio of at least 1:750* (Healthy People 2010, 2000, 7-17). (See Chapter 4 activities for more information.

Some infectious diseases can have more than one type of agent, such as hepatitis A, B, C (and actually two others), all of which are viral infections of the liver. Influenza has three types with type A capable of **genetic shifting,** the ability of an agent to develop subtypes or **strains** at irregular intervals. HIV/AIDS is another disease of which there is more than one viral strain.

Biological agents demonstrate various characteristics. One characteristic is **communicability,** which is the ability of an agent to be easily transmitted from a source host or environment to a new host. Another characteristic is **immunogenicity,** which is the ability to elicit an immune defense response, including immunity, in a host. More specifically, the biological agent, which acts as an **antigen,** stimulates the immune defense system to produce antibodies, white blood cells, and other cells that counteract the antigen. This characteristic is seen more often in viral agents. **Infectivity,** or infectibility, is the ability of the agent to enter and multiply within a host. Epidemiologists can ascertain an agent's infectivity by counting cases of disease occurring in a group after the first case was reported. **Pathogenicity** is the ability of the agent to produce signs and symptoms of disease. This characteristic is determined by comparing the number of diagnosed persons with those exposed to the agent. **Virulence** refers to the agent's ability to produce severe, possibly life-threatening signs and symptoms. Virulence is the degree of pathogenicity expressed by the agent. Some biological agents are responsible for **zoonosis,** which are human diseases acquired from another vertebrate animal. There are about 150 known zoonotic diseases, many of which are common in currently developing countries throughout the world and represent a major threat to public health. There are certainly plentiful cases of zoonotic diseases in the United States, e.g., anthrax, rabies, etc.

Agent characteristics of **rabies** are stark. Historically, rabies has been a notorious infectious disease. Recently, it has reemerged as a matter of public health concern. The *Lyssavirus* causes this highly pathogenic and virulent zoonosis. Although more prevalent in wildlife carnivores, *Lyssavirus* can be transmitted via saliva by the bite of the animal source host to domestic animals such as dogs and cats. Pet infection, of course, increases the risk of exposure to human hosts. During infectivity, which lasts anywhere from ten to fifty days, the virus grows in number while attacking the central nervous system. Characteristic signs and symptoms mark pathogenicity: depression, restlessness, fatigue, fever, excitability, excessive salivation, and convulsions. Due to dehydration and difficulty swallowing, the sight of water by the infected host triggers painful, sudden, involuntary contractions of the throat muscles. This sign is sometimes mistakenly labeled **hydrophobia,** or fear of water. All signs and symptoms intensify leading to death in about ten days. Being the most virulent infectious disease to vertebrate animals and humans, practically all diagnosed cases result in death from paralysis and suffocation. For the record, there are only two known cases of survival. Once the symptoms of rabies appear in humans, no treatment of the disease is possible except for invasive surgery into the cranium to relieve brain tissue swelling (Virginia Department of Health, 1998).

CHEMICAL AGENTS

Chemical agents of disease are pollutants and toxic substances. **Pollutants** are those that degrade environmental quality and threaten personal and public health. Some chemical agents not only pollute, but their poisonous, corrosive, or flammable characteristics qualify them as **toxic substances.** Most toxic substances are human-made and are sometimes called hazardous substances. Other toxic substances are found naturally. They could be in the form of allergens or poisons from industrial plants and animals. Pollutants and toxic substances are present in air, water, and soil. For instance, the Clean Air Act of 1972 (amended in 1991) regulates and restricts the release of criteria air pollutants:

1. **Carbon monoxide** (CO) is a colorless, odorless gas that is produced from incomplete combustion of carbon-containing fuels. CO reduces the blood's ability to carry oxygen.
2. **Lead** is a metallic element used in manufacturing processes that pollutes the environment through dust and fumes released by industrial plants. Long-term exposure can affect red blood cell

production and damage vital organs such as the brain, liver, and kidneys.

3. **Ozone** (O_3), or ground-level ozone, is a form of oxygen that is a highly reactive gas resulting primarily from the chemical reaction of sunlight on hydrocarbons and nitrogen oxides emitted in fuel combustion. As an air pollutant, ozone reacts chemically (oxidizes) and breaks down synthetic materials such as rubber compounds, and irritates living tissue such as the respiratory tract.

4. **Particulate matter** (PM 10) is a complex and varying mixture of substances that includes carbon-based particles, dust, and acid aerosols that are emitted primarily from transportation sources.

5. **Nitrogen** and **sulfur oxides** are oxygen-based compounds that usually result from the combustion of fossil fuels. These compounds can impede oxygen absorption by the human body as well as diminish the defensive capabilities of the upper respiratory tract.

6. **Radon** is a colorless, odorless gas that is a product of decaying uranium and occurs naturally in soil and rock. As radon gas breaks down it becomes a carcinogen of the respiratory tract. Radon is both an air and water pollutant. Concern about indoor air pollution necessitated U.S. Congress to pass the Indoor Radon Abatement Act of 1988.

Outdoor Air Quality

The public and environmental health problem of air pollution is responsible for premature death, cancer, and long-term damage to respiratory and cardiovascular systems. Air pollution also reduces visibility, damages crops and buildings, and deposits pollutants in the soil and in bodies of water where they affect the chemistry of the water and the organisms living there. Approximately 113 million people live in U.S. areas designated as nonattainment areas by the EPA for one or more of the six commonly found air pollutants: carbon monoxide, lead, ozone, particulate matter, nitrogen oxide, and sulfur oxide. Although efforts have been successful in regulating and reducing levels of these criteria air pollutants, ground level ozone is the largest problem, as determined by the number of people affected and the number of areas not meeting federal standards (EPA, 1997, pp. 5-7, 17).

This relates to Healthy People 2010 Objective 8-1: *Reduction in the proportion of persons exposed to air that does not meet the U.S. Environmental Protection Agency's health-based standards for harmful air pollutants* (Healthy People 2010, 2000, 8-15). (See Chapter 4 activities for more information.)

To maintain environmental quality in surface water areas, the Clean Water Act of 1972 and subsequent amendments have been responsible for decreasing levels of

- sewage contaminants such as bacteria;
- toxic substances such as metals, oils, and other substances; and
- eutrophicates such as phosphates and nitrates in fertilizers.

Accordingly, the Safe Drinking Water Act of 1974 and subsequent amendments set standards for the amount of lead allowable in drinking water and forbade the use of lead solder in drinking water pipes in new homes. This same legislation has improved methods for testing and treating disease-causing microorganisms in drinking water (e.g., fecal coliform).

The Comprehensive Environmental Response, Compensation, and Liability Act of 1980 and later amendments has been a governmental effort to clean up hazardous waste sites (through Superfund) and enforce the proper storage and disposal of these substances. Through this legislation, the Environmental Protection Agency (EPA) created a priority list of ten toxic substances that human hosts are able to ingest, inhale, or absorb through the skin:

- Arsenic
- Lead
- Mercury
- Vinyl chloride
- Benzene
- PCBs (polychlorinated biphenyls)
- Cadmium
- PAHs (polycyclic aromatic hydrocarbons)
- Chloroform
- Trichloroethylene

There have been international efforts at addressing pollutants and hazardous substances. For example, Earth Summit, a United Nation's sponsored conference, has been responsible for many nations adopting strict control of the following:

- Carbon dioxide and methane gas emissions that contribute to the greenhouse effect and global warming
- **Chlorofluorocarbons** (CFCs), which are refrigerants and insulators, destroy the ozone layer in the upper atmosphere, allowing more ultraviolet radiation that damages plants and greatly increases people's risk of skin cancer (World Resources Institute, 1998, p. 10).

Whereas the EPA identifies many toxic substances in the environment, the general public overlooks what might be considered the most toxic consumer product—tobacco. Besides containing the psychotropic drug **nicotine,** which can stimulate both the sympathetic and parasympathetic portions of the autonomic nervous system, tobacco contains the known carcinogen, **tar.** To make matters worse, tobacco also boasts of the following ingredients that are on the top ten of EPA's most toxic priority list: lead, benzene, cadmium, and PAHs. The toxic substances in tobacco products act as risk factors to the following diseases: cardiovascular and cerebrovascular disease, cancer, hypertension, unintentional injuries, chronic obstructive pulmonary disease, back pain, headaches, gastrointestinal ulceration, and addiction.

PHYSICAL AGENTS

Physical agents of disease and other morbid conditions represent naturally or human-made features of the physical environment that could also act as pollutants. They also represent agents of force and energy. Examples are:

1. **Solid waste** including refuse from households, agriculture, and businesses such as trash, grass clippings, tree trimmings, manure, excess stone generated from mining, and steel scraps from automobile plants. Solid waste can contain biological agents of infectious disease as well as chemical agents of noninfectious disease.
2. Energy products can produce excessive heat, electricity, radiation, or noise. Thermal pollution happens when water has been

used to cool industrial processes yet has not been allowed to resume its natural temperature before returning it to its source. High intensity electrical power lines have been implicated in child leukemia cancer clusters. Long-term exposure to low radiation is correlated with cancer; short-term exposure to high radiation levels results in tissue damage. Hearing loss (difficulty in detecting pitch) as well as elevated blood pressure are effects from excessive noise exposure.

3. Physical objects, when combined with force, are agents to unintentional and intentional injuries. One could argue that it is necessary to have a social or behavioral agent (e.g., aggressiveness) combined with the necessary factor of a weapon to explain the occurrence of a morbid condition (e.g., inflicted injury).

4. The operation of mechanical equipment is implicated not only in unintentional injuries, but also self-inflicted injuries such as repetitive motion and overuse syndrome.

5. Natural disasters involving weather conditions and related catastrophes.

SOCIAL AGENTS

Social agents of disease and other morbid conditions represent human-made features of the social environment that are experienced by groups of persons: depressed socioeconomic conditions, lack of education, lack of employment opportunities, psychosocial influences from media or peers, discrimination, severe civil unrest, and war. Unsafe products and services would also fall in this category. The recently recognized phenomenon of road rage is a behavioral expression of frustration arising from sundry social agents including overused transit systems, poor driver training for the general population, etc. Considerable concern and attention has been directed at gang behavior, domestic violence, and suicide as social agents to intentional injuries and death. Strategies for reducing violence should begin early in life, before violent beliefs and behavioral patterns can be adopted.

BEHAVIORAL AGENTS

Behavioral agents of some infectious and many noninfectious diseases are represented by unhealthy life practices by persons:

- Under- or overnutrition
- Physical inactivity
- Poor coping with stress
- Unsafe practices resulting in unintentional or intentional injuries
- Excessive or inappropriate psychoactive substance involvement
- Poor infection control (e.g., unsafe sexual acts)

These practices imply that a person can self-subject behavioral agents to affect himself or herself. Of course there are instances when the actions of one person can result in diseases and other conditions in another. For example, unsafe practices, called **misactions,** of one party can lead to harmful contact incidents, intentional or unintentional injuries, in a second party. Likewise, poorly executed practices of a professional can result in an **iatrogenic** condition, one created by the practice of medicine in the course of health care delivery. An intriguing example of an iatrogenic condition recently appeared in the popular press. The well-known comedian Dana Carvey is suing his physician for allegedly incorrectly operating on his coronary arteries. It is claimed that the surgeon operated on the wrong artery. This apparent "botched" surgery resulted in Carvey's continued high health risk and morbid condition. Since malpractice by the health care provider is alleged, a behavioral agent, an example of an iatrogenic condition is illustrated. To correct the mistake, an **angioplasty,** widening of artery via inserted balloons, was necessary, and Carvey is believed to have since recovered.

GENETIC AGENTS

Genetic agents are chemical instructions within genetic material that cause or contribute to disease or other morbid conditions. Some of these diseases are inherited, such as **hemophilia,** a blood-clotting disorder, **sickle cell anemia,** a red-blood-cell abnormality, and **phe-**

nylketonuria, an amino acid enzyme deficiency disorder. Genetic as well as other agents are responsible for **congenital diseases,** which are disorders present at birth. Genetic agents can also be indirectly responsible for predisposing persons to other diseases. Presently, the **Human Genome Project,** an international scientific program, has successfully mapped all of the chemical instructions found in genetic material that control human heredity. This health information will help provide a greater understanding of genetic agents of disease.

SUMMARY

Various kinds of agents have a role in disease occurrence. Biological agents are responsible for infectious diseases, many of which need to be reported to local health departments upon discovery. They are bacterial, viral, rickettsial, protozoan, and metazoan in nature. Pollutants and toxic substances represent chemical agents. A human-made toxic substance is called a hazardous substance. The Environmental Protection Agency monitors the population's exposure to these substances. Physical agents comprise naturally and human-made features of the physical environment including sources of force and energy (e.g., radiation). Social agents pertain to human-made features of the social environment that affect groups of persons (e.g., poverty). Behavioral agents are composed of unhealthy practices, such as overnutrition and physical inactivity. Last, genetic agents are hereditary bases to various diseases.

REVIEW QUESTIONS

1. What is an agent to disease? Which kind of agent is responsible for an infectious disease? Which kinds are responsible for non-infectious diseases?
2. Do you know the definitions of the important terms in bold print throughout this chapter?
3. What are examples of biological agents? Which biological agents cause which notifiable infectious disease(s)? What role do physicians, nurses, and other health professionals play in notifying public health departments about infectious disease cases?

4. What does it mean that biological agents can have more than one type? Can you explain the various characteristics of biological agents? Do you know the agent characteristics of the *Lyssavirus* (rabies)?
5. What are the two kinds of chemical agents? What is a toxic substance? A hazardous substance? What are the criteria air pollutants and how do they affect health? Which air pollutant is probably the largest problem faced by the EPA? Which chemical agents in water are of primary concern these days?
6. Could you recognize examples of toxic substances that have made the EPA's top ten priority list? Which of these substances are also found in tobacco products?
7. Which chemical agents have been recognized as international health concerns?
8. What are the various kinds of physical, social, behavioral, and genetic agents? Could you identify examples?
9. Do you know the answers to the following chapter activity questions based on objectives from Healthy People 2010 focus areas 7 and 8?

WEB SITE RESOURCES

Agency for Toxic Substance and Disease Registry
<http://atsdr1.atsdr.cdc.gov>

Medical Information on Diseases
<http://galaxy.einet.net/galaxy/Medicine.html>

National Institute on Mental Health (on depression and other mental disorders)
<http://www.nimh.nih.gov/publicat/>

National Tuberculosis Center
<http://www.umdnj.edu/ntbcweb/>

WebMD Health
<http://my.webmd.com/>

REFERENCES

Centers for Disease Control (1994). Notifiable diseases update. *Morbidity and Mortality Weekly Report,* 43(1): 43.

EPA (1997). National air quality and trends report. Washington, DC: Environmental Protection Agency, Office of Air and Radiation.

Healthy People 2010 (2000). *Healthy People 2010: Objectives for improving health.* Washington, DC: U.S. Department of Health and Human Services, Office for Disease Prevention and Health Promotion.

Kann, L., Collins, J.L., and Pateman, B.C. (1995). The school health policies and programs study (SHPPS): Rationale for a nationwide status report on school health programs. *Journal of School Health* 65(8): 291-294.

Last, J.M. (1988). *A dictionary of epidemiology.* New York: Oxford University Press.

Moore, P. (2001). *Killer germs and rogue diseases of the 21st century.* London, England: Carlton Books.

Stone, D.B., Armstrong, W.R., Macrina, D.M., and Pankau, J.W. (1996). *Introduction to epidemiology.* Madison, WI: Brown and Benchmark.

Timmreck, T.C. (1998). *An introduction to epidemiology* (Second edition). Sudbury, MA: Jones and Bartlett Publishers.

Virginia Department of Health (1998). Human rabies, Virginia 1998. *Epidemiology Bulletin,* (3)5: 1-4.

World Resources Institute (1998). *World resources: A guide to the global environment, the urban environment, 1996-1997.* Oxford, United Kingdom: Oxford University Press.

Purpose: (1) to acquaint the reader with Healthy People 2010 targets for improvement and (2) present examples of epidemiology as the underlying science to health promotion and disease prevention.

Directions: Check out your knowledge of these Healthy People 2010 focus areas by taking the following tests (answers follow in a separate section).

FOCUS AREA 7: EDUCATIONAL
AND COMMUNITY-BASED PROGRAMS

This focus area's goal is to increase the quality, availability, and effectiveness of educational and community-based programs designed to prevent disease and improve health and quality of life.

School Setting

7-1. *Increase in high school completion.* As of 1998, what percent of eighteen to twenty-four year olds completed high school?
a. 25 percent
b. 45 percent
c. 65 percent
d. 85 percent

7-2. *Increase in the proportion of middle, junior high, and senior high schools that provide school health education to prevent health problems in the following areas: unintentional injury; violence; suicide; tobacco use and addiction; alcohol and other drug use; unintended pregnancy and HIV/AIDS and other STD infection; unhealthy dietary patterns; inadequate physical activity; and environmental health. As of 1994,*

what percent of middle, junior high, and senior high schools provide all of the aforementioned health education units to the students?
a. 8 percent
b. 28 percent
c. 48 percent
d. 68 percent

7-3.   *Increase in the proportion of college and university students who receive information from their institution on each of the six priority health-risk behavior areas.* As of 1995, what percent of undergraduate students received information about unintentional/intentional injuries, tobacco consumption, psychoactive substance involvement, risky sexual behavior, unhealthy eating, and inadequate physical activity?
a. 6 percent
b. 26 percent
c. 46 percent
d. 66 percent

7-4.   *Increase in the proportion of the nation's elementary, middle, junior high, and senior high schools that have a nurse-to-student ratio of at least 1:750.* What is the targeted percentage of schools to have this nurse-to-student ratio?
a. 10 percent
b. 30 percent
c. 50 percent
d. 70 percent

Work Site Setting

7-5.   *Increase in the proportion of work sites that offer a comprehensive employee health promotion program to their employees.* What is the targeted proportion of work sites offering this kind of programming to their employees?
a. 25 percent
b. 50 percent
c. 75 percent
d. 100 percent

7-6. *Increase in the proportion of employees who participate in employer-sponsored health promotion activities.* As of 1994, what proportion of employees participate in these activities?
a. 21 percent
b. 41 percent
c. 61 percent
d. 81 percent

Health Care Setting

7-7. *Increase in the proportion of health care organizations that provide patient and family education (developmental).* All of the following are correct about patient and family education in health care settings except:
a. The right to comprehensive patient and family education is included in Consumer's Bill of Rights and Responsibilities.
b. Improved health is a primary objective.
c. Health care providers generally are considered credible sources of information.
d. Patient education and counseling have positive and clinically important effects on persons with acute and chronic conditions.

7-8. *Increase in the proportion of patients who report that they are satisfied with the patient education they receive from their health care organization (developmental).* Related to this objective, why is it important to examine patient satisfaction with health promotion programs in health care organizations?
a. Patient satisfaction is an indicator of performance by managed care organizations.
b. Patient satisfaction is a prevention-oriented indicator of managed care organizations.
c. Patient satisfaction is significant to marketing managed care organizations.
d. All of the above are correct.

7-9. *Increase in the proportion of hospitals and managed care organizations that provide community disease prevention and* health promotion activities that address the priority health needs identified by their community (developmental). Related to this objective, which of the following is correct?

    a. Community health promotion services provided by hospitals and managed care organizations are growing.

    b. Even though hospitals and managed care organizations differ on objectives and strategies, they share a mutual interest in improving the health of communities.

    c. Collaboration between private hospitals, managed care organizations, and public health agencies makes sense, considering how they share the same health promotion objectives.

    d. All of the above are correct.

Community Setting and Select Populations

7-10. *Increase in the proportion of tribal and local health service areas or jurisdictions that have established a community health promotion program that addresses multiple Healthy People 2010 focus areas (developmental).* Related to this objective, which of the following is correct?

    a. There should be a specific model for program planning, implementing, and evaluating.

    b. There should be community member involvement in planning, implementing, and evaluating the program.

    c. Programming should be directed at communities rather than at individuals in the population.

    d. All of the above are correct.

7-11. *Increase in the proportion of local health departments that have established culturally appropriate and linguistically competent community health promotion and disease prevention programs.* Related to this objective, which of the following is correct?

    a. Over the next ten years the U.S. population will continue to become more culturally diverse.

    b. Mainstream health promotion and disease prevention activities are often unsuccessful in reaching select communities within the population.

    c. By not reaching select and disadvantaged communities, the persons making up these communities might not meet health status indicators comparable to the overall U.S. population.

    d. All of the above are correct.

7-12. *Increase in the proportion of older adults who have partici-pated during the preceding year in at least one organized health promotion activity.* As of 1998, what proportion of this population has participated in this kind of programming in the past year?

    a. 11 percent

    b. 31 percent

    c. 51 percent

    d. 71 percent

FOCUS AREA 8: ENVIRONMENTAL HEALTH

This focus area's goal is to promote health for all through a healthy environment.

Outdoor Air Quality

8-1. *Reduction in the proportion of persons exposed to air that does not meet the U.S. Environmental Protection Agency's health-based standards for harmful air pollutants.* What is the targeted proportion of persons not being exposed to air pollutant levels exceeding EPA levels?

    a. 0 percent

    b. 20 percent

    c. 40 percent

    d. 60 percent

8-2. *Increase in the use of alternative modes of transportation to reduce motor vehicle emissions and improve the nation's air quality.* Which is considered an alternative mode of transportation for improving air quality?

    a. Double trips made by bicycling

    b. Trips made by walking

c. Trips made by transit
d. All of the above

8-3.   *Improvement in the nation's air quality by increasing the use of cleaner alternative fuels.* As of 1997, cleaner alternative fuels represented what percent of U.S. motor fuel consumption?
a. 2.7 percent
b. 22.7 percent
c. 44.7 percent
d. 66.7 percent

8-4.   *Reduction in toxic air emissions to decrease the risk of adverse health effects caused by airborne toxins.* How much of an improvement is targeted in reducing toxic air emissions?
a. 25 percent improvement
b. 50 percent improvement
c. 75 percent improvement.
d. 100 percent improvement

Water Quality

8-5.   *Increase in the proportion of persons served by community water systems who receive a supply of drinking water that meets the regulations of the Safe Drinking Water Act.* As of 1995, what percent of persons were served drinking water from community water systems that were within federal regulations for safety?
a. 25 percent
b. 45 percent
c. 65 percent
d. 85 percent

8-6.   *Reduction in waterborne disease outbreaks arising from water intended for drinking among persons served by community water systems.* On the average, how many outbreaks originating from community water systems are reported by the states annually?
a. Three outbreaks
b. Six outbreaks

c. Nine outbreaks
d. Twelve outbreaks

8-7. *Reduction in per capita domestic water withdrawals.* Related to this objective, what is a per capita domestic water withdrawal?
   a. The number of gallons of water delivered per day for each person served by a community water system
   b. A toilet flush
   c. The amount of water in a car wash
   d. The amount of water actually consumed by an individual in a given day

8-8. *Increase in the proportion of assessed rivers, lakes, and estuaries that are safe for fishing and recreational purposes (developmental).* What proportion of assessed surface water is unsafe for fishing and recreational purposes?
   a. 20 percent
   b. 40 percent
   c. 60 percent
   d. 80 percent

8-9. *Reduction in the number of beach closings that result from the presence of harmful bacteria (developmental).* What is the targeted percentage of coastal water sites for swimming that will support healthy aquatic communities?
   a. 25 percent
   b. 50 percent
   c. 75 percent
   d. 100 percent

8-10. *Reduction in the potential human exposure to persistent chemicals by decreasing fish contaminant levels (developmental).* Related to this objective, which is an environmental contaminant in fish?
   a. Organochlorine persistent chemicals
   b. Organophosphate insecticides
   c. Carbamate insecticides
   d. All of the above

Toxics and Wastes

8-11. *Elimination of elevated blood lead levels in children.* Related to this objective, all of the following are correct except:
   a. There has been in incline in childhood lead poisoning in the United States.
   b. Lead is a toxic substance that can affect vital organs and the brain.
   c. Reduction of lead poisoning takes place by identifying those at risk, conducting broad-base screenings, and cleaning up substandard housing.
   d. The risk for childhood lead poisoning is high for those of lower income, living in older housing, and belonging to certain racial and ethnic groups.

8-12. *Minimization of the risks to human health and the environment posed by hazardous sites.* Related to this objective, what is a hazardous substance?
   a. Any substance that possesses properties that can cause harm to human health and ecologic systems
   b. A toxic substance or toxicant
   c. Any substance not produced by a living organism that can cause harm to human health and ecologic systems
   d. All of the above

8-13. *Reduction in pesticide exposures that result in visits to a health care facility.* How much of an improvement is targeted by this objective?
   a. 10 percent improvement
   b. 30 percent improvement
   c. 50 percent improvement
   d. 70 percent improvement

8-14. *Reduction in the amount of toxic pollutants released, disposed of, treated, or used for energy recovery (developmental).* What is a way to accomplish this objective?
   a. Reduce pollution at the source through manufacturing process modifications
   b. Shifting to less polluting ingredients
   c. Make packaging changes
   d. All of the above

8-15.   *Increase in recycling of municipal solid waste.* What percent-
         age of total municipal waste is being targeted for recycling?
         a. 18 percent
         b. 38 percent
         c. 58 percent
         d. 78 percent

Health Homes and Health Communities

8-16.   *Reduction in indoor allergen levels.* Related to this objective,
         which is a source of an indoor allergen?
         a. House dust mites
         b. Cockroaches
         c. Mold
         d. All of the above

8-17.   *Increase in the number of office buildings that are managed
         using good indoor air quality practices.* Related to this objec-
         tive, which of the following is correct?
         a. A building's indoor air quality impacts the comfort and
            health of the occupants.
         b. Compared to outdoor air, indoor air has higher levels of
            pollutants.
         c. On the average, a majority of people spend over 90 percent
            of the time indoors.
         d. All of the above are correct.

8-18.   *Increase in the proportion of persons who live in homes
         tested for radon concentrations.* As of 1998, what percent of
         persons lived in homes tested for radon?
         a. 17 percent
         b. 37 percent
         c. 57 percent
         d. 77 percent

8-19.   *Increase in the number of new homes constructed to be radon
         resistant.* How much of an improvement is targeted for in-
         creasing new homes that are radon resistant?
         a. 10 percent improvement
         b. 20 percent improvement

c. 50 percent improvement
d. 70 percent improvement

8-20. *Increase in the proportion of the nation's primary and secondary schools that have official school policies ensuring the safety of students and staff from environmental hazards, such as chemicals in special classrooms, poor indoor air quality, asbestos, and exposure to pesticides (developmental).* Related to this objective, what is a special classroom?
a. A classroom having a substandard structure
b. A classroom such as laboratories and art rooms
c. A classroom for students with developmental, physical, or learning disabilities
d. A classroom identified as a hazardous waste site

8-21. *Assurance that state health departments establish training, plans, and protocols and conduct annual multi-institutional exercises to prepare for response to natural and technological disasters.* Related to this objective, which of the following is correct?
a. A disaster can result in a humanitarian emergency due to the event's negative effect on basic human needs (i.e., food, shelter, and water).
b. A disaster can be the release of radiation or chemical or biological substances whose occurrence overwhelms a population's ability to respond.
c. A disaster can be hurricanes, wind storms, earthquakes, volcanic eruptions, or floods overwhelming a population's ability to respond.
d. All of the above are correct.

8-22. *Increase in the proportion of persons living in pre-1950s housing that has been tested for the presence of lead-based paint.* As of 1998, what proportion of persons living in homes built before 1950 reported their homes had been tested for lead-based paint?
a. 16 percent
b. 36 percent
c. 56 percent
d. 76 percent

8-23. *Reduction in the proportion of occupied housing units that are substandard.* How much improvement is targeted in this objective?
a. 12 percent improvement
b. 32 percent improvement
c. 52 percent improvement
d. 72 percent improvement

Infrastructure and Surveillance

8-24. *Reduction in exposure to pesticides as measured by urine concentrations of metabolites.* In our efforts to reduce this kind of exposure, how much improvement is targeted?
a. 10 percent improvement
b. 30 percent improvement
c. 50 percent improvement
d. 70 percent improvement

8-25. *Reduction in exposure of the population to pesticides, heavy metals, and other toxic chemicals, as measured by blood and urine concentrations of the substances or their metabolites (developmental).* Related to this objective, all of the following are correct except:
a. Exposure to toxic substances can take place only with substances that are in current use.
b. Exposure to toxic chemicals can be a suspected or known cause of cancer.
c. Exposure to toxic substances can be a known or suspected cause of birth defects.
d. Exposure to toxic substances can be a known or suspected cause of other diseases in people.

8-26. *Improvement in the quality, utility, awareness, and use of existing information systems for environmental health (developmental).* Which environmental health information systems are available for use and can be accessed through the Internet?
a. EPA's Toxics Release Inventory
b. Environmental Defense Fund
c. TOXLINE
d. All of the above

8-27.   *Increase in or maintenance of the number of territories, tribes, and states, and the District of Columbia that monitor diseases or conditions that can be caused by exposure to environmental hazards.* Which diseases or morbid conditions would be included in this monitoring system?
   a. Lead poisoning
   b. Pesticide poisoning
   c. Mercury poisoning
   d. All of the above

8-28.   *Increase in the number of local health departments or agencies that use data from surveillance of environmental risk factors as part of their vector control programs (developmental).* Related to this objective, what is vector control?
   a. Unplanned and inefficient development of open land
   b. Control of any object, organism, or thing that transmits disease from one host to another
   c. Collection of online information on drugs and other chemicals maintained by the National Library of Medicine
   d. Classrooms with special characteristics, such as laboratories and art rooms, in which particular environmental hazards may be found

Global Environmental Health

8-29.   *Reduction in the global burden of disease due to poor water quality, sanitation, and personal and domestic hygiene.* How much of an improvement is targeted in terms of reducing this burden of disease?
   a. 20 percent improvement
   b. 40 percent improvement
   c. 60 percent improvement
   d. 80 percent improvement

8-30.   *Increase in the proportion of the population in the U.S.-Mexico border region that have adequate drinking water and sanitation facilities.* How much of an improvement is targeted in terms of increasing this proportion of this population?
   a. 10 percent improvement
   b. 30 percent improvement
   c. 50 percent improvement
   d. 70 percent improvement

TEST ANSWERS

Focus Area 7

7-1.   (d) 85 percent. The target is for 90 percent of persons aged eighteen to twenty-four years completing high school. Dropping out of school places youth at risk of delayed employment opportunities, poverty, and poor health.

7-2.   (b) 28 percent. The target is 70 percent of schools providing all of these health education units.

7-3.   (a) 6 percent. The target is for 25 percent of undergraduate students receiving information from their college or university on unintentional/intentional injuries, tobacco consumption, psychoactive substance involvement, risky sexual behavior, unhealthy eating, and inadequate physical activity.

7-4.   (c) 50 percent. Presently, about 28 percent of schools at all levels have a nurse-to-student ratio of 1:750. The school health nurse assesses students' health and development, assists families to access medical services, and acts as a link between families and community/clinical health services.

7-5.   (c) 75 percent. This target pertains to work sites of all sizes (number of employees). A comprehensive employee health promotion program comprises health education, socially and physically supportive work environments, program incorporation into the organization's administrative structure, and coordination with related employee services programs.

7-6.   (c) 61 percent. The target for improvement is 75 percent of employees aged eighteen years and older participating in employer-sponsored health promotion activities.

7-7.   (a) The right to comprehensive patient and family education is included in the Consumer's Bill of Rights and Responsibilities. All of the remaining answers are correct, however, there is noticeable variability in the health promotion and disease prevention activities delivered to members of managed care organizations.

7-8.   (d) All of the above are correct. Managed care plans rely on health plan employer data and information sets to record performance, prevention, and marketing indicators. Part of the collected data is patient satisfaction.

7-9.   (d) All of the above are correct. Besides collaborating on health promotion programming, these entities are now collaborating on clinical preventive services, surveillance, and research.

7-10   (d) All of the above are correct. The answer is obvious. Just as obvious is the less-than-ideal way many local community health programs attempt to address Healthy People 2010 objectives.

7-11.   (d) All of the above are correct. A majority of excess deaths among U.S. communities, especially African Americans and Hispanics or Latinos, can be prevented. Efforts at culturally and linguistically appropriate programming should address these leading causes of death: cancer, cardiovascular disease, cirrhosis, diabetes, HIV or AIDS, homicide, and unintentional injuries.

7-12.   (a) 11 percent. The targeted improvement is 90 percent of older adults participating during the preceding year in at least one organized health promotion activity.* Probably more so than other age groups, older adults desire health information and will commit to making personal changes to ensure health and independence. Addressing modifiable behaviors that are age appropriate, programming would comprise education, counseling, screening/chemoprophylaxis, environmental enhancements, and protective services.

Focus Area 8

8-1.   (a) 0 percent. This target pertains to air pollutants: carbon monoxide, nitrogen dioxide, sulfur dioxide, and lead. Similar targets pertain to ozone for the year 2012, and particulate matter for the year 2018.

8-2.   (d) All of the above. Automobile emissions are the primary contributant to air pollution in many U.S. communities, so electing alternative means of travel will improve air quality.

8-3.   (a) 2.7 percent. The target is for 30 percent of motor fuel consumption to be from cleaner alternatives such as ethanol-blended fuels.

---

* Ages adjusted to the year 2000 standard population.

8-4.   (c) 75 percent improvement. Toxic air pollutants are known or suspected causes of cancer and other morbid conditions (e.g., birth defects). They are also responsible for adverse environmental effects.

8-5.   (d) 85 percent. The target is 95 percent of persons to receive safe drinking water through public water supplies. Smaller municipal water systems (serving 25 to 3,300 persons) are more widespread yet reach only 10 percent of the U.S. population. These smaller systems also account for a majority of the EPA drinking water violations (usually due to the presence of disease-causing agents).

8-6.   (b) Six outbreaks. The target is two outbreaks reported annually by each state. The average is now about six per year. Smaller community water systems account for a majority of these outbreaks.

8-7.   (a) The number of gallons of water delivered per day for each person served by a community water system. In an era of water-demand, management, and conservation, the nation has to continue active water conservation efforts such as the installation of additional meters and water-conserving plumbing features.

8-8.   (b) 40 percent. According to the EPA, about 40 percent of the nation's streams, lakes, and estuaries are too polluted for fishing, swimming, or other designated uses. A primary reason is inappropriate release of or inadequately treated human, industrial or agricultural wastes that comprise the water's quality for human use.

8-9.   (c) 75 percent. The EPA will be developing a nationwide beach-closing survey to monitor water quality in U.S. swimming beaches (not including small streams, private lakes, and ponds).

8-10.   (d) All of the above. A surveillance system has been established, the Biomonitoring of Environmental Status and Trends (BEST), to assess and monitor the effects of environmental contaminants on biological resources such as fish.

8-11.   (a) There has been in incline in childhood lead poisoning in the United States. This statement is incorrect. At one point during the 1980s, between 2 to 3 million children six months to five years old had blood lead levels exceeding 15 mg/dl of blood, and that number has declined to fewer than 900,000. Reduction efforts at identifying and screening those at risk, as well as cleaning up substandard housing, need to continue to eradicate this environmental health problem.

8-12.   (d) All of the above. All of the listed choices mean hazardous substance. To minimize the risk from hazardous substance sites, the EPA identifies waste sites requiring clean up which are eligible for federal assistance. These sites must maintain a safe and appropriate way to manage and dispose of these wastes. One needed effort is identifying and eliminating the risk of underground tank leakage into the groundwater and soil. Attention is also directed at "brownfields," abandoned or little-used property whose (re)development is jeopardized by real or perceived environmental contamination.

8-13.   (c) 50 percent improvement. A surveillance system known as the American Association of Poison Control Centers monitors health care visits due to exposures to pesticides, disinfectants, fungicides, herbicides, insecticides, moth repellants, and rodenticides.

8-14.   (d) All of the above. All are source reduction methods. Moreover, all pollutants released, treated, and/or disposed of should be measured.

8-15.   (b) 38 percent. As of 1996, 27 percent of total municipal solid waste generated was recycled and this includes composting.

8-16.   (d) All of the above. Indoor air allergens also arise from the presence of pets. These allergens can aggravate the symptoms of respiratory conditions such as asthma.

8-17.   (d) All of the above are correct. Indoor air quality is the overall state of the air inside a building as reflected by the presence of pollutants, such as dust, fungi, animal dander, volatile organic compounds, carbon monoxide, and lead.

8-18.   (a) 17 percent. The target is 50 percent of persons living in homes to be tested for radon concentrations. This represents a 20 percent improvement.

8-19.   (c) 50 percent improvement. Radon-resistant construction comprises affordable and simple techniques that, when incorporated during construction of a new home, reduce indoor radon levels by preventing radon entry and providing a means for venting radon to the outdoors.

8-20.   (b) A classroom such as laboratories and art rooms. This kind of classroom has special characteristics within which particular environmental hazards may be found.

8-21.   (d) All of the above are correct. Disaster preparedness through organizational and community plans and protocols is receiving more attention nationally as well as globally.

8-22.   (a) 16 percent. The target is for 50 percent of persons living in homes built before 1950 reporting that their homes have been tested for the presence of lead-based paint. Lead-based paint on walls, trim, floors, and ceilings is a hazardous substance source. There is also household lead dust, which are very fine particles containing lead caused by the deterioration of lead paint.

8-23.   (c) 52 percent improvement. As of 1995, about 6.2 percent of occupied housing units in the country had moderate to severe physical problems, and the target is to reduce this number to 3 percent.

8-24.   (b) 30 percent improvement. Pesticides like carbaryl, methyl parathion and parathions, chlorpyrifos, and propoxur. These pesticides inhibit cholinesterase, an enzyme found in the human body. These pesticides are among those commonly used in the home and garden, agriculture, and industry.

8-25.   (a) Exposure to toxic substances can take place only with substances that are in current use. Actually, toxic substances have been banned from manufacturing and use since the 1970s such as polychlorinated biphenyls (PCBs) whose presence linger in the environment.

8-26.   (d) All of the above. Besides these information systems, there are also: integrated risk information system (IRIS), registry of toxic effects of chemical substances (RTECS), HazDat, and aerometric information retrieval system (AIRS).

8-27.   (d) All of the above. In addition, the following diseases and conditions would be monitored: arsenic poisoning, cadmium poisoning, methemoglobinemia, acute chemical poisoning, asthma, hyperthermia, skin cancer, and birth defects.

8-28.   (b) Control of any object, organism, or thing that transmits disease from one host to another. More specifically, the diseases are transmitted to people by organisms, such as insects.

8-29.   (a) 20 percent improvement. Providing access to clean water and improving sanitation and hygiene will decrease incidence of diarrheal disease, alleviate human distress, and lengthen life expectancy.

8-30.   (a) 10 percent improvement. This area of the country faces a serious water pollution problem due to deficiency in wastewater treatment, disposal of untreated sewage, and inadequately operated water treatment plants.

Chapter 5

Person, Place, and Time

INTRODUCTION

Recall the definition of epidemiology—the study of the occurrence and distribution, cause and control, treatment and prevention of disease and other morbid conditions. In explaining the occurrence of disease and other morbid conditions, epidemiologists rely on the principle known as the epidemiological triad. Within this triad is the necessary factor or agent as well as the sufficiency factors of host and environment. Although the triad is useful in explaining disease occurrence, it is limited in explaining disease distribution.

Rarely are cases of disease completely or evenly distributed throughout an exposed population. Not all persons develop a disease after exposure to agents or risks. Some cases follow the full disease process while others are inapparent. Still, other cases express full pathogenicity and virulence, hence the distribution of disease becomes staggered. The reason for the variance in case distribution has a lot to do with personal characteristics of exposed hosts. Likewise, features of their surroundings, also known as place characteristics, can come into play. The factor of time also needs to be considered. Hence, disease distribution is better explained by exploring what are known as person-place-time characteristics. These characteristics are considered detailed levels or features of the sufficiency factors to disease.

Factors and Characteristics

Disease can occur in a single case or more likely in a group of cases. When describing occurrence in a single case, the term factor is used. In a group of cases, the term characteristic is used. In a single case, the factors are:

- Agent
- Host
- Environment
- Time

In a group of cases, the characteristics are:

- Risk
- Person
- Place
- Time

Each characteristic has levels:

Risk	Person	Place	Time
Low	Age	Biological	Periodicity
Moderate	Gender	Physical	Time of year
High	Race	Sociocultural	Disease length
		Occupation	Incubation
		Other	Other

Disease Distribution

Before exploring person, place, and time characteristics, it should be mentioned that epidemiologists have developed mathematical models and formulas for calculating present and projecting future case distribution within a population. The distribution of present cases of disease can be graphically depicted in an **epidemic curve** (see Fig. 3.2), a charting of the case appearance during an epidemic along a time line (as discussed in Chapter 3).

There are means of calculating future distribution of disease cases. A course in introductory statistics covers such analyses as Poisson distribution as well as the negative binomial. Even with these techniques of depicting and calculating case distribution, the questions remain: What person, place, and time characteristics are at work? What varying characteristics of the person, place, or time influence how a disease spreads through a group or population? To answer these questions, the specific kinds of characteristics will be examined.

PERSON CHARACTERISTICS

Person characteristics are inherited qualities or personal activities that determine who is at risk for disease and negative behavioral conditions. They are best depicted as demographic variables. Age is the chief person characteristic; gender is next in importance. Other person characteristics are race and ethnicity, socioeconomic status, marital status, religion, occupation, and lifestyle. If age is the chief person characteristic, then it is necessary to explore further explanations. Foremost, there are periods during the life cycle (early and later ages) during which persons are more susceptible to the infectivity of agents. This probably has to do with either underdeveloped or compromised immune defense systems. Another reason is the longer one's life cycle, the greater the exposure to agents of all kinds. Whereas older persons have developed active immunity to many viral infections, during the same time they have accumulated exposures to chemical, physical, and behavioral agents. The body's physiological activity in the event of illness or injury is another factor in the age equation. Older persons tend to have less efficient physiological activity. Examples of the age characteristic having a significant influence on disease distribution include:

- The incidence and prevalence of childhood diseases such as measles, mumps, pertussis, and others that are inoculated against is higher among younger age groups. These infectious conditions tend to be early age-specific diseases due to immature immune defense systems. However, other place and time characteristics could contribute to "children's diseases" distributions (e.g., attending schools in more dense groups of persons compared to staying at home in less dense groups).
- The incidence and prevalence of chronic degenerative diseases increase proportionately with age. This is probably due to the cumulative effects of exposure to chemical, physical, social, and behavioral agents over the life cycle. A good example of this

characteristic is musculoskeletal conditions, which represent the major causes of disability in the United States. **Arthritis** and other rheumatic conditions are inflammatory and possibly degenerative diseases of the joints, muscles, fascia, tendons, bursa, ligaments, and other connective tissues of the body. **Osteoporosis** is a bone disease characterized by a reduction of bone mass and a deterioration of the microarchitecture of the bone leading to bone fragility. **Chronic back conditions** refers to back pain and other conditions affecting only the back. These musculoskeletal conditions significantly impact personal and public health. With more persons reaching and exceeding sixty-five years of age, these conditions will be taking their toll on quality of life, especially for persons wishing to continue working past this age point. Arthritis is second only to heart disease as a cause of work disability (LaPlante, 1988).

Given the significant influence of age on disease distribution, most epidemiologists age-adjust any incidence of disease. This will be further explained in Chapter 7.

Gender is the second most important person characteristic. In general, males have higher mortality rates whereas women have higher morbidity rates. Obviously, there are some diseases that are gender-specific, such as certain types of cancer affecting the various reproductive organs. Other examples of the gender characteristic having a significant influence on disease distribution include:

- Behavioral disorders such as mood and anxiety disorders are more common in females.
- Annual gonorrhea incidence rates are generally higher in males than in females, whereas annual chlamydia rates are higher in females than in males. Both are sexually transmitted bacterial diseases that primarily involve the urogenital tract.
- Although cardiovascular disease (CVD) remains the leading cause of death in females over the age of thirty, mortality rates from this disease—a collection of disorders of the heart tissue/valves or the blood vessels vasculating the organ—are higher in males than in females.

Person Factors and Adolescent Pregnancy

In the United States, the rate of adolescent pregnancy is much higher than in many other developed countries. To ensure the optimum potential of females, and the proper growth and development of newborns, the pregnancy rate among fifteen- to seventeen-year-old females should be reduced, whereas the number of pregnancies in females under fifteen years of age should be zero. Most adolescent pregnancies (78 percent) take place outside of marriage, a trend that has increased since the 1970s. Nearly two-thirds of young adolescent pregnancies end in induced abortion or fetal loss. The probability of low birth weight children is also a matter of concern (Ventura, Martin, and Curtin, 1999).

This relates to Healthy People 2010 Objective 9-7: *Reduction in pregnancies among adolescent females* (Healthy People 2010, 2000, 9-19). (See Chapter 5 activities for more information.)

It should be noted that few diseases appear race or ethnicity specific. However, examples include:

- Higher incidence rates of **sickle-cell anemia,** a genetic disorder that forms abnormal hemoglobin and limits the oxygen-carrying capacity of red blood cells, occur in the African-American population.
- **Tay-Sachs,** a rare genetic disease causing neurological damage and death, primarily occurs in infants of eastern European Jewish descent.
- Higher than expected rates of **diabetes,** an endocrine disorder that disrupts insulin production or absorption in the body, are noted among Hispanics.
- Immigration and emigration studies have presented evidence that white people tend to maintain higher rates of heart disease morbidity than other races; the same observation has been made with African Americans and hypertension; and some Asian populations and gastrointestinal tract cancers.

During mortality surveillance, epidemiologists have observed a phenomenon known as the **crossover effect.** This means that a characteristically high rate of mortality in one group decreases as persons in that group progress through the life cycle, while other groups in the same population experience increases in mortality rates. This has been seen in African American and white populations. A literal interpretation for African Americans is "the older you get, the older you get." But for whites, "the older you get, the more likely you are to meet your Maker." To confirm this phenomenon, researchers conducted a prospective study (types of studies are covered in Chapter 9). They followed 4,136 men and women (1,875 whites and 2,261 blacks) living in North Carolina for nine years. Mortality rates and ratios (studied in Chapter 7) were calculated and adjusted according to age and other characteristics. African Americans had higher mortality rates than whites at young-old age (sixty-five to eighty years) but had significantly lower mortality rates after age eighty. Black persons aged eighty or older had a significantly lower risk of all-cause mortality, specifically heart disease. The epidemiologists concluded that racial differences in mortality are affected by the age characteristic. This phenomenon might take place because of the selective survival of the healthiest persons, or perhaps it is due to biomedical factors affecting longevity after age eighty (Corti et al., 1999).

Marital status also appears to have a significant influence on disease and death distribution. Mortality rates for each gender are lower for married persons compared to those for widowed or divorced persons. Of course, there are other variables to consider, such as the possibility that some persons may not marry because of existing health problems or limitations.

Occupation as a person characteristic is also intriguing. To begin, just being employed is associated with a higher health status compared to being unemployed. This is known as the **healthy worker effect.** In general, a person's occupational category (manager, professional, laborer, etc.) does not seem to influence illness or death patterns in the worker population. For example, laborers with college degrees have comparable health status to professionals with college degrees (Miller, Golaszewski, Pfeiffer, and Edington, 1990). However, specific job positions might involve exposure to biological, chemical, or physical agents. Whereas there are OSHA standards to protect workers from health and safety risks, it cannot be overlooked that certain occupations have greater incidents of morbidity and mortality. For example, a pattern of unintentional injuries is more likely to be observed among construction workers.

Lifestyle as a person characteristic also has direct bearing on disease distribution. Upon examining the leading causes of death, it is worth noting how a majority of cases are associated with an unhealthy lifestyle. Comprising an unhealthy lifestyle are the following behavioral agents or risk practices:

- Any tobacco use, and inappropriate or excessive alcohol and other drug use
- Overnutrition resulting in hypercholesterolemia (an elevated cholesterol level of ≥220 mg/dL blood) or obesity (20 percent or more greater than recommended body weight)
- Physical inactivity
- Poorly managing stress
- Unsafe practices resulting in unintentional or intentional injuries
- Not practicing self-examination (i.e., skin, breast, or testicle)
- Poor infection control (e.g., unsafe sexual acts, unsafe food preparation, etc.)

The Person Factor of Infection Control During Food Preparation

Only about 72 percent of consumers practice the person factor of infection control during food preparation. That is why public health officials have launched the FightBAC! campaign. This food safety campaign centers on key food safety practices conveyed through four simple messages: clean—wash hands and surfaces often; separate—do not cross-contaminate; cook—cook to proper temperatures; and chill—refrigerate promptly (Altekruse, Street, and Fein, 1996).

This relates to Healthy People 2010 Objective 10-5: *Increase in the proportion of consumers who follow key food safety practices* (Healthy People 2010, 2000, 10-14). (See Chapter 5 activities for more information.)

Person Characteristic Interaction

It is unclear as to the influence of socioeconomic status on disease distribution, since this person characteristic is interwoven with other variables such as level of education, occupational category, living arrangements, access to health care, and lifestyle. For instance, it is now known that adult males of lower socioeconomic status have high annual rates of mortality, but this group is also poorly educated, unskilled, and less likely to pursue health care compared to other adult males in higher socioeconomic status. About 47 percent of homeless persons have chronic health problems whereas 34 percent have mental health disorders, according to a study conducted for the Department of Housing and Urban Development (Lam and Rosenheck, 1999).

Religion is another person characteristic whose influence on disease distribution is complicated by other variables. Demographically, there is a wide variety of persons within any major religion. However, some religious groups advocate specific health practices such as alcohol refrainment. Still, alcohol abstinence (whether advocated by a religious faith or not) does not appear to stand out as a notable influence on a person's morbidity and mortality when compared to other persons who choose not to follow this life practice. Studies are under way examining the linkage between spiritual health—one's state of health as affected by transcending material existence and interconnecting with others—and morbidity and mortality rates.

Looking further at the interaction of person characteristics, there are evident examples of its influence on disease distribution. **Tuberculosis** comes to mind. This bacterial disease of the respiratory tract tends to have higher incidence rates in younger, nonwhite persons. Another example is **suicide,** which is intentional self-inflicted injury leading to death. Annual mortality rates are highest among white males under the age of twenty-five. Still another example is AIDS-related opportunistic diseases, which account for more deaths in twenty-five to forty-four-year-old black females than any other cause of death. There are several other illustrations of person characteristic interaction and its influence on disease distribution.

PLACE CHARACTERISTICS

Place characteristics are inherent in the three kinds of environments: physical, biological, and sociocultural. The **physical environment** represents natural or human-made structures and conditions of the natural surroundings. The **biological environment** is comprised of living things and their surroundings. These living things interact as functional units or ecosystems. The **sociocultural environment** involves human-made conventions and constructs of the surroundings. These environments play the dual role of being the source of disease agents as well as the context of disease formation.

Lyme disease is a compelling example of how the biological environment capitalizes on the interaction of living things to influence disease occurrence and distribution. Next to HIV disease, Lyme disease is the fastest-growing infectious disease in the United States (Meltzer, Dennis, and Orloski, 1999). Each year, state health departments are notified of about 13,000 cases of Lyme disease. Surveillance systems have noted a twenty-five-fold increase in the annual number of cases reported since 1982, with the disease occurring in new geographic areas. Because Lyme disease is a multistage, multisystem, bacterial infection, epidemiologists consider its occurrence a classic example of the environment-as-ecosystem concept, meaning that the spread of the disease to humans is dependent upon the interaction of various living things—the changes in one affect the others. Lyme disease is caused by the spirochete *Borrelia burgdorferi*. Symptoms include a rash at the site of infectivity with resulting flulike symptoms such as headache, muscular aches and pains, and fatigue. Pathogenicity and virulence include arthritis (40 to 60 percent of untreated cases), heart problems (8 percent), and neurological problems (15 to 20 percent). Lyme disease bacteria are transmitted by a vector, the black-legged tick of the *Accedes* genus, and the primary reservoir is the white-footed mouse. Once a tick feeds on the blood of an infected mouse, each subsequent stage of development exhibits a preference for a particular host to infect. For example, the tick's larvae prefer to continue to feed on white-footed mice and other small rodents in forested or wooded areas. But once the larvae molt, the nymphs that emerge retain the infection and are able to transmit it to other hosts such as larger mammals, birds, and humans. Most human cases of Lyme disease can be attributed to bites from the nymph. But what does this have to do with the ecosystem? Consider the life stages of the tick. After larval and nymphal stages, the adult tick prefers to feed on deer. In fact, in order for the tick population to flourish in nature, it requires the presence of deer. Therefore, the proliferation of Lyme disease-carrying ticks is a direct result of burgeoning deer populations, because adult ticks are able to find hosts more easily (Meltzer, Dennis, and Orloski, 1999).

Place characteristics are implicated in disease occurrence when age-adjusted sickness or death rates increase for immigrants into a place, and decrease for emigrants out of that place. There have been a number of studies on **multiple sclerosis** (a neurological disease in which nerve fiber covering is damaged from an unknown agent) gastrointestinal tract cancer, and heart disease demonstrating how people from high-risk places reduce their sickness and death rates by moving to low-risk places. Likewise, the risk of developing these diseases increases when persons immigrate to places that have existing high rates of these diseases. Still, it is necessary to be cautious and not commit **ecological fallacy,** presuming physical environmental characteristics are the direct explanation of disease, when it could likely be a sociocultural environmental influence from a previous location transported to a new location. People tend to bring their customs and diseases with them when immigrating to a new place (Gordis, 1996).

By physical or geographic location alone, there are distinct distributions of diseases throughout the globe. For example, warmer, moist climatic conditions of the tropics are the primary place characteristics for malaria. Despite efforts at malaria control through pesticides and other means, the only way to successfully eradicate the disease is to develop the land through settlements, thus significantly reducing the volume of standing surface water areas that support breeding mosquitoes.

Variations in disease distribution have been observed between nations. An evident example would be waterborne diseases (e.g., shigellosis, cholera) being prevalent in developing countries lacking adequate sewage disposal and treatment systems. In another example, nutritional deficiencies (e.g., lack of iron and anemia, lack of vitamin D and rickets) can be explained by a country's dependence upon local agriculture which furnishes an inadequate range of nutrients. Other countries suffer from overnutrition in terms of excess saturated fats and simple sugars in the diet acting as risk factors to heart disease. In other sites around the world, a combination of place characteristics is at play. Certain cancers might be prevalent in more developed countries not only because of the population's sustained long-term exposure to industrial-related pollutants, but also due to the prevalence of risky behaviors, such as tobacco use.

There are variations in disease distribution observed between regions within a nation. Population density is a key to the spread of many infectious diseases, such as influenza. Warmer climate explains tickborne disease distribution as well as the native vegetation and wildlife necessary for transmission. In the United States, **Rocky Mountain spotted fever,** a tickborne rickettsial disease that causes fever, rash, and discomfort, is prevalent along the East Coast and south central part of the United States. Lyme disease exists in the northeast, mid-Atlantic, north central, and Pacific coast regions.

Regional differences in noninfectious disease distribution are more challenging to explain. If a disease trend is truly due to place characteristics, it is considered a **factual difference.** If, however, the regional difference is better explained by human error in measurement or interpretation, it is considered an **artifactual difference.**

Place Characteristic Interaction

Already discussed is how individual person characteristics can interact, and their combined influence is observed in disease distribution. This can also be seen in place characteristic interaction. For example, the physical and biological characteristics of the environment help determine the occurrence of waterborne diseases. Also, the physical occupational environment can expose workers to many agents and risk factors for injuries, cancer, and other specific diseases. This risk can be exacerbated in a stressful sociocultural work environment. Although traditional medical professionals question the relationship between stress and disease, many epidemiologists agree that, minimally, stressful environmental conditions will amplify the effect of exposure to physical or chemical agents.

Place and Environmental Health

Personal and public health depend on conservation of the environment. A separate discipline, **ecology,** studies the interrelationships of organisms and their environment. The environment plays a direct/indirect role in disease development. Directly, the environment is the origin of infectious diseases. Indirectly, it is the context of illnesses of all kinds. In fact, the environment can explain the geographic distribution of many infectious and some noninfectious diseases.

Although it is difficult for epidemiologists to establish the degree to which risk factors and exposures cause illness and death, the environment is the context of all risk factors and agents. It is a formidable task to search for environmental causes of disease for several reasons:

- *Source:* In many cases of exposure to environmental health hazards, it is difficult to determine the source, especially if it is a **nonpoint source,** a dispersed source of exposure usually distant from the originating or **point source.** For example, the originating source of contaminated runoff water might be a distant pasture. The local air breathed might have traveled from a distant site fraught with pollutants.
- *Exposure:* There are varying degrees of exposure among persons in the same place who inhale, consume, or come in contact with the same substance. This has a lot to do with individual breathing cycles, actual amount of agent taken in, etc.
- *Concentration:* Environmental health hazards vary in concentration as they disperse through air, water, or soil.
- *Accumulation:* Many toxic substances are absorbed into fatty tissues of the body; hence, the higher one's body fat composition, the greater the accumulation. Also, persons vary in the length of time they have been exposed (age) which allows for accumulation.
- *Interaction:* During exposure, individual environmental health pollutants or chemicals are likely to interact; and the results are unpredictable.
- *Latency of environmental diseases:* All of these diseases are noninfectious and many are chronic with long latency periods. Therefore, it would be difficult to discern the present-day cause for a disease that does not become clinically apparent until years or decades later.

Despite the complex relationships between environmental exposures and ill effects on human health, there is a call to establishing causality. Given the billions of dollars spent annually on cleaning up and managing hazardous U.S. waste sites, a noticeably smaller proportion of funding is allocated to determining the health risk of chronic, low-level exposures to hazardous substances. If anything, government officials should want to know if clean up efforts have made a significant impact on the health of those most likely to be exposed (NRC, 1991). Therefore, the complex relationship between human health and the acute and long-term effects of environmental exposures must be studied so prevention measures can be designed. Epidemiological surveillance systems need to track exposures to toxic substances (e.g., pesticides and heavy metals). These systems should use **biomonitoring data,** which provide measurements of toxic substances in the human body.

TIME CHARACTERISTICS

Time characteristics involve incubation/latency time, length of disease process, time of occurrence, and trends and cycles. Chapter 6 will cover the disease process and, within it, the incubation/latency phase. The length of a disease outbreak is discussed in Chapter 7. In this chapter there is a focus on the time of occurrence, trends, and whether the disease displays **periodicity**—which is when cases recur during intervals.

Time of occurrence is customarily noted during an epidemiological investigation. Cases are charted on an epidemic curve. Recall that an epidemic curve offers clues to the kind of epidemic being experienced. If cases appear as a spiked curve, the investigators suspect a point epidemic, a short-term dramatic increase in disease occurrence indicative of a common source epidemic. The disease is likely infectious with a short incubation period. Commonly, foodborne bacterial diseases have these characteristics. If the epidemic curve is flattened (known as platykurtic) or wavy (known as leptokurtic), a propagated epidemic is suspected.

Epidemiologists will also examine cases of infectious/noninfectious diseases in reported time periods of either less than or greater than a year. Commonly, surveillance systems use this time frame for collecting case data, calculating rates, and reporting. All are indicators of the population's health status. Epidemiologists are interested in month-to-month comparisons of reported disease cases as well as the overall annual rate. Within the reporting period, epidemiologists might observe seasonal variations, when cases are distributed according to the four natural divisions of a year. For example, epidemiologists have observed these short-term trends in disease occurrence:

- Aseptic or viral meningitis cases peak yearly, usually during the late summer months.

- Tuberculosis has higher incidence reports in the early winter months.
- Encephalitis occurs during the summer months.
- Influenza peaks in January and February.
- Varicella cases generally occur during winter/spring months.
- Hypercholesterolemia is observed in particular occupational categories during certain times of year (e.g., accountants during income tax filing season).
- Suicide rates are tied into times of year with higher rates in adults during winter and higher rates in youth during late spring and early summer.
- Heart attacks are linked to days of week (Sunday and Monday) and geographic places where climate changes are great.

Cyclical variations can be observed when cases are distributed according to sociocultural designations of the year (i.e., when children return to school). Epidemiologists have even noted periodicity in weekly periods. **Secular trends** of disease are long term (greater than one year), and are also of interest to epidemiologists. For example, cancer death rates for all body sites combined decreased about 0.6 percent annually from 1990 to 1996. This decrease was mainly seen in male lung, female breast, prostate, and colorectal cancers (Wingo et al., 1999). The following are other long-term trends in disease occurrence noted by epidemiologists:

- Hepatitis A outbreaks have a seven-year cycle.
- Measles outbreaks generally occur about every two years.
- Syphilis cases seem to rise and fall in five-year cycles, although there has been a general decline in cases since 1990.
- Hospital admissions show long-term as well as short-term cycles.

Time Interactions and Clusters

Clustering is when a closely grouped series of events or cases of a disease or morbid condition with well-defined patterns, occur in relation to time, place, or both. The term is normally used to describe aggregation of relatively uncommon events or diseases, e.g., leukemia, multiple sclerosis.

Similar to person and place, there are time characteristic interactions. For example, an epidemic curve depicts the time of occurrence of one case in relation to another. Whether a common source or propagated, the number of cases eventually wanes as the outbreak progresses. However, the length of the outbreak can be influenced by a short- or long-term time characteristic. For instance, time of year (e.g., warmer-weather months) might sustain an outbreak of encephalitis. In this example, the role of the physical environment— weather/climatic conditions—can be spotted.

The periodic nature of some long-term trends can also sustain an epidemic, but the explanation for this is complex. When cases are first detected through epidemiological surveillance (studied in Chapter 7), the place and time of each case are noted. That information alone might provide answers to the cause and spread of the disease. Accordingly, epidemiologists conduct an investigation (see Chapter 8) and gather information from cases and their associates (those without the disease) regarding person characteristics. As the number of cases rises and then falls, it is probably more a matter of infectivity of the agent, meaning the agent cannot be transmitted from a source host to a potential infected host if the latter is not susceptible to the agent. Susceptibility, therefore, can hinge on a number of factors. After an epidemic, the affected host population contains a sufficiently small proportion of susceptible individuals. This is because a large number of persons in the population had a disease experience and subsequently developed active immunity. In other words, the host population is now immune to a possible future epidemic disease. This is called **herd immunity.**

During the time after an epidemic, however, the host population tends to revert to susceptibility because they lose individual immunity, they lose immune individuals due to death from other causes and from members migrating out of the population. Concurrently, more susceptible persons are born.

After awhile, the population becomes susceptible. The time between succeeding epidemics varies, but many times will demonstrate periodicity. Sometimes when place and time characteristics interact, a phenomenon known as clustering happens. The clustering of disease cases can be depicted through spot mapping. The cases are geographically identified according to location of exposure, or by site of clinical manifestation.

A tragic example of the interaction between person, place, and time factors can be seen in the recent increases in Latino pedestrian fatalities. Of the 270 pedestrians who died in 1998 from collisions with motor vehicles in the Washington, DC, metropolitan area, at least 43 (16 percent) were Hispanic. These numbers are disproportionately high considering the Latino representation in the total population is about 8 percent. The explanation seems to be a combination of person, place, and time factors. The higher-than-expected mortality cases tend to occur in suburban areas. Epidemiologists have reported that most victims are immigrants living in concentrated apartment complexes proximal to heavily traveled thoroughfares (Surface Transportation Policy Project, 1999). Many of the immigrants came from countries whose roadways were more conducive to slower and less concentrated traffic. Given the increased trends in immigration as well as the general Washington, DC, metropolitan population increase throughout the 1990s, this was an automobile versus immigrant culture clash in the making. Many immigrants might not be able to purchase an automobile and, therefore, choose to walk. Epidemiologists have urged an organized response to this public health concern in the Hispanic population, and professionals have responded through pedestrian and traffic safety education programs (NHTSA, 1998, pp. 22-23).

SUMMARY

Person, place, and time characteristics are used to describe and understand the distribution of disease. Person characteristics are features of the biological, physical, and sociocultural environments. Time characteristics can be sequential aspects of the disease as well as trends and cycles of disease/condition occurrence and distribution. Each characteristic has its respective (variable) levels. One characteristic can interact with another to explain the occurrence and distribution of diseases and other conditions. One can refer to the examples provided in this chapter for each kind of characteristic as well as for characteristic interactions.

REVIEW QUESTIONS

1. What are person, place, and time characteristics and how can they be used to explain disease occurrence and distribution? How are person, place, and time characteristics different from other factors of disease?
2. Do you know the definitions of important terms in bold print throughout this chapter?
3. Can you identify and describe person characteristics? Can you give examples? Which is the most important person characteristic? Second most important?
4. Can you identify and describe place characteristics and give examples? How does the occurrence of Lyme disease exemplify the environmental characteristic known as ecosystem?
5. Can you identify and describe time characteristics and give examples?
6. What are characteristic interactions? What are clusters?
7. Can you spot person, place, and time characteristics if given examples (e.g., alcohol involvement in fatal motor vehicle crashes)?
8. Do you know the answers to the following chapter activity questions based on objectives from Healthy People 2010 focus areas 9 and 10?

WEB SITE RESOURCES

Biomonitoring of Environmental Status and Trends (BEST) program
<http://www.best.usgs.gov>

EPA Program on Beach Closing
<http://www.epa.gov/ost/beaches>

Morbidity and Mortality Weekly Report
<http://www.cdc.gov/mmwr>

Natural Resources Defense Council
<http://www.nrdc.org>

Renewable Fuels Association
<http://www.ethanolrfa.org.>

Toxics Release Inventory
<http:/www.epa.gov/tri/>

TOXNET
<http://toxnet.nlm.nih.gov/>

U.S. Department of Energy Clean Cities Program
<http://www.ccities.doe.gov/>

U.S. Department of Interior, U.S. Geological Survey (USGS).
<http://water.usgs.gov/watuse>

WHO—World Health Organization
<http://www.who.int/home-page/>

REFERENCES

Altekruse, S.F., Street, D.A., and Fein, S.B. (1996). Consumer knowledge of foodborne microbial hazards and food-handling practices. *Journal of Food Protection,* 59(2): 287-294.

Corti, M.C., Guralnik, J.M., Ferrucci, L., Izmirlian, G., Leveille, S.G., Pahor, M., Cohen, H.J., Pieper, C., and Havli, R.J. (1999). Evidence for a black-white crossover in all-cause and coronary heart disease mortality in an older population: The North Carolina EPESE. *American Journal of Public Health* 89(3): 308-314.

Gordis, L. (1996). *Epidemiology.* Philadelphia, PA: W.B. Saunders Company.

Healthy People 2010 (2000). *Healthy People 2010: Objectives for improving health.* Washington, DC: U.S. Department of Health and Human Services, Office for Disease Prevention and Health Promotion.

Lam, J.A. and Rosenheck, R. (1999). Street outreach for homeless persons with serious mental illness: Is it effective? *Medical Care,* 37(6): 894-907.

LaPlante, M.P. (1988). Data on Disability from the National Health Interview Survey, 1983–1985. Washington, DC: National Institute on Disability and Rehabilitation Research, U.S. Department of Education.

Meltzer, M.I., Dennis, D.T., and Orloski, K.A. (1999). The cost effectiveness of vaccinating against Lyme disease. *Emerging Infectious Diseases,* 5(3): 321-328.

Miller, R.E., Golaszewski, T.G., Pfeiffer, G., and Edington, D.W. (1990). Significance of the lifestyle system to employee wellness and assistance. *Health Values,* 14(2): 41-49.

NHTSA (1998). *Traffic Safety Facts 1998: Pedestrians.* Washington, DC: National Highway Traffic Safety Administration.

NRC (1991). *Environmental epidemiology: Public health and hazardous wastes* (Volume 1). National Research Council. Washington, DC: National Academy Press.

Surface Transportation Policy Project (1999). Washington, DC. Accessed online: <http://www.transact.org/stpp.htm>.

Ventura, S.J., Martin, J.A., Curtin, S.C. (1999). Births: Final data for 1997. *National Vital Statistics Reports,* 47(18): 1-17.

Wingo, P.A., Ries, L.A.G., Giovino, G.A. (1999). Annual report to the nation on the status of cancer, 1973–1996, with a special section on lung cancer and tobacco smoking. *Journal of the National Cancer Institute* 91(8): 675-690.

Purpose: (1) to acquaint the reader with Healthy People 2010 targets for improvement and (2) present examples of epidemiology as the underlying science to health promotion and disease prevention.

Directions: Check out your knowledge of these Healthy People 2010 focus areas by taking the following tests (answers follow in a separate section).

FOCUS AREA 9: FAMILY PLANNING

This focus area's goal is to improve pregnancy planning, spacing, and prevent unintended pregnancy.

9-1.   *Increase the proportion of pregnancies that are intended.* As of 1995, what proportion of all pregnancies among females aged fifteen to forty-four years was intended?
a. 11 percent
b. 31 percent
c. 51 percent
d. 71 percent

9-2.   *Reduce the proportion of births occurring within twenty-four months of a previous birth.* Related to this objectives, what is the health concern regarding births occurring within twenty-four months of a previous birth?
a. Increase risk of low birth weight
b. Increase risk of preterm birth
c. Increase risk of small-for-size gestational age
d. All of the above

9-3.   *Increase the proportion of females at risk of unintended pregnancy (and their partners) who use contraception.* As of 1995, what proportion of females (and their partners) within this risk group used contraception?
a. 33 percent
b. 53 percent
c. 73 percent
d. 93 percent

9-4.   *Reduction in the proportion of females experiencing pregnancy despite use of a reversible contraceptive method.* Related to this objective, what is a reversible contraceptive method?
a. Tubal ligation
b. Oral contraceptive pill
c. Vasectomy
d. Abortion

9-5.   *Increase in the proportion of health care providers who provide emergency contraception (developmental).* All of the following are correct about emergency contraception except:
a. Physicians are aware of and willing to prescribe the use of emergency postcoital contraception.
b. Emergency contraception is not widely known by the public.
c. Emergency contraceptive pills can reduce the risk of subsequent pregnancy by about 75 percent.
d. Emergency contraception can be specified regimens of oral contraception pills taken within seventy-two hours of coitus.

9-6.   *Increase in the male involvement in pregnancy prevention and family planning efforts (developmental).* Which of the following represents this kind of involvement in pregnancy prevention and family planning efforts?
a. Addressing the possibility of unintended pregnancy
b. Recognizing condom use as the most effective way of preventing HIV/STD transmission
c. Accepting responsibility in welfare and child support enforcement
d. All of the above

9-7. *Reduction in pregnancies among adolescent females.* Related to this objective, which of the following is correct?
a. The rate of teenage pregnancy rate in United States is about the same as other developed countries.
b. Most adolescent childbearing by adolescents occurs inside marriage.
c. Only about one-third of pregnancies in females under fifteen years of age end in induced abortion or fetal loss.
d. Consensus is widespread that all pregnancies in females under fifteen years old are inappropriate and that ideally the target number should be zero.

9-8. *Increase in the proportion of adolescents who have never engaged in sexual intercourse before age fifteen years.* What is the target proportion of adolescents ages fifteen to nineteen to not engage in sexual intercourse before age fifteen?
a. 28 percent of females, 28 percent of males
b. 48 percent of females, 48 percent of males
c. 68 percent of females, 68 percent of males
d. 88 percent of females, 88 percent of males

9-9. *Increase in the proportion of adolescents who have never engaged in sexual intercourse.* As of 1995, what proportion of adolescents has never engaged in sexual intercourse?
a. 22 percent of females, 17 percent of males
b. 42 percent of females, 37 percent of males
c. 62 percent of females, 57 percent of males
d. 82 percent of females, 77 percent of males

9-10. *Increase in the proportion of sexually active, unmarried adolescents aged fifteen to seventeen years who use contraception that both effectively prevents pregnancy and provides barrier protection against disease.* As of 1995, what proportion of sexually active unmarried females and males under eighteen years of age used a condom during first sexual intercourse?
a. 27 percent of females, 32 percent of males
b. 47 percent of females, 52 percent of males
c. 67 percent of females, 72 percent of males
d. 87 percent of females, 92 percent of males

9-11.   *Increase in the proportion of young adults who have received formal instruction before turning age eighteen years on reproductive health issues, including all of the following topics: birth control methods, safer sex to prevent HIV, prevention of sexually transmitted diseases, and abstinence.* As of 1995, what proportion of young adult females had received this formal instruction before turning eighteen years old?
   a. 24 percent
   b. 44 percent
   c. 64 percent
   d. 84 percent

9-12.   *Reduction in the proportion of married couples whose ability to conceive or maintain a pregnancy is impaired.* As of 1995, what proportion of married couples have an impaired ability to conceive or maintain a pregnancy?
   a. 13 percent
   b. 33 percent
   c. 53 percent
   d. 73 percent

9-13.   *Increase in the proportion of health insurance policies that cover contraceptive supplies and services (developmental).* Related to this objective, many privately insured females who need contraceptive care:
   a. Must go out of plan and pay for it themselves
   b. Might choose to use over-the-counter methods that may be less effective than prescribed methods
   c. Might choose not to use any method at all
   d. All of the above

FOCUS AREA 10: FOOD SAFETY

This focus area's goal is to reduce foodborne illnesses.

10-1.   *Reduction in infections caused by key foodborne pathogens.* How much of an improvement is targeted in terms of reducing infections from specific foodborne pathogens?
   a. 10 percent improvement
   b. 30 percent improvement

c. 50 percent improvement
d. 70 percent improvement

10-2. *Reduction in outbreaks of infections caused by key foodborne bacteria.* How much of an improvement is targeted in terms of reducing outbreaks of infections from specific foodborne bacteria?
a. 10 percent improvement
b. 30 percent improvement
c. 50 percent improvement
d. 70 percent improvement

10-3. *Prevention of the increase in the proportion of isolates of salmonella species from humans and from animals at slaughter that are resistant to antimicrobial drugs.* Related to this objective, which of the following is correct about antimicrobial drug resistance?
a. Known pathogens such as salmonella are resistant to multiple important antimicrobial drugs.
b. The general trend toward increased resistance by microorganisms to multiple antimicrobial agents heightens public health concerns about treatment options and health care costs.
c. Of particular concern is the potential for transmission of antimicrobial-resistant pathogens to humans through the food supply.
d. All of the above are correct

10-4. *Reduction in deaths from anaphylaxis caused by food allergies (developmental).* All of the following are correct about anaphylaxis caused by food allergies except:
a. Anaphylaxis is a severe allergic reaction commonly caused by certain foods resulting in hives, itching, skin swelling, blood vessel collapse, shock, and often life-threatening respiratory distress.
b. Food allergy is the least frequent cause of anaphylaxis occurring outside of the hospital, and the least common cause for emergency department visits for anaphylaxis.
c. Foods and their products are most likely to cause allergic reactions: milk, eggs, peanuts, tree nuts, soybeans, fish, shellfish, cereals containing gluten, and seeds.

    d. Besides research and education, clear food ingredient labeling information is critical for managing food allergies.

10-5. *Increase in the proportion of consumers who follow key food safety practices.* Which is one of these safety practices?
    a. Wash hands and surfaces often
    b. Do not cross-contaminate
    c. Cook to proper temperatures as well as refrigerate promptly afterward
    d. All of the above

10-6. *Improvement in food employee behaviors and food preparation practices that directly relate to foodborne illnesses in retail food establishments (developmental).* Which is the most commonly reported food preparation practice that contributes to foodborne disease?
    a. Improper holding temperature
    b. Poor personal hygiene
    c. Inadequate cooking
    d. Food obtained from an unsafe source

10-7. *Reduction in human exposure to organophosphate pesticides from food (developmental). Related to this objective.* All of the following are correct about organophosphate pesticides except:
    a. The EPA is currently reassessing existing standards for pesticides used on food crops.
    b. Organophosphates pesticides are low priority in the standards reassessment.
    c. Organophosphate pesticides are used on fruits and vegetables important in the diet of children.
    d. The EPA considers the risk of pesticides used on food, water, and for lawn care as well as any special sensitivities for children.

TEST ANSWERS

Focus Area 9

9-1.   (c) 51 percent. The target is 70 percent. There has been a significant decline in the rate of unintended pregnancy in the United States, although the rate remains higher than in other countries such as Canada and the Netherlands. Unintended pregnancy is a matter of concern among all reproductive age groups.

9-2.   (d) All of the above. Females not spacing their births run the risk of the aforementioned perinatal adverse outcomes. As of 1995, about 11 percent of females aged fifteen to forty-four years old had two consecutive births within twenty-four months. The target is a reduction to 6 percent.

9-3.   (d) 93 percent. The target is for 100 percent of those females at risk for unintended pregnancy to be using contraception. Unintended pregnancy is a general term that includes pregnancies a woman reports as either mistimed or unwanted at the time of conception. If an unintended pregnancy occurs and is carried to term, the birth may be a wanted one, but the pregnancy would be classified as unintended. Inadequate or nonexistent contraceptive use are the main reasons for unintended pregnancy.

9-4.   (b) Oral contraceptive pill. Tubal ligation and vasectomy are sterilizations of females and males respectively, and are considered permanent contraception. Abortion is not considered a contraceptive method. As of 1995, 13 percent of females aged fifteen to forty-four years experienced pregnancy despite use of a reversible contraceptive method and the target is a reduction to 7 percent.

9-5.   (a) Physicians are aware of and willing to prescribe the use of emergency postcoital contraception. Unfortunately, this is still not correct. Since 1997, the Food and Drug Administration has reported that a regulated administration of oral contraceptive pills can act as postcoital contraception. However, physicians and patients need to increase their knowledge about the availability of this method. Recently, the FDA approved a progestin-only pill that can act as a postcoital means of contraception.

9-6.   (d) All of the above. Although these represent ways for greater male involvement, information is scant on the actual amount of male participation in these matters. As of 1995, it appeared that males represented somewhere between 6 and 10 percent of the client base in family planning clinics. Programs promoting increased male involvement should be culturally and linguistically appropriate.

9-7.   (d) Consensus is widespread that all pregnancies in females under fifteen years old are inappropriate and that ideally the target number should be zero. The other three responses are incorrect. U.S. teenage pregnancy rate is practically twice as high as other developed countries. Most adolescent childbearing occurs outside marriage, and this trend has been on the rise. Nearly two-thirds of pregnancies in the under fifteen year old age group end in induced abortion or fetal loss.

9-8.   (d) 88 percent of females, 88 percent of males. As of 1995, about 79 percent of males and 81 percent of females who were sexually active during their fifteen-to-nineteen-years age range reported not having sexual intercourse before age fifteen.

9-9.   (c) 62 percent of females, 57 percent of males. The target for this objective is to increase to 75 percent of adolescent females and 75 percent of adolescent males not having sexual intercourse. Adolescent sexual interaction increases the risk of unintended pregnancy and exposure to sexually transmitted diseases.

9-10.   (c) 67 percent of females, 72 percent of males. A contraceptive that includes birth control and barrier protection elements reduces risks of unintended pregnancy and exposure to sexually transmitted diseases. A certain way to prevent both health concerns is through abstinence. Still, the high proportion of sexually active adolescents necessitates instructing them about proper condom use and its greater ability to prevent STD transmission compared to hormonal methods of contraception. The target for this objective is 75 percent of unmarried, adolescent females, and 82 percent unmarried, adolescent males using a condom during first intercourse.

9-11.   (c) 64 percent. The 1995 data pertain to females, since data on males were not available. The target proportion for both genders in this objective is 90 percent. The education should be developmentally as well as culturally and linguistically appropriate. It has to be medically accurate, involve parents, and align with conscious, informed, and responsible decision making.

9-12.   (a) 13 percent. This was the baseline in 1995. The target is to reduce this to 10 percent of married couples with wives aged fifteen to forty-four years having an impaired ability to conceive or maintain a pregnancy. A woman is classified as having impaired fecundity if it is impossible for her (or her husband or cohabiting partner) to have a baby for any reason other than a sterilizing operation; it is difficult or dangerous to carry a baby to term; or she and her partner have not used contraception and have not had a pregnancy for three years or longer.

9-13.   (d) All of the above. As of 1993, only about half of indemnity (fee-for-service) insurance plans covered costs for reversible contraceptives; however, over 90 percent of HMOs did provide coverage. The plans covering this cost are inconsistent in eligible contraceptive expense with a pronounced bias toward covering permanent surgical methods.

Focus Area 10

10-1.   (c) 50 percent improvement. To accomplish this objective, it will be necessary to reduce the incidence rates of the following pathogens: campylobacter (from 24.6 to 12.3 cases per 100,000 persons), *E. coli* (from 2.1 to 1.0 cases per 100,000 persons), listeria (from .5 to .25 cases per 100,000 persons), salmonella (from 13.7 to 6.8 cases per 100,000 persons), and others.

10.2.   (c) 50 percent improvement. To accomplish this objective, it will be necessary to reduce the number of yearly outbreaks reported by the states of the following pathogens: *E. coli* (from 22 to 11 outbreaks per year), salmonella (from 44 to 22 outbreaks per year).

10-3.   (d) All of the above are correct. For all of these reasons, National Antimicrobial Resistance Monitoring System, a surveillance system, will increase testing to identify and monitor changes in patterns and trends of antimicrobial resistance in both human and animal populations.

10-4.   (b) Food allergy is the least frequent cause of anaphylaxis occurring outside of the hospital and the least common cause for emergency department visits for anaphylaxis. In fact, it is just the opposite: this kind of allergy is most likely to cause anaphylaxis outside of the hospital as well as the most likely cause of anaphylactic-related visits to emergency departments. The severity of this condition and the widespread presence of these food allergens (even in trace amounts) necessitates more research, education, and better food labeling.

10-5.   (d) All of the above. These are the key food safety practices in the FightBAC! campaign messages: clean—wash hands and surfaces often; separate—do not cross-contaminate; cook—cook to proper temperatures; and chill—refrigerate promptly. The target for this objective is to have 79 percent of consumers follow these food safety practices. The FightBAC! campaign works in conjunction with FoodNet, a federal agency surveillance system to produce better national estimates of foodborne disease.

10-6.   (a) Improper holding temperature. The second most common practice is poor personal hygiene and the least common practice is food obtained from an unsafe source. Other practices of concern are inadequate cooking and contaminated equipment. To help control these practices and behaviors, the CDC has published the *Food Code* for state public health officials. This is a text of recommendations such as use of time-temperature control, prevention of hand contact with food, training of food handlers, demonstration of knowledge by retail food managers, and institution of consumer advisories on the risks of eating raw or undercooked animal foods.

10-7.   (b) Organophosphate pesticides are low priority in the standards reassessment. This is incorrect because actually these pesticides are first priority in the standards reassessment. The standards reassessments are mandated by the Food Quality Protection Act of 1996, and are to be completed by the year 2006.

Chapter 6

Disease Process

DISEASES AND MORBID CONDITIONS

Having learned there are agents and risk factors to disease and other morbid conditions, and that occurrence and distribution are subject to the interaction of person, place, and time characteristics, it is time to look more closely at the dynamics of the disease process. This will shed light on what causes disease and identify opportunities for its control.

To begin, it is important to know that there is **taxonomy of disease,** an orderly classification of diseases into appropriate categories based on relationships among them. The most widely used taxonomy is the *International Classification of Diseases* (ICD), now in its tenth revision (WHO, 2000a). Every disease is coded and organized into seventeen divisions within which are further subdivisions. Some of the divisions are etiologic, such as infective and parasitic conditions. Other divisions represent bodily systems, such as the nervous system, and other divisions relate to classes of conditions such as neoplasm (cancer) and injuries (unintentional and intentional).

As previously discussed, disease can be classified as either infectious or noninfectious. Most practicing epidemiologists classify infectious disease either by agent (as described in Chapter 4) or mode of transmission: airborne, intestinal discharge, skin sores, zoonosis, or fomite. For example, the protozoan infection known as **giardiasis** is an infectious disease whose mode of transmission is intestinal discharge and consumption of contaminated food and water (fomites). Signs and symptoms are gastrointestinal problems. Although the disease is self-limiting, its long duration of weeks to months necessitates treatment in most cases. None of the therapeutic medications is 100 percent effective, so prevention is the best measure. For example, people using water recreationally for sport or leisure (e.g., swimming, water-skiing, and white-water boating) have to be careful about possible exposure to contaminated water. There have been instances of lap swimmers contracting giardia from fecally contaminated pools. Outdoor recreation participants (e.g., hiking, rock climbing, mountain biking) should be cautious about consuming surface water for refreshment. Given the limited access to comfort stations, it not uncommon for water sources to become inadvertently contaminated (Backer, 2000).

Regarding noninfectious disease, a general classification system is as follows:

- *Congenital* and *heredity,* such as birth defects, respiratory distress syndrome, hemophilia, and others
- *Allergic* and *inflammatory,* such as food allergy, chronic joint inflammation, arthritis, and others
- *Degenerative* or *chronic,* such as back disorders, chronic obstructive pulmonary diseases, chronic kidney disease, and others
- *Metabolic,* such as diabetes, iron deficiency and anemia, obesity, and others
- *Neoplasmic,* such as various kinds of cancer, benign tumors, and other cellular growths

An epidemiological principle examined in Chapter 3 was the disease process. Recall that it represents a pathological progress starting with a susceptibility phase, exposure to an agent, through subclinical and clinical phases, and ultimately to a stage of full, partial, or no recovery. Now it is time to look at the process in greater detail and apply it to infectious and noninfectious diseases (see Figure 6.1).

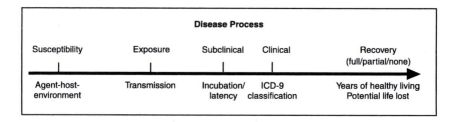

FIGURE 6.1. Disease process in greater detail (*Source:* Adapted from CDC, 1992, p. 43)

INFECTIOUS DISEASE APPLICATION

In the susceptibility phase of the disease process, agent, host, and environment factors are conducive to disease occurrence. Various agents—among which are biological agents—are responsible for infectious diseases. Physical, chemical, social, behavioral, and genetic agents are more likely to explain noninfectious disease occurrence. During the susceptibility phase, questions can be posed regarding the host and his or her person characteristics, such as: Does the host have immunity to the biological agent? A host can have either active or passive immunity. Active immunity is attained as a result of exposure to a highly immunogenic agent, or inoculation against the agent. Passive immunity is the borrowing of antibodies from another host or from a serologic preparation. If not immune, can the host overcome the biological agent through immune defense? Here is where T cells, lymphocytes produced in the thymus gland, and B cells, lymphocytes produced in bone marrow, act as antibodies attacking and destroying the biological antigen.

The demographic profile of the host in terms of age and gender might also place him or her at greater risk of susceptibility. In addition, a person's physical fitness might also place him or her at greater risk of infectious disease. There is a growing body of epidemiological data to support regular, moderate exercise's enhancement of the immune defense system. This enhancement appears to be temporary, but if exercise is performed regularly, it is possible to periodically give the body "booster shots" of immune function enhancement. However, researchers emphasize that the positive effect is not discernible along a dose-response J-shaped curve. Still, more exercise scientists promulgate that nutrition, hygiene, exercise, environmental, and pharmacological strategies can lower a person's risk of infection, especially from viruses such as the common cold. Others point out that regular exercisers are at lower risk for developing colon cancer. Persons who have systemic or bodywide symptoms and signs of disease should not be competing or engaging in intense competition or heavy training (Shephard and Shek, 1999).

Environmental factors can also coincide and thus increase susceptibility. One overlooked environment is within the womb, **in utero.** The unborn grows within the amniotic sac submerged in a water medium known as **amniotic fluid.** This fluid contains important antibodies borrowed from the mother. It might also contain biological (e.g., rubella virus) and chemical agents (e.g., toxic substances) of disease that have passed through the placenta from the mother's circulatory system.

At the point of exposure in the disease process, several dynamics are at work. To begin, it is necessary to know if transmission is direct or indirect. **Direct transmission** takes place when the agent is passed from a source host to another host, or from a source environment to a host. **Indirect transmission** takes place when an intermediary, or vehicle is necessary for passing the agent from a source to another host. A **vehicle** is a mechanism for transmitting an infectious agent from a reservoir. The vehicle can be person to person, foodborne, or vectorborne. An inanimate vehicle is sometimes called a **fomite.** It is usually a contaminated article such as clothing, a handkerchief, a drinking glass, etc. An animate vehicle, usually an arthropod or small rodent, is called a **vector.** A vector transports an infectious agent from a source host or its waste products to the new host. The agent might or might not pass through developmental stages while thriving within the vector. A related term is **reservoir,** which is a medium for storage and growth of a biological agent (e.g., human or animals, the physical environment). Any person, animal, arthropod, plant, soil, or substance, or a combination of these can be a reservoir in which an infectious agent normally lives and multiplies, on which it depends primarily for survival, and where it reproduces itself in such a manner that it can be transmitted to a susceptible host. One such example is **droplet nuclei,** dried or congealed nasal and/or throat discharges that act as reservoirs for biological agents.

During the **subclinical phase** of the disease process, pathological changes occur in the host, and his or her immune defense is activated in response to growing numbers of agent. This phase is also known as the **incubation period** for infectious diseases, which is the time interval between invasion by an infectious agent and appearance of the first sign or symptom of the disease. It is during this phase that an agent displays its infectivity. For the most part, the host is asymptomatic until the clinical phase has been reached in the disease process.

Another related term is **carrier,** which is an infected host who is progressing through the disease process but many times does not display signs or symptoms. Known as a healthy carrier, he or she is capable of transferring the biological agent to other hosts. There are carriers who, during incubation and clinical stages, continue to transmit agents to susceptible hosts. An example would be hepatitis C carriers who are experiencing preliminary liver complications, yet unknown to others, are spreading the disease.

When describing the subclinical phase of the disease process, it is important to mention **quarantine,** a disease control strategy involving detaining and isolating known source hosts from potential hosts. It is derived from the Latin language expression for "forty days." The strategy started in fourteenth-century Europe and Asia during the Black Death bubonic plague epidemic. **Bubonic plague** is a bacterial disease transmitted from rodents to human hosts through a flea vector that if untreated has a case fatality of 60 to 90 percent. Although exposure through a vector was unknown at the time, health officials were still concerned that any infected sea traveler might transmit the disease to their potential hosts. Therefore, ships at port were inspected for sick sailors or passengers. Symptoms were fever and delirium, vomiting, muscle ache, and the presence of buboes (swollen lymph nodes). All on board were kept from contacting people on shore during quarantine. Whether or not the inspectors conceived the concept of incubation period, which for bubonic plague is about six days, it was an effective strategy for protecting the community. Quarantine not only allowed time to detect plague cases that were incubating, but also permitted active cases to progress through the disease process (which is about seven days) until their contagiousness period had past (McNeil, 1997).

During the clinical phase of the disease process, **pathogenicity** takes place, wherein the agent produces signs and symptoms of disease. Sometimes, pathogenicity is referred to as the power an organism has to produce disease. As previously mentioned, diagnosed diseases are assigned three-digit codes according to the *International Classification of Diseases* or ICD-10 (Tenth Edition), which is under the direction of the World Health Organization (WHO, 2000a). The classification system is comprised of seventeen divisions containing subdivisions arranged according to etiology, body systems affected, and classes of morbid conditions. For instance, infectious and parasitic diseases have a code between 001 to 139. Other diseases, injuries, and causes of death have their own respective codes. Another related WHO system of disease and morbid condition classification is the *International Classification of Health Problems in Primary Care* (WHO, 2000b).

Also during the clinical phase, a disease is treated via a variety of methods. For example, bacterial diseases are normally treated with **antibiotics,** substances (e.g., penicillin) derived from bacteria, fungi, and other organisms that destroy or inhibit bacterial growth.

During the recovery phase of the disease process there will be no degree or some degree of recuperation from the disease. During the clinical stage the agent displays **virulence,** which is the ability of an organismim to produce severe, possibly life-threatening signs and symptoms. Hopefully, the host convalesces, recovers from disease.

Another classification by WHO (2000c) is the *International Classification of Impairments, Disabilities, and Handicaps,* which furnishes a systematic taxonomy of the consequences of injury and disease. Through this classification, **impairment** is considered any loss or abnormality of psychological, physiological, or anatomical structure or function. Impairment represents abnormalities of body structure, appearance, and with organ or system function resulting from any cause. In principle, impairments represent disturbances at the organ level within any body system (e.g., muscular, skeletal, endocrine, etc.). A **disability** is any restriction or lack (resulting from impairment) of ability to perform an activity in a manner or within a range considered normal for a human being. The term disability reflects the consequences of an impairment in terms of lost functional performance and activity by the individual. A **handicap** is a disadvantage for a given individual, resulting from an impairment or disability that limits or prevents the fulfillment of a role that is normal (depending on age, sex, and social and cultural practice) for that individual. The term thus reflects interaction with, and adaptation to, the individual's surroundings.

Health Care Providers and Communication

During the disease process, it is important that communication between health care providers and patients be satisfactory, especially in the clinical stage of the disease. Unfortunately, many patients report difficulty in communicating with their providers, stating that the professionals do not give them enough information even though they highly value the information and want to know more. Clear, candid, accurate, culturally and linguistically competent provider-patient communication is essential for the prevention, diagnosis, treatment, and management of health concerns. Presently, efforts are under way to train health care professionals in good personal interactive and communication skills (Rosenberg, Lussier, and Beaudoin, 1997).

This relates to Healthy People 2010 Objective 11-6: *Increase in the proportion of persons who report that their health care providers have satisfactory communication skills (developmental)* (Healthy People 2010, 2000, 11-17). (See Chapter 6 activities for more information.)

One indicator of recovery is the host's resumption of **activities of daily living,** which include the ability to function independently in basic living areas: grooming, dressing, feeding, toileting, etc., with special equipment if needed. This can be measured through assessments of a person's mobility, self-care, grooming, etc. The extent and duration of this daily life functioning is measured in terms of **years of healthy living.** Unfortunately, if the outcome is death, then epidemiologists rely on **years of potential life lost,** which is calculated by subtracting the person's actual age in years from his or her expected lifetime in years. Potential years of life lost is a measure of the relative impact of diseases and other lethal conditions in a population— the sum of years the person would have lived had they experienced normal life expectations.

A more detailed application of the disease process can be seen in **hepatitis B,** also called serum hepatitis, a viral disease that affects the liver. The disease is fairly common, although incidence in the general population has declined due to an available vaccine, routine screening, and more careful organ donor exchanges. The incidence of hepatitis B has increased in sexually active heterosexuals, homosexual men, and injection drug users. Hepatitis B virus is transmitted directly through blood and body fluids. Besides the vaccine, there is a hepatitis B immune globulin for people who have been exposed to the virus. Once exposed, it takes about one to three months before symptoms appear: tiredness, poor appetite, fever, vomiting, and occasionally joint pain, abdominal pain, hives, or rash. Urine may become darker in color, and then **jaundice** (a yellowing of the skin and whites of the eyes) may appear. Some individuals may experience few or no symptoms. The virus can be found in blood and other body fluids several weeks before symptoms appear and generally persist for several months afterward. Approximately 6 to 10 percent of infected adults become long-term carriers of the virus. This percentage is much higher (70 to 90 percent) for children infected very early in life. Usually, no special medicines or antibiotics are prescribed to treat a person once symptoms appear. Generally, bed rest is all that is needed for uncomplicated cases. However, it should be known that about 4 to 5 percent of infected persons require hospitalization, since hepatitis B can result in cirrhosis and liver cancer. With this in mind it should also be emphasized that about 2 percent of all hepatitis B cases result in death.

NONINFECTIOUS DISEASE APPLICATION

Even though the disease process is more often applied to infectious diseases, the principle does have application for noninfectious diseases, though it is a bit more challenging. To start, the susceptibility stage relies more on the contemporary rather than the traditional epidemiological triad. In this model, explanation of factors takes the form of explanation of characteristics. Remember that the traditional epidemiological triad explains disease occurrence in individuals, whereas the contemporary triad focuses on groups of people. By having an understanding of which characteristics place groups of persons at risk for developing a noninfectious disease, the susceptibility stage can be detailed.

For noninfectious diseases, unlike infectious diseases, the exposure to risk factors generally takes place over an extended period of time. That is why it is difficult to narrow down specific factors to a disease. In fact, a number of noninfectious chronic diseases, such as hypertension, asthma, and many cancers, do not have an identified cause.

The subclinical phase for a noninfectious disease is called the **latency period.** Just as exposure to an infectious agent takes considerable time to manifest, so does the latency period in many noninfectious diseases. Of course, signs and symptoms represent the clinical phase and, in many noninfectious diseases, can persist for a considerable period. What then follows is an exerted effort at treatment, support, and recovery. Treating and curing noninfectious diseases tend to be more difficult compared to infectious diseases. Long-term disability is more likely associated with noninfectious diseases.

Automatic External Defibrillators in Sport, Recreation, and Fitness Areas

During the heart disease process, cardiac arrest and other compelling symptoms and signs can mark the clinical stage. Sport, recreation, and fitness areas can be points of emergency care provision in the form of automatic external defibrillators. Although a cardiac event is rare among young, healthy athletes (usually from ventricular fibrillation associated with underlying cardiovascular disease or as a result of blunt impact to the chest wall), there are others who are at risk such as officials, coaches, and fans. The use of on-site automatic external defibrillators to treat cardiac arrest is becoming more popular because traditional emergency medical service might not be able to address this need adequately. Of chief concern is the time between patient collapse and defibrillation, because each minute of delay lowers chances of survival about 7 to 10 percent. A majority of patients survive cardiac arrest if their defibrillation takes place within three minutes of collapse (National Heart Attack Alert Program Committee, 1998).

This relates to Healthy People 2010 Objective 12-5: *(Developmental) Increase the proportion of eligible persons with witnessed out-of-hospital cardiac arrest who receive their first therapeutic electrical shock within 6 minutes after collapse recognition* (Healthy People, 2010, 2000, 12-17). (See Chapter 6 activities for more information.)

An example of a noninfectious disease process is **kidney disease.** This disease most likely manifests in successive, irreversible stages from subclinical to clinical: chronic renal insufficiency, chronic renal failure, and end-stage renal disease. These stages represent a continuum of increasing renal dysfunction and decreasing glomerular filtration rate. Chronic renal insufficiency tends to be asymptomatic. Chronic kidney failure means renal function has deteriorated, leaving the door open to other conditions that might appear (e.g., anemia, bone disease, acidosis, and salt and fluid retention). End-stage renal disease necessitates renal replacement therapy, dialysis, or kidney transplantation to sustain life. About 10 million persons aged twelve years and older have some form of chronic kidney disease with most

of them progressing through three stages of disease process. Therefore, epidemiologists and other health professionals are challenged to
implement prevention programs to detect kidney disease in its earliest stages (Jones, McQuillan, and Kusek, 1998).

MORBID CONDITION APPLICATION

The disease process can also be applied to morbid conditions. This
application might be even more challenging than applying the principle to noninfectious diseases. The reason for this is because the phase
of susceptibility contains numerous agents and risk factors—most
likely not biological. Attention has to be directed at the multitude of
person, place, and time characteristics whose interchange acts as a
"special recipe" for morbid condition formation. Exposure to these
factors and characteristics can vary in duration and amount. Similar
to noninfectious disease, the subclinical phase for a morbid condition
is also called **latency period,** and it varies in length of time depending on the condition. Once signs and symptoms present, the clinical
phase has begun and can remain for quite some time. However, descriptive features of the condition might not be classifiable according
to the ICD codes. For example, there is no code for violent behaviors.
Similar to diseases, a phase of treatment, support, and recovery follows. Treating and curing morbid conditions are possible, although
some are more challenging than others. Three prevalent morbid conditions in the U.S. population are obesity, violence, and substance
abuse.

Obesity is a condition characterized by excessive body fat,
whereas being overweight is excess body weight. There has been a
notable increase in the number of obese and overweight persons. Several social, behavioral, and genetic agents seem to mix to explain this
condition in an individual. The person eats more calories from food
(energy) than he or she expends, for example, through physical activity. This process carries on for months to years resulting in body mass
index of greater than twenty-five for adults. **Body mass index,** or
BMI, is weight (in kilograms or pounds) divided by the square of
height (in meters or inches) multiplied by 704.5. Because it is readily
calculated, BMI is the measurement of choice as an indicator of being

of a healthy weight, being overweight, and being obese. Obesity or overweightness in children and youth is assessed via other means (height-weight charts, etc.). There is the presumption that an obese or overweight person is unhealthy and that his or her body composition has a direct effect on health status. However, it is more likely that an overweight person's health status is under bombardment from a constellation of concurrent unhealthy behaviors—rather than just a greater amount of adipose tissue or body weight. The list of diseases associated with obesity, especially, is extensive: cardiovascular, some cancers, diabetes, chronic kidney disease, muscular disorders, etc. Obesity and overweightness are treated through dietetic counseling, guided physical activity, support from others, and possible medical intervention (e.g., medications, liposuction). Dieting (caloric restriction) alone is successful in about 2 percent of obese/overweight persons who wish to lower their body weight. Healthy food substitution for hypercaloric foods combined with physical activity seems to be the winning combination as the person sets out on a lifelong weight management plan.

Violence is pervasive in the United States and can affect the quality of living. Reports of children killing children in schools are shocking and cause parents to worry about the safety of their children. Reports of gang violence make persons wonder about their safety. Although suicide rates began decreasing in the mid-1990s, prior increases among youth ages ten to nineteen years and adults ages sixty-five years and older have raised concerns about the vulnerability of these population groups. Intimate partner violence and sexual assault threaten people in all walks of life. Youth continue to be involved as both perpetrators and victims of violence. Elderly persons, females, and children continue to be targets of both physical and sexual assaults, which are frequently perpetrated by individuals they know. Examples of general issues that impede the public health response to progress in this area include the lack of comparable data sources, lack of standardized definitions and definitional issues, lack of resources to establish adequately consistent tracking systems, and lack of resources to fund promising prevention programs. Understanding injuries allows for development and implementation of effective prevention interventions. Some interventions can reduce injuries from both unintentional and violence-related episodes. For example, proper firearm storage is believed to be associated with reduced intentional/unintentional shootings in the home. Higher alcoholic beverage taxes are believed to be associated with reduced fatal car crashes.

Substance abuse is the inappropriate and/or excessive involvement with a psychoactive substance that results in personal, family, social, and work problems. Much has been reported about drug and alcohol abuse among youth, but inappropriate and excessive substance involvement cuts across all age groups. The perceptual distortion from alcohol/drugs is a safety risk, whereas intensive and extensive substance abuse is a mental and physical health hazard. Given the dependency-producing potential of most psychoactive substances, the continued abuse wreaks havoc in the person's family, community, and work life. For most substance users, care is required in the form of individual and group therapy, self-help, and restoration of physical health. The prospect of substance abuse recovery is good if a minimization of relapses are observed in an idividual. Recovery is a lifelong process, which is why a person in such circumstances is referred to as "recovering."

SUMMARY

Ways in which diseases are categorized include two main categories—infectious and noninfectious diseases—and are better understood by using the principle of the disease process. When applied to infectious diseases, a number of important points arise during each phase of the process: characteristics of susceptibility, means of transmission, subclinical and clinical phases, and what constitutes recovery. Application of this process to noninfectious disease is more challenging because the occurrence and distribution of disease is presented in terms of multiple risk factors as well as person, place, and time characteristics. In addition, the process is usually lengthened in terms of latency period and clinical stage. Simarily, the disease process can also be applied to morbid conditions, but again, challenges need to be faced. The susceptibility, exposure, and subclinical stages are complex given the interaction of risk factors and person, place, and time characteristics. The clinical stage, however, might not display signs and symptoms easily classified by ICD-10 codes.

REVIEW QUESTIONS

1. How are diseases categorized? Can you give examples?
2. Can you describe the disease process in greater detail? Can you explain dynamics taking place during susceptibility, exposure, subclinical and clinical phases, and some degrees of recovery?
3. Do you know the definitions of the important terms in bold print throughout this chapter?
4. What is the role of quarantine and where does it fit into the disease process?
5. Can you apply the disease process to infectious diseases? Noninfectious diseases? Morbid conditions?
6. Do you know the answers to the following chapter activity questions based on objectives from Healthy People 2010 focus areas 11 and 12?

WEB SITE RESOURCES

Centers for Disease Control and Prevention, Health Topics A-Z
<http://www.cdc.gov/health/diseases.htm>

Centers for Public Health Research and Evaluation
<http://www.battelle.org/cphre/>

John Hopkins University Research
<http://www.hopkins-id.edu/>

Michigan Public Health Institute
<http://www.mphi.org/>

Sickle Cell Information Center
<http://www.cc.emory.edu/PEDS/SICKLE/>

REFERENCES

Backer, H.D. (2000). Giardiasis: An elusive cause of gastrointestinal distress. *The Physician and Sportsmedicine* 28(7): 1-6.

CDC (1992). *Principle of Epidemiology.* Atlanta, GA: Centers for Disease Control and Prevention.

Healthy People 2010 (2000). *Healthy People 2010: Objectives for improving health*. Washington, DC: Office of Disease Prevention and Health Promotion, U.S. Department of Health and Human Services.

Jones, C.A., McQuillan, G.M., and Kusek, J.W. (1998). Serum creatinine levels in the U.S. population: Third National Health and Nutrition Examination Survey. *American Journal of Kidney Diseases* 32: 992-999.

McNeil, H. (1997). *Plagues and people*. New York: Anchor Books/Doubleday.

National Heart Attack Alert Program Coordinating Committee, Access to Care Subcommittee (1998). Access to timely and optimal care of patients with acute coronary syndromes—Community planning considerations: Report by the the National Heart Attack Alert Program. *Journal of Thrombosis and Thrombolysis*, 6(1): 119-146.

Rosenberg, E.E., Lussier, M.T., and Beaudoin, C. (1997). Lessons for clinicians from physician-patient communication literature. *Archives of Family Medicine*, 6(2): 279-283.

Shephard, R.J. and Shek, P.N. (1999). Exercise, immunity and susceptibility to infection. A J-shaped relationship? *The Physician and Sportsmedicine* 27(6): 6-7.

World Health Organization (2000a). *International Classification of Disease*, 10th revision. Zurich, Switzerland: World Health Organization.

World Health Organization (2000b). *International Classification of Health Problems in Primary Care*. Zurich, Switzerland: World Health Organization.

World Health Organization (2000c). *International Classification of Impairments, Disabilities, and Handicaps*. Zurich, Switzerland: World Health Organization.

Purpose: (1) to acquaint the reader with Healthy People 2010 targets for improvement and (2) present examples of epidemiology as the underlying science to health promotion and disease prevention.

Directions: Check out your knowledge of these Healthy People 2010 focus areas by taking the following tests (answers follow in a separate section).

FOCUS AREA 11: HEALTH COMMUNICATION

This focus area's goal is to use communication strategically to improve health.

11-1.　*Increase in the proportion of households with access to the Internet at home.* What is the targeted proportion of households with Internet access?
　　a. 20 percent
　　b. 40 percent
　　c. 60 percent
　　d. 80 percent

11-2.　*Improvement in the health literacy of persons with inadequate or marginal literacy skills (developmental).* Related to this objective, all of the following are correct except:
　　a. Approximately 90 million U.S. adults have inadequate or marginal literacy skills.
　　b. Written information is the only way to communicate about health.
　　c. A great deal of health education and promotion are organized around printed materials customarily written for a tenth-grade-level readership.
　　d. Health education and promotion materials have little utility to persons with limited literacy skills.

11-3. *Increase in the proportion of health communication activities that include research and evaluation (developmental).* Related to this objective, research:
  a. Provides the ideas and tools to design and carry out formative, process, and outcome evaluations to improve health communication efforts
  b. Certifies the degree of change that has occurred as a result of the health communication effort
  c. Identifies health communication programs or elements of these programs that are not working
  d. All of the above

11-4. *Increase in the proportion of health-related World Wide Web sites that disclose information that can be used to assess the quality of the site (developmental).* What is a current initiative at improving the quality of Web sites?
  a. Professional associations are issuing guidelines and recommendations.
  b. Federal agencies are actively monitoring and sanctioning owners of Web sites that are false or misleading.
  c. Developers and purchasers of online health resources are being urged to adopt standards for quality assurance.
  d. All of the above are true.

11-5. *Increase in the number of centers for excellence that seek to advance the research and practice of health communication (developmental).* A center for excellence would be responsible for:
  a. Promoting health communication theories and practices in health promotion and disease prevention
  b. Developing and disseminating quality standards
  c. Coordinating initiatives to develop a consensus research agenda
  d. All of the above

11-6. *Increase in the proportion of persons who report that their health care providers have satisfactory communication skills (developmental).* Related to this objective, which of the following is correct?
  a. Patients find communicating with their health care providers easy.

b. Patients report that providers give them enough information.
c. Patients highly value the information from providers and want to know more.
d. All of the above are correct.

FOCUS AREA 12: HEART DISEASE AND STROKE

This focus area's goal is to improve cardiovascular health and quality of life through the prevention, detection, and treatment of risk factors; early identification and treatment of heart attacks and strokes; and prevention of recurrent cardiovascular events.

Heart Disease

12-1.   *Reduction in coronary heart disease deaths.* How much of an improvement is targeted in the reduction of coronary heart disease deaths?
a. 20 percent improvement
b. 40 percent improvement
c. 60 percent improvement
d. 80 percent improvement

12-2.   *Increase in the proportion of adults ages twenty years and older who are aware of the early warning symptoms and signs of a heart attack and the importance of accessing rapid emergency care by calling 911 (developmental).* Related to this objective, all of the following are correct except:
a. About 1.1 million persons experience a heart attack (acute myocardial infarction) each year in the United States.
b. The vast majority of persons dying from heart attack is male while a small minority is female.
c. More than 50 percent of heart attack deaths occur suddenly, within one hour of the first symptoms, outside the hospital.
d. Survivors of a heart attack who are subject to a delay in treatment can experience damage to the heart muscle and poorer outcomes.

12-3. *Increase in the proportion of eligible patients with heart attacks who receive artery-opening therapy within an hour of symptom onset (developmental).* Related to this objective, which of the following would be most likely administered within an hour of symptom onset?
   a. Balloon angioplasty
   b. Coronary stenting
   c. Clot-dissolving agents
   d. Coronary artery bypass surgery

12-4. *Increase in the proportion of adults ages twenty years and older who call 911 and administer cardiopulmonary resuscitation (CPR) when they witness an out-of-hospital cardiac arrest (developmental).* Related to this objective, how does the bystander recognize a possible collapse from cardiac arrest? The bystander notices that the affected individual:
   a. Is unresponsive
   b. Has slowed or stopped breathing
   c. Lacks a detectable pulse
   d. All of the above

12-5. *Increase in the proportion of eligible persons with witnessed out-of-hospital cardiac arrest who receive their first therapeutic electrical shock within six minutes after collapse recognition (developmental).* Early access to emergency health care services is also a critical determinant of outcomes for victims of out-of-hospital cardiac arrest. Related to this objective, all of the following are correct except:
   a. The sooner CPR is given to a person in cardiac arrest, the greater the chances of survival.
   b. Effective response to an out-of-hospital cardiac arrest is minimizing the time between recognized collapse and delivery of a short burst of therapeutic electrical current.
   c. A majority of persons having an out-of-hospital cardiac arrest receive therapeutic electrical shock early enough to benefit from it.
   d. The public should develop and maintain programs for easier identification and treatment of individuals with out-of-hospital cardiac arrest.

12-6. *Reduction in hospitalizations of older adults with congestive heart failure as the principal diagnosis.* Related to this objective, what is congestive heart failure?
   a. When a blood vessel bringing oxygen and nutrients to the brain bursts or is clogged by a blood clot
   b. When narrowed or clogged coronary arteries interfere with blood flow to the heart, possibly causing pain and resulting in heart muscle damage
   c. When insufficient blood flow in coronary arteries weakens the heart so it cannot pump enough blood to meet the needs of the body's other organs
   d. When narrowed blood and lymph vessels to leg and arm muscles cause pain or ulcers

Stroke

12-7. *Reduction in stroke deaths.* How much of an improvement is targeted in the reduction of stroke deaths?
   a. 20 percent improvement
   b. 40 percent improvement
   c. 60 percent improvement
   d. 80 percent improvement

12-8. *Increase in the proportion of adults who are aware of the early warning symptoms and signs of a stroke (developmental).* Related to this objective, which of the following is correct?
   a. Stroke is also called cerebrovascular disease or "brain attack."
   b. Stroke affects the blood vessels supplying blood to the brain, and when that part of the brain has impaired circulation, nerve cells die.
   c. Health care providers can counsel about symptoms and signs of stroke, the importance of accessing emergency medical services, and how to control risk factors.
   d. All of the above are correct.

Blood Pressure

12-9. *Reduction in the proportion of adults with high blood pressure.* What is the targeted proportion of adults with high blood pressure?
a. 16 percent
b. 36 percent
c. 56 percent
d. 76 percent

12-10. *Increase in the proportion of adults with high blood pressure whose blood pressure is under control.* What is the targeted proportion of adults with high blood pressure whose condition is under control?
a. 10 percent
b. 30 percent
c. 50 percent
d. 70 percent

12-11. *Increase in the proportion of adults with high blood pressure who are taking action (for example, losing weight, increasing physical activity, or reducing sodium intake) to help control their blood pressure.* As of 1998, what proportion of persons with high blood pressure were taking action to control it?
a. 22 percent
b. 42 percent
c. 62 percent
d. 82 percent

12-12. *Increase in the proportion of adults who have had their blood pressure measured within the preceding two years and can state whether their blood pressure was normal or high.* What is high blood pressure?
a. A systolic blood pressure of 80 mmHg or greater or a diastolic pressure of 30 mmHg or greater
b. A systolic blood pressure of 100 mmHg or greater or a diastolic pressure of 50 mmHg or greater
c. A systolic blood pressure of 120 mmHg or greater or a diastolic pressure of 70 mmHg or greater
d. A systolic blood pressure of 140 mmHg or greater or a diastolic pressure of 90 mmHg or greater.

Cholesterol

12-13. *Reduction in the mean total blood cholesterol levels among adults.* What is the mean total blood cholesterol level among adults?
a. 186 mg/dL
b. 206 mg/dL
c. 226 mg/dL
d. 246 mg/dL

12-14. *Reduction in the proportion of adults with high total blood cholesterol levels.* As of 1994, what is the proportion of U.S. adults with high total blood cholesterol levels of 240 mg/dL or greater?
a. 1 percent
b. 21 percent
c. 41 percent
d. 61 percent

12-15. *Increase in the proportion of adults who have had their blood cholesterol checked within the preceding five years.* What is the targeted proportion of adults having their blood cholesterol checked within past five years?
a. 20 percent
b. 40 percent
c. 60 percent
d. 80 percent

12-16. *Increase in the proportion of persons with coronary heart disease who have their LDL-cholesterol level treated to a goal of less than or equal to 100 mg/dL (developmental).* Related to this objective, which is correct about low density lipoprotein (LDL) cholesterol?
a. LDL is sometimes called the good cholesterol.
b. LDL inhibits blood cholesterol being carried to the tissues and organs of the body, including the arteries.
c. Cholesterol from LDL is the main source of damaging buildup and blockage in the arteries.
d. The lower the level of LDL in the blood, the greater the risk of coronary heart disease.

TEST ANSWERS

Focus Area 11

11-1.   (d) 80 percent. As of 1998, 26 percent of households have Internet access. Since many health-related organizations and agencies utilize the Internet to channel their information and services, it is essential that the public be able to tap into these valuable health resources.

11-2.   (b) Written information is the only way to communicate about health. Obviously, this is incorrect. Given the large number of U.S. adults having inadequate or marginal literacy skills, there is a gap here because so many health education and promotion materials are in printed format and designed at a tenth-grade reading level. This gap means many persons are denied the full benefits of health information and services.

11-3.   (d) All of the above. Research and evaluation are used to design, implement, and improve the overall quality of health communication efforts.

11-4.   (d) All of the above are true. There is a concern about the quality of health information released at World Wide Web sites regarding products and services. Web users can browse the Internet for many health-related reasons such as purchasing medications and consulting with providers.

11-5.   (d) All of the above. Besides these responsibilities, there are others: developing systems to identify and assess health communication research, evaluating communication strategies, messages, materials, and resources; fostering networking and collaboration among health communicators, health educators, and other health professionals; promoting health communication skills training for health professionals; and promoting research and dissemination activities among specific population groups.

11-6.   (c) Patients highly value information from providers and want to know more. Recent studies reveal that patients find communicating with providers difficult, and that patients do not receive sufficient information even though they value it and want more. Therefore, the providers have to communicate more clearly, candidly, accurately, and in a culturally and linguistically appropriate manner.

Focus Area 12

12-1.   (a) 20 percent improvement. As of 1998, there were 208 deaths per 100,000 population and the target is 166 deaths per 100,000 population.*

12-2.   (b) The vast majority of persons dying from heart attack is male while a small minority is female. This is incorrect. In 1996, of the 476,000 persons who died from heart attacks about 51 percent were males and 49 percent were females.

12-3.   (c) Clot-dissolving agents. Epidemiological studies have demonstrated that clot-dissolving (thrombolytic) agents are effective in opening affected coronary arteries during a heart attack. Although these agents should be administered within an hour of symptom onset, they have some effectiveness up to twelve hours after symptoms appear. Balloon angioplasty, coronary stenting, and coronary artery bypass surgery are other acute interventions for a heart attack.

12-4.   (d) All of the above. After recognizing the collapse, the by-stander should call 911 or the local emergency number and, if qualified, administer CPR.

12-5.   (c) A majority of persons having an out-of-hospital cardiac arrest receive therapeutic electrical shock early enough to benefit from it. This is incorrect since it is really a minority of witnessed out-of-hospital cardiac arrest cases receiving therapeutic electrical shock and other interventions in time for them to be effective.

12-6.   (c) When insufficient blood flow in coronary arteries weakens the heart so it cannot pump enough blood to meet the needs of the body's other organs. This is congestive heart failure. When a blood vessel bringing oxygen and nutrients to the brain bursts or is clogged by a blood clot, the person has had a stroke. When narrowed or clogged coronary arteries interfere with blood flow to the heart, possibly causing pain and resulting in heart muscle damage, coronary heart disease has

---

*Ages adjusted to the year 2000 standard population.

set in. Peripheral vascular disease is when narrowed blood and lymph vessels to leg and arm muscles cause pain or ulcers.

12-7.   (a) 20 percent improvement. As of 1998, there were sixty deaths per 100,000 population and the target is forty-eight deaths per 100,000 population.

12-8.   (d) All of the above are correct. Stroke is a kind of cardiovascular disease and the third leading cause of death in the United States. It has the same risk factors as coronary heart disease: elevated cholesterol levels, high blood pressure, tobacco use, and physical inactivity. A form of stroke is transient ischemic attacks or small strokelike events that are symptoms of cerebrovascular disease.

12-9.   (a) 16 percent improvement. Between 1988 and 1994, 28 percent of adults twenty years and older had high blood pressure, and the target is a reduction to 16 percent.

12-10.   (c) 50 percent. Between 1988 and 1994, 18 percent of adults twenty years and older with high blood pressure had it under control. The target is 50 percent.

12-11.   (d) 82 percent. As of 1998, 82 percent of adults aged eighteen years and older with high blood pressure were managing risk factors such as losing weight, increasing physical activity, or reducing sodium intake. The target for improvement is to increase this proportion to 95 percent.

12-12.   (d) A systolic blood pressure of 140 mmHg or greater or a diastolic pressure of 90 mmHg or greater. With high blood pressure, the heart has to work harder, resulting in an increased risk of a heart attack, stroke, heart failure, kidney and eye problems, and peripheral vascular disease.

12-13.   (b) 206 mg/dL. Between 1988 and 1994, the baseline mean total blood cholesterol level for U.S. adults twenty years and older was 206 milligrams per deciliter of blood. The target is a reduction to 199 mg/dL.

12-14.   (b) 21 percent. Between1988 and 1994, 21 percent of United States adults ages twenty years and older had total blood cholesterol levels of 240 mg/dL or greater. The target is to reduce this proportion to 17 percent.

12-15.   (d) 80 percent. As of 1998, 67 percent of adults eighteen years of age and older had a blood cholesterol check within past five years, and the goal is to increase this proportion to 80 percent.

12-16. (c) Cholesterol from LDL is the main source of damaging buildup and blockage in the arteries. All of the other responses are incorrect. LDL is the so-called bad cholesterol. LDL contains most of the cholesterol in the blood and carries it to the tissues and organs of the body, including the arteries. The higher the level of LDL in the blood, the greater the risk for coronary heart disease.

Chapter 7

Surveillance

INTRODUCTION

Recall that epidemiology is the study of the occurrence and distribution, cause and control, and treatment and prevention of disease and other morbid conditions. Epidemiologists rely on surveillance not only to spot the occurrence and distribution of disease, but to act as the baseline of data needed during investigations into the cause and control of outbreaks. **Surveillance** is the monitoring of a population's morbidity and mortality through data collection, analysis, interpretation, and reporting. Surveillance results are used in health promotion and disease prevention programs. It is a primary activity of international, federal, state, and local-level public health agencies. Foremost, surveillance identifies indicators of **endemic** and **epidemic** diseases. The former means the usual incidence and prevalence of disease and other behaviors affecting health status; the latter represents the greater than expected incidence or sudden increase in prevalence of disease or other behaviors affecting health status (Lilienfeld and Stolley, 1994).

Surveillance is a delineable, sentinel function of public health agencies. For example, cases of disease at the local level are reported to the state, which operates a notifiable disease surveillance system. The data on cases are then forwarded to the U.S. Centers for Disease Prevention and Control and prepared for public release through the U.S. Center for Health Statistics. Ultimately, the data reach the World Health Organization (WHO). In addition to notifiable disease reporting, epidemiologists use other sources of morbidity information: surveying animal populations, inspecting environmental conditions, monitoring drug/biological utilization, examining laboratory results, and supporting incident reporting systems in student and employee populations.

A whole other system of surveillance involves **vital statistics.** Public health agencies collect, analyze, and summarize data on major life events such as births, deaths, marriages, and divorces. Although all four vital statistics are significant indicators of a population's health, epidemiologists pay particular attention to mortality data, which comes from death certificate registrations. Data are systematically tabulated based on the registration of these vital events.

Surveillance transcends routine data collection systems by supporting epidemiological investigators and researchers. During a disease outbreak, epidemiologists undertake the investigative method: determining the needs of a disease control program, designing appropriate interventive and preventive health services, and responding to the usual or unusual presence of a disease in a population. A more detailed explanation of the investigative method can be found in a five-step problem-solving protocol for controlling epidemics (see Chapter 8). Within these steps, investigators use surveillance data to compare disease rates of the local population studied with rates in the overall U.S. population. During research studies (see Chapters 9 through 12), again, epidemiologists tap existing surveillance systems for baseline data on a population's disease rates, especially when these rates are apt to change during the course of the research study.

Public Health

Before proceeding with surveillance, attention should be focused on public health. With their mission of protecting, promoting, and restoring the population's health and environment, **public health agencies** assure safe food and water, adequate sanitation, preventive health services, and the formulation of relevant legislation—all within the context of health promotion and disease prevention. Public health has been called a social institution, a discipline, and a practice (Last, 1988). In light of changing technology and social values, public health combines sciences, skills, and beliefs to maintain and improve the health of all people through collective actions. The successes are the reduction of disease, morbid conditions such as disability, and premature death.

At the international level is the **World Health Organization (WHO),** located in Zurich, Switzerland. Founded in 1942, this United Nations agency conducts worldwide campaigns to control such diseases as malaria, tuberculosis, and venereal diseases. The agency helps establish pure-water supplies and sanitation systems in developing countries especially. It also provides community health education, health care planning assistance, and health professional training.

At the national level are the **Centers for Disease Prevention and Control (CDC),** a U.S. public health agency located in Atlanta, Georgia. Founded in 1946, the agency is comprised of centers dealing with epidemiology, international health, laboratory improvement, prevention services, environmental health, occupational health, infectious diseases, and professional development. Each center works nationally and in cooperation with WHO. Although the CDC has many varied activities and accomplishments, some of the more well-known include the establishment of a notifiable disease reporting system implemented at the state level, research into causation of disease outbreaks such as Legionnaires' disease and toxic shock syndrome, vaccine effectiveness studies and immunization standards, guidelines for comprehensive school health programming, clean drinking water standards, and the current research agenda regarding HIV disease. Within the CDC is the **National Center for Health Statistics** whose main responsibilities are collecting, analyzing, and reporting surveillance-related data, especially with regard to vital statistics. Besides maintaining morbidity and mortality data systems, data for which are furnished from the states, this national center conducts periodic surveys of the general public.

At the state level are the respective health departments, known as **official health agencies.** These agencies conduct the core functions of assessing and assuring health, and developing policies. Essentially, state health departments can make and enforce public health law, which of course is approved through the legislative process. They usually have jurisdiction over local health departments such as approving administrative assignments in county health departments. Within the state health department are various offices or bureaus, which include infectious disease prevention and control, chronic disease prevention and control, laboratory services, and environmental health. Public health surveillance of diseases and other morbid conditions are usually conducted in these units.

At the local level are regional, county, and city health departments which provide direct health services to the public. Essentially, local departments implement the health policies established at the state level. Examples of this include routine food service inspections, immunization clinic operation, sexually transmitted disease testing and treatment, public sanitation, health promotion programming, and others. Among these services are collection of data from vital events (e.g., death certificates), infectious disease occurrence, occupational health and safety incidents, among others. These surveillance data are collected and reported to the state health department by local departments.

SURVEILLANCE SYSTEMS

School Population Surveillance

Several surveillance systems operate within school-age populations. The Centers for Disease Prevention and Control routinely administer the Youth Risk Behavior Survey, a representative school-based survey that measures the prevalence of health risk behaviors among adolescents. In fact, there is a counterpart for postsecondary school students called the National College Health Risk Behavior Survey. At the local level, epidemiologists rely on procured data from school absenteeism records, especially during influenza outbreaks.

Workplace Population Surveillance

Diseases and other morbid conditions resulting from exposure to agents on the job are considered **occupational diseases.** Surveillance systems are in place to detect incidents of exposure as well as incidence of disease. In fact, such systems are required thanks to 1970 federal legislation. The **Occupational Safety and Health Administration (OSHA)** was founded in the U.S. Department of Labor to ensure healthy and safe working conditions. OSHA applies to every employer whose business is involved in interstate commerce. OSHA collaborates with the **National Institute of Occupational Safety and Health (NIOSH),** which through research establishes workplace health and safety standards. OSHA also responds to claims that health and safety standards are not being maintained at work sites. NIOSH's research is focused on allowable limits of exposure to biological, chemical, and physical agents. Many times, one of these agents works in conjunction with another in a process known as **synergism** to cause disease.

Examples of biological agents encountered in the workplace include hepatitis B and HIV in health care workers, and anthrax in agricultural workers. Examples of chemical agents are the halogenated hydrocarbons used in pesticides, herbicides, industrial solvents, refrigerants, and plastics, which in addition to being carcinogenic, cause liver and neural damage. Particulate matter in the forms of coal, silica, and cotton dust cause lung disorders. Physical agents such as noise, radiation, extreme temperatures, and vibration also represent direct hazards to workers' health, including working conditions that require repetitive motion. This can oftentimes result in repetitive stress injury, symptoms of which include severe pain in the hands or arms and sometimes a partial loss of function. In 1988, practically half of all reported occupational illness cases were of this type of injury.

General Public Surveillance Systems

As previously mentioned, the National Center for Health Statistics maintains morbidity and mortality data systems and conducts periodic surveys of the general public. These data are either procured directly from persons through surveys, interviews, and examinations, or are taken from existing medical, health, and vital statistics records and registrations. Examples of these systems include:

- National Ambulatory Medical Care Survey
- National Employer Health Insurance Survey
- National Health Care Survey
- National Health Interview Surveys
- National Health and Nutrition Examination Survey
- National Hospital Ambulatory Medical Care Survey
- National Hospital Discharge Survey
- National Immunization Survey
- National Maternal and Infant Health Survey
- National Mortality Followback Survey
- National Survey of Family Growth
- National Vital Statistics System

Surveillance for asthma provides insight into these various systems. Asthma is a common, noninfectious, chronic disease in the United States. This respiratory disorder's symptoms include breathing difficulty caused by temporary constriction of the bronchi (the airways connecting the trachea to the lungs). Although there is no single surveillance system for asthma, several individual systems operated by the National Center for Health Statistics collect asthma-related data. The National Health Interview Survey asks about self-reported asthma prevalence. The National Ambulatory Medical Care Survey inquires about asthma office visits, while the National Hospital Ambulatory Medical Care Survey collects information on asthma emergency room visits. The National Hospital Discharge Survey surveys asthma hospitalizations, and asthma death information is collected as state vital statistics (i.e., death certificates). Over the past twenty years there has been an increase in self-reported asthma prevalence rates and asthma death rates. In addition, asthma hospitalization rates have increased in the Northeast and decreased in the Midwest and West regions of the country. Furthermore, asthma-related death rates were highest in the Northeast and Midwest, although rates varied substantially among states within the same region. Data such as these can be used to design more effective treatment and prevention strategies (NHLBI, 1999). Other examples of general public surveillance systems can be found in the Web Site Resources section at the end of this chapter.

Other Surveillance Systems

Besides the human population, epidemiologists conduct surveillance on animal populations. An example of this was presented in Chapter 3 regarding rabies. Suspected incidents are brought to the attention of animal control specialists, who report cases to infectious disease control specialists in their local health department. Aside from rabies, other examples would include surveillance for encephalitis, West Nile virus, and other arboviral diseases transmitted by mosquitoes. Essentially, public health specialists rely on surveys of wild or domestic bird populations to detect the presence of these viral diseases within a locality. Similarly, deer tick samples are procured for the purpose of detecting the presence of Lyme disease bacteria (Stone et al., 1996).

RATES

To investigate, control, and prevent illness and death, epidemiologists need to gather data and calculate rates. Rate calculations are based on a **generic rate formula,** of which the number of cases or events (N) is divided by a representative number or sample of a population, and the quotient is multiplied by some power of ten, which represents the rate of occurrence per $10^{(n)}$ individuals (see Figure 7.1). A rate is calculated within a specified period of time, for example, a twelve-month period, and usually measured against 100, 1,000, or 10,000 or higher number of individuals divisible by 10.

Morbidity Rates

Morbidity rates pertain to disease occurrence and are calculated as attack, incidence, and prevalence usually measured against 100, 1,000 or 10,000. Since N is the total number of cases, they have to be diagnosable, meaning that the disease or condition has apparent classifiable symptoms according to the ICD-10. The denominator is a count of those in the population who were at risk for developing the disease. Someone with immunity to a viral disease should not be counted in the denominator because he or she would never become a case. However, this exclusion is impractical, especially when calculating rates in large populations.

To help illustrate, an example of rate calculations for selected diseases from the Commonwealth of Virginia is provided (see Table 7.1). The state health department's notifiable disease surveillance system accepts incident reports from health care professionals and certified laboratory sites. During rate calculations, the state health department will rely on the same population count (6,758,567) in the denominator regardless of the immunogenicity of the agent, meaning that the true number of susceptible persons varies, just as the number of at-risk people will change throughout the reporting year. Yet for 1998, the estimated population at risk was approximated to the midpoint of that reporting period.

$$\text{rate} = \frac{N}{\text{Population}} \times 10^{(n)}$$

FIGURE 7.1. Generic rate formula

TABLE 7.1. Reported cases and rate per 100,000 population (6,758,567) for selected diseases in Virginia, 1998

Disease	Number of Cases	Rate
AIDS	963	14.25
Amebiasis	31	0.46
Aseptic meningitis	240	3.55
Bacterial meningitis	57	0.84
Campylobacteriosis	700	10.36
Chicken pox	1,115	16.50
Chlamydia (STD)	13,370	197.82
Encephalitis, primary	17	0.25
Giardiasis	503	7.44
Gonorrhea	9,215	136.35
H. influenzae infection	19	0.28
Hepatitis A	226	3.34
Hepatitis B	109	1.61
Hepatitis non-A non-B	13	0.19
Histoplasmosis	6	0.09
HIV infection	825	12.21
Influenza	1,160	17.16
Kawasaki syndrome	36	0.53
Legionellosis	27	0.40
Lyme disease	73	1.08
Malaria	61	0.90
Measles	2	0.03
Meningococcal infection	49	0.73
Mumps	13	0.19
Pertussis	56	0.83
Rabies in animals	549	–
Rocky Mountain spotted fever	14	0.21
Salmonellosis	1,135	16.79
Shigellosis	200	2.96
Syphilis, early	379	5.61
Tuberculosis	339	5.02
Typhoid fever	7	0.10

Source: Office of Epidemiology, 1998, pp. 3-4.

The surveillance system records new cases, and therefore calculates **incidence rates.** In the incidence rate formula, as in the generic, the numerator is the total number of new cases and the denominator represents persons exposed to the risk of that disease within a given reporting period. Since Table 7.1 displays new cases occurring during 1998, the annual incidence rate for each disease was calculated. A **period incidence rate** is a subset based on new cases within a specified length of time within a year. During an outbreak, epidemiological detectives will likely calculate incidence rates during even shorter periods of time, such as a month, week, or a day, especially during the length of an episodic outbreak. Such short periods of measurement would be considered **point incidence.** Another related rate calculation is **infection rate,** in which the numerator includes both new cases and inapparent infection cases—persons who start a disease process but do not display symptoms.

AIDS Surveillance in the United States

The HIV/AIDS Surveillance System, operated by the Centers for Disease Control, collects, analyzes and reports notifiable disease data on AIDS cases. For example, as of 1998, there were 19.5 new cases of AIDS per 100,000 persons, a decline in rate from the previous two years. By 2010, the target annual rate is 1.0 new cases of AIDS per 100,000 persons. This target is achievable not only due to advances in prevention and treatment, but also from the simple fact that the length of time between HIV diagnosis and AIDS diagnosis has lengthened. The number of new AIDS cases per year, although decreasing, no longer represents an accurate estimate of the current HIV epidemic. Even though AIDS may occur much later than infection with HIV, only AIDS cases are currently reported by all state health departments. Because tracking HIV infection is more accurate for tracking the status of the epidemic, states are making progress in reporting HIV infection by establishing key baseline data about HIV (CDC, 1998, pp. 2-7).

This relates to Healthy People 2010 Objective 13-1: *Reduce AIDS among adolescents and adults* (Healthy People 2010, 2000, 13-13). (See Chapter 7 activities for more information.)

A specific kind of incidence can be expressed as an **attack (or case) rate,** in that only persons exposed to an identified agent or risk factor can be included in the denominator (population). Related, there is the **secondary attack rate,** within which anyone exposed to the first case of a disease is included in the denominator, although the numerator must be reduced in count by one because the initial case is excluded.

Prevalence rates are calculated using existing cases during a specified time—which would include cases that began before but then extended into the reporting year as well as any new case that develops during the time period. Most times, the prevalence rates for specific diseases and other morbid conditions are calculated during a cross-sectional or prevalence study (described in Chapter 8). Similar to incidence, epidemiologists can calculate annual, period, and point prevalence rates. There is even a subset known as **lifetime prevalence,** where the total number of persons ever having a disease at some time in their life acts as the numerator, and the population at risk remains included in the denominator.

Mortality Rates

Mortality rates pertain to death occurrences and are calculated as crude, disease-specific, age-specific, maternal, and natal, with the power of ten usually set at 10,000 or 100,000. This calculation provides an estimate of the proportion of the population that dies during a specified period within the circumstances mentioned. In keeping with the generic rate formula, the numerator (N) is the number of people dying, and each must be a certified death from a primary cause with a corresponding ICD-10 code. These data are derived from death certificates filed with the local health department by primary care providers. The denominator corresponds to those in the population who were at risk for dying during the specified time period, and is an approximation of the area's census at the midpoint of a given reporting year. Hence, the general mortality rate of a population could actually be considered a **crude rate.** For example, during an epidemiological study, the population might be expressed as **years of life lived,** which denotes a population member's age in countable time within the census year. For instance, a person living in a population for six months would have a half year of life lived for the purposes of the study.

Disease-specific (or cause of death) mortality rates are commonly reported statistics. As the name denotes, deaths from a specific cause represent the numerator. For example, if the number of mortal cases of heart disease (N = 725,790) is divided by the approximate U.S.

population (267,000,000) and then multiplied by 100,000, one gets 271.2. That means out of every 100,000 people who lived during 1997, 271 passed away due to heart disease (National Center for Health Statistics, 1999, p. 13). (See Table 7.2, which also contains ICD-10 codes.) There are also age-specific death rate calculations wherein the numerator counts disease-specific deaths and the denominator, that is, the population, refers to a specified age group. Epidemiologists usually break ages down according to these levels (Timmreck, 1998, p. 315):

- 0-4 years old
- 5-14 years old
- 15-24 years old
- 25-44 years old
- 45-64 years old
- 65-84 years old
- 84 + years old

Age-specific death rates are needed calculations when epidemiologists are comparing two populations regarding disease occurrence and distribution.

A more specific kind of mortality rate is maternal death rate, of which the numerator corresponds to death cases associated with childbirth and the denominator accounts for live births within a specified time, all multiplied by 1,000. Another related category is known as natality rates, and pertain to fetal (>20 or 28 weeks of gestation), perinatal (>28 weeks of gestation plus postnatal deaths), postneonatal (between 28 days and 1 year old), neonatal <28 days old), and infant (<1 year of age), death rates. Each natality rate refers to deaths occurring at specific stages of fetal or early life development in proportion to live births (fetal deaths are included with live births in fetal and perinatal rates). These rates are usually measured against 1,000.

Two other mortality rates are fatality rate and case fatality rate. The former refers to the rate in a designated series of persons exposed to or affected by a simultaneous event such as a disaster. Sometimes, this rate is confused with case fatality rate, which is the proportion of cases of a specific disease or condition that are fatal within a specified period.

TABLE 7.2. U.S. deaths and death rates (per 100,000 population) for all ages on the ten leading causes of death with ICD-10 codes (included)

Rank	Cause of Death	Number	Rate
	All causes	2,314,729	864.9
1	Diseases of heart (390-398, 402, 404-429)	725,790	271.2
2	Malignant neoplasms, including neoplasms of lymphatic and hematopoietic tissues (140-208)	537,390	200.8
3	Cerebrovascular diseases (430-438)	159,877	59.7
4	Chronic obstructive pulmonary diseases and allied conditions (490-496)	110,637	41.3
5	Accidents and adverse effects (E800-E949)	92,191	34.4
	Motor vehicle accidents (E810-E825)	42,420	15.8
	All other accidents and adverse effects (E800-E807, E826-E949)	49,772	18.6
6	Pneumonia and influenza (480-487)	88,383	33.0
7	Diabetes mellitus (250)	62,332	23.3
8	Suicide (E950-E959)	29,725	11.1
9	Nephritis, nephrotic syndrome, and nephrosis (580-589)	25,570	9.6
10	Chronic liver disease and cirrhosis (571)	24,765	9.3
	All other causes (residual)	458,069	171.2

Source: National Center for Health Statistics, 1997.

Rate Adjustment

Many times morbidity or mortality rates as well as ratios are adjusted through a direct or indirect method of standardization. In addition, there are other techniques of adjustment such as regressional analysis. Adjustment is necessary whenever the population appears to be overrepresented by a host factor (e.g., age) in comparison to the U.S. standard population. Thus, epidemiologists suspect that differing age distribution within two populations being compared might affect the calculated rates of disease or death.

It is commonplace to see charts of disease occurrence with the footnote, "rates age-adjusted" (see Figure 7.2). Most likely, the data

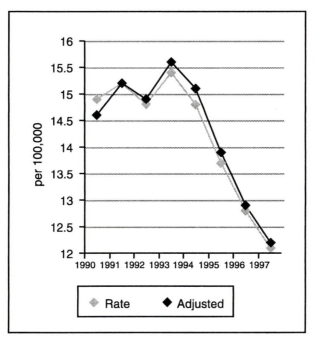

FIGURE 7.2. U.S. death rates for injury by firearms (*Source:* Healthy People 2010, 2000, p. 15-8).

were subjected to the direct method of rate adjustment. In this method, cases within each age group of the local population (the population under observation) are multiplied by the standardized population's age-specific case rate. The resulting products at each age level are thus an adjusted number of cases, and the total of these cases acts as the numerator in the generic rate formula. Sometimes this is called weighted averaging. The U.S. standardized population acts as the denominator and the resulting quotient is multiplied by 100,000.

The indirect method of rate adjustment is more likely to be used when epidemiologists are faced with a relatively rare occurrence of disease, and hence there is not a sufficient (or stable) age-specific disease rate they can use from the standard population. Another time this method is preferred is when epidemiologists wish to compare small groups of people, such as one neighborhood against another, who are experiencing a disease outbreak. Therefore, the number of cases of disease in the standard population is multiplied by the age-specific rate of that disease in the local population, and the resulting products are summarized as expected cases and inserted into the generic rate formula. In this case, the count of persons in the local population acts as the denominator. One additional step to the indirect method is calculating a standardized mortality ratio, which is the observed (actual) cases in the study population divided by the expected number, which is then multiplied by 100.

If rate adjustment appears complex, just think of it as a way of leveling the playing field when two groups are being studied for disease occurrence. Usually the older group's rate is adjusted down while the younger group's rate is adjusted up. Considering that there are two ways of adjusting or standardizing rates, the direct method is merely a transposition of the indirect method. It should be emphasized, however, that the calculated age-adjusted rate of one method should not be used in combination or comparison with another method.

Ratios

Similar to rates are ratios. Epidemiologists use ratios as further calculations of disease occurrence and distribution, and they are also calculated using the generic formula. Quotients are usually multiplied by 100. Technically, persons representing the numerator should not be contained within the denominator, since ratios express instances per 100, or the likelihood of occurrence, not the rate of occurrence in a specific population. At times, ratio results are expressed as percentages (Timmreck, 1998). Here are the more commonly calculated ratios in epidemiology:

- **Case fatality ratio** (or rate) represents persons who die from a disease or condition divided by those who were diagnosed with the condition. The ratio is attained where the quotient is multiplied by 100. Sometimes case fatality is expressed as a rate when the quotient is multiplied by a higher power of ten. This ratio was mentioned earlier in the examples of untreated persons who do not recover from diseases such as plague, rabies, and hepatitis B.

- **Proportionate mortality** (and morbidity) **ratio** (or rate) refers to the number of deaths (or illness cases) from a specific cause divided by the total number of deaths is a selected group of persons. When expressed as a rate, the quotient is multiplied by 100.
- **Relative risk** is the incidence of disease in exposed persons divided by incidence of disease in nonexposed persons. An estimate of relative risk calculates the odds of an occurrence from an epidemiological two-by-two table, where the persons without the disease have been controlled. Recall from Chapter 3, a risk calculation allows epidemiologists to say: "The risk of developing 'such and such disease' is 'so many' times more likely in persons exposed to 'such and such factor.' " Relative risk ratios are calculated during epidemiological investigations and studies.
- **Standardized morbidity** (mortality) ratio figures the number of events expected in an observed local population (study population), if the study population had the same specific rates as the standared population. Again, the quotient is multiplied by 100. This ratio is calculated using the indirect method of rate adjustment.

Measurement Issues

A rate or ratio is only as good as the quality of the surveillance data placed in the numerator and denominator of the generic formula. If either part of the formula is inaccurate due to human error, it is considered an **artifactual difference.** The potential for artifactual difference has already been recognized when epidemiologists attempt to describe the occurrence and distribution of diseases according to person, place, and time characteristics. The rule of thumb is that mortality-related rates and ratios are more valid and reliable when they rely on standardized data collected from death certificates and population censuses. Morbidity-related rates and ratios might not be as accurate and dependable because of insufficient surveillance systems. For instance, the notifiable disease reporting system in Virginia is only as good as the dependability of health care professionals reporting incidents of disease.

Why the Meningitis Epidemic in College Students?

During the past few years, tragic cases of bacterial meningitis have occurred in the U.S. college student population. To presume that college students have person characteristics (e.g., other than age) that make them more susceptible to bacterial meningitis is false. What seems to be the explanation is that advances in immunizations for *haemophilus influenzae* have dramatically decreased the rate of bacterial meningitis in young children. Whereas bacterial meningitis cases typically occurred by age two, the median age has shifted to the early to mid-twenties age group. The emergence of these new cases is alarming, yet somewhat predictable given the success of earlier age-group inoculation. This explanation is not meant to minimize the seriousness of this disease in college-age persons—the disease process in this case can progress to coma, severe deformity, and even death. College students who live on campus appear more likely to be exposed to this disease and can contract the bacteria through sharing food, beverages, and other fomites (e.g., cigarettes) that come in contact with the mouth. There are at least five different bacteria responsible for this disease and current vaccines address only two of them. Clinical trials are being conducted to perfect a conjugate vaccine that provides protection against all five bacteria (Harrison et al., 1999).

This relates to Healthy People 2010 Objective 14-7: *Reduce meningococcal disease* (Healthy People 2010, 2000, 14-20). (See Chapter 7 activities for more information.)

Other measurement tactics used by epidemiologists need addressing. One is the **life table,** which uses deaths in a population, profiled by demographic variables, to project the possibility of persons in a particular age group dying during a specified year. The life table data (sometimes called survival data) are time-specific and cumulative probabilities of survival for an age group, and are used in generating age-specific mortality rates. Life insurance companies rely on life tables to determine appropriate premium rates for policy coverage. It should be mentioned that the life table method can be applied to other morbidity if epidemiologists are studying the end point of a particular disease. Epidemiologists take life table information, called **actuarial data,** to determine life expectancy, the projected average number of years of living for a birth cohort (or group), if the mortality rates at that time continue. So, epidemiologists can predict the mean age of a birth group's mortality, known as **life expectancy.** Incidentally, these projections are also used in health risk appraisals through which a person's life expectancy can be delayed based on two adjustments: the current mortality (disease-specific and age-specific) rates as well as the adoption of healthy life practices. When a person completes a health risk appraisal, self-reported healthy habits or behavioral agents are factored-in, and a calculated appraised age is computed. When comparing appraised age to actual age, the person is presented an estimated life expectancy depending on his or her health status. Subsequently, if the person adopts healthy habits, he or she can actually increase individual life expectancy. For example, a birth cohort in 1952 had a life expectancy of sixty-two years. However, if an individual from that cohort incorporates lifelong healthy practices, the individual's personal life expectancy is likely to exceed sixty-two years.

According to the National Center for Health Statistics, life expectancy for the 1997 birth cohort (or group) increased to 76.5 years in 1997—an all-time high—primarily due to decreases in mortalities resulting from HIV/AIDS, heart disease, cancer, stroke, and homicide. White females continue to have the highest life expectancy, 79.9 years; followed by black females, 74.7 years; white males, 74.3 years; and black males, 67.2 years—a record high for each group. Life expectancy for Asians and Hispanics will be calculated and reported after Census 2000 is completed. Overall, the largest gain in life expectancy between 1980 and 1997 was for white males, 3.6 years, followed by black males, 3.4 years, to narrow the gap between men and women to 5.8 years.

Some epidemiologists have been interested in life expectancy specific to occupation. For example, the on-field death a few years ago of a veteran Major League Baseball (MLB) umpire raised the issue of whether professional umpires are at greater risk of earlier mortality compared to the general population. To address this, the ages of death of MLB umpires were collected and the differences from the overall population were noted. While looking at the data, it was necessary to make age adjustments because the older the umpire was, the more likely he or she was to meet mortality. Other variables considered during data analysis were how long they umpired and the average age of mortality for umpires during each year of the period of study. The results showed no significant differences between the average age of MLB umpire deaths and that of the overall population. Still, there might be risks unique to umpiring that, if properly addressed, could actually increase the life expectancy of "the man or woman behind the plate" (Cohen et al., 2000, p. 4).

Related to life expectancy is **life expectancy free from disability,** which is an estimate of life expectancy adjusted for activity limitations.

SUMMARY

Epidemiologists surveil and systematically collect, analyze, and report on data pertaining to the occurrence and distribution of illnesses and death. Surveillance systems operate at local, state, national, and international levels, and are directed at school-age persons, workers, and the general population. While analyzing the data, rates and ratios are calculated to illustrate occurrence and distributions. There are many kinds of rates, but nearly all use a generic rate calculation formula. Given the influence of the person characteristic of age on disease distribution, rates are usually age adjusted. Ratios, which are used to express risk, also rely on a generic formula. Other measurement issues include the quality of data collected, life tables, and life expectancy.

REVIEW QUESTIONS

1. Explain what epidemiological surveillance is. Can you identify examples of surveillance performed in schools, workplaces, and general populations?
2. Are you aware of the various public health agencies that conduct surveillance?
3. Do you know the definitions of terms in bold print in this chapter?
4. What is a morbidity rate? A mortality rate? How is each based on the generic formula? If given examples, could you recognize a morbidity or mortality rate calculation?
5. What is rate adjustment? Could you explain how rates are adjusted according to age using either the direct or indirect method?
6. Do you know the more common ratios: standardized mortality (morbidity), case fatality, and relative risk?
7. Explain this idea: "A rate or ratio is only as good as the quality of surveillance data that are placed in the numerator and denominator of the generic formula."

8. Do you understand how life table data as well as life expectancy are considered when completing a health risk appraisal?
9. Do you know the answers to the following chapter activity questions based on objectives from Healthy People 2010 focus areas 13 and 14?

WEB SITE RESOURCES

Assisted Reproductive Technology Success Rates
<http://www.cdc.gov/nccdphp/drh/>

Birth Defects Surveillance
<http://www.cdc.gov/nceh/cddh/bd/>

Cancer Registries Program
<http://www.cdc.gov/cancer/npcr/>

CDC, Publications and Software
<http://www.cdc.gov/epo/pub_sw.htm>

CDC, Scientific Data, Surveillance, and Injury Statistics
<http://www.cdc.gov/ncipc/osp/mortdata.htm>

CDC, Suicide Deaths and Rates Per 100,000
<http://www.cdc.gov/ncipc/data/us9794/Suic.htm> November 23, 1999.

CDC WONDER
<http://wonder.cdc.gov/>

HIV/AIDS Surveillance Report
<http://www.cdc.gov/hiv/dhap.htm>

National Center for Health Statistics
<http://www.cdc.gov/nchs/>

Pregnancy Risk Assessment Monitoring System
<http://www.cdc.gov/nccdphp/drh/srv_prams.htm>

Sexually Transmitted Diseases
<http://www.cdc.gov/nchstp/dstd/>

Tuberculosis Surveillance Reports
<http://www.cdc.gov/nchstp/tb/>

U.S. Bureau of the Census
<http://www.census.gov/>

World Health Organization
<http://www.who.int/home-page/>

Youth Risk Behavior Surveillance System
<http://www.cdc.gov/nccdphp/dash/yrbs/>

REFERENCES

CDC (1988). *HIV/AIDS surveillance report,* 10(2): 2-7. Atlanta, GA: Centers for Disease Control and Prevention.

Cohen, R.S., Celia A. Kamps, C.A., Kokoska, S., Segal, E.M., and Tucker, J.B. (2000). Life expectancy of major league baseball umpires. *The Physician and Sportsmedicine* 28(5): 1-6.

Harrison, L.H., Dwyer, D.M., Maples, C.T., and Billmann, L. (1999). Risk of meningococcal infection in college students. *JAMA,* 281(20): 762-769.

Healthy People 2010 (2000). *Healthy People 2010: Objectives for improving health.* Office of Disease Prevention and Health Promotion, U.S. Department of Health and Human Services, Washington, DC.

Last, J.M. (1998). *A dictionary of epidemiology.* New York: Oxford University Press.

Lilienfeld, D.E. and Stolley, P.D. (1994). *Foundations of epidemiology* (Second edition). New York: Oxford Press.

National Center for Health Statistics (1997). *Leading causes of death for U.S. population.* Atlanta, GA: U.S. Centers for Disease Control and Prevention.

National Center for Health Statistics (1998). *Leading causes of death for U.S. population.* Atlanta, GA: U.S. Centers for Disease Control and Prevention.

NHLBI (1999). *Data fact sheet: asthma statistics.* Bethesda, MD: National Heart, Lung, and Blood Institute, National Institutes of Health, U.S. Public Health Service.

Office of Epidemiology (1998). *Reported cases and rates for selected diseases in Virginia.* Richmond, VA: Commonwealth of Virginia Health Department.

Stone, D.B., Armstrong, W.R., Macrina, D.M., and Pankau, J.W. (1996). *Introduction to epidemiology.* Madison, WI: Brown and Benchmark.

Timmreck, T.C. (1998). *An introduction to epidemiology* (Second edition). Sudbury, MA: Jones and Bartlett Publishers.

Purpose: (1) to acquaint the reader with Healthy People 2010 targets for improvement and (2) present examples of epidemiology as the underlying science to health promotion and disease prevention.

Directions: Check out your knowledge of these Healthy People 2010 focus areas by taking the following tests (answers follow in a separate section).

FOCUS AREA 13: HIV

This focus area's goal is to prevent HIV infection and its related illness and death.

13-1. *Reduction in AIDS among adolescents and adults.* Related to this objective, persons reported with AIDS will increasingly represent those who:
   a. Were diagnosed too late for them to benefit from treatments
   b. Neither sought nor had access to care
   c. Failed treatment
   d. All of the above

13-2. *Reduction in the number of new AIDS cases among adolescent and adult men who have sex with men.* How much of an improvement is targeted in the reduction of new AIDS cases among this population?
   a. 5 percent improvement
   b. 25 percent improvement
   c. 45 percent improvement
   d. 65 percent improvement

13-3. *Reduction in the number of new AIDS cases among females and males who inject drugs.* How much of an improvement is

targeted for the reduction of new AIDS cases in this population?
a. 5 percent improvement
b. 25 percent improvement
c. 45 percent improvement
d. 65 percent improvement

13-4. *Reduction in the number of new AIDS cases among adolescent and adult men who have sex with men and inject drugs.* Related to this objective, all of the following are correct about prevention programs for these at-risk groups except:
a. Prevention programs should focus on both adolescent and adult males in these at-risk groups.
b. Prevention programs should focus on both HIV-infected and uninfected members of these at-risk groups.
c. Prevention programs should focus on reaching only those persons who identify themselves as either homosexual or bisexual.
d. Prevention programs should focus on representatives of certain racial and ethnic groups whose proportions of total AIDS cases are greater than the percentage of AIDS cases in the overall U.S. population.

13-5. *Reduction in the number of cases of HIV infection among adolescents and adults (developmental).* Related to this objective, what is the relationship between HIV infection and AIDS?
a. Persons infected with HIV are said to have AIDS when they get certain opportunistic infections.
b. Persons infected with HIV are said to have AIDS when their CD4+ cell count drops below 200.
c. AIDS is the most severe phase of HIV infection.
d. All of the above are true.

13-6. *Increase in the proportion of sexually active persons who use condoms.* What is the targeted proportion of sexually active persons using condoms?
a. 10 percent
b. 30 percent
c. 50 percent
d. 70 percent

13-7. *Increase in the number of HIV-positive persons who know their serostatus (developmental).* Related to this objective, what is serostatus?

    a. Serostatus is the result of a blood test for the antibodies that the immune system creates to fight specific diseases.

    b. Serostatus is the set of guidelines and procedures to protect health care workers from exposure to infection from blood and other body fluids.

    c. Serostatus is something that guards against or prevents disease.

    d. Serostatus is an opportunistic disease.

13-8. *Increase in the proportion of substance abuse treatment facilities that offer HIV/AIDS education, counseling, and support.* As of 1997, what proportion of such facilities offer this kind of education, counseling, and support?

    a. 18 percent

    b. 38 percent

    c. 58 percent

    d. 78 percent

13-9. *Increase in the number of state prison systems that provide comprehensive HIV/AIDS, sexually transmitted diseases, and tuberculosis (TB) education (developmental).* Why is it significant to provide these kinds of services to the incarcerated population?

    a. Incarceration provides an environment in which early interventions and risk-reduction behaviors can be taught

    b. Incarceration provides an environment in which early interventions and risk-reduction behaviors can be reinforced over time.

    c. Incarceration represents an opportunity to provide the education, support, and continuity of care needed when incarcerated persons are released and return to their home communities.

    d. All of the above are true.

13-10. *Increase in the proportion of inmates in state prison systems who receive voluntary HIV counseling and testing during incarceration (developmental).* Related to this objective, all of the following are correct except:

a. All state prison systems are required to provide HIV testing to all inmates before discharge.

b. HIV testing to inmates upon intake allows for sufficient medical care and necessary follow-up.

c. Discharge planning and formal linkages with community-based HIV care should be offered to all HIV-positive inmates just prior to or upon release.

d. Early access to care reduces both immediate and long-term health care costs for correctional institutions and the community.

13-11. *Increase in the proportion of adults with tuberculosis (TB) who have been tested for HIV.* As of 1998, what proportion of adults with TB were tested for HIV?
a. 15 percent
b. 35 percent
c. 55 percent
d. 75 percent

13-12. *Increase in the proportion of adults in publicly funded HIV counseling and testing sites who are screened for common bacterial sexually transmitted diseases (STDs) (chlamydia, gonorrhea, and syphilis) and are immunized against hepatitis B virus (developmental).* Related to this objective, which of the following is correct?
a. Being infected with one STD makes it easier to get and give HIV therefore increasing the risk of HIV transmission.
b. Treating other STDs reduces the spread of HIV.
c. STD vaccines can minimize the probability of infection and an effective vaccine for hepatitis B is widely available.
d. All of the above are correct.

13-13. *Increase in the proportion of HIV-infected adolescents and adults who receive testing, treatment, and prophylaxis consistent with current public health service treatment guidelines.* Related to this objective, which represents an effective treatment of HIV infection?
a. HAART
b. Pandemic
c. Universal infection control precautions
d. C4+ cells

13-14. *Reduction in deaths from HIV infection.* Related to this objective, which of the following is correct?
   a. New drug therapies appear to delay progression of HIV to AIDS.
   b. New drug therapies appear to delay progression of AIDS to death.
   c. New drug therapies appear to explain the decline in deaths attributed to HIV.
   d. All of the above are correct.

13-15. *Extend the interval of time between an initial diagnosis of HIV infection and AIDS diagnosis in order to increase years of life of an individual infected with HIV (developmental).* To accomplish this objective, the HIV-infected person should be identified early and referred to appropriate services for:
   a. Preserving his or her health and extending the quality of living
   b. Helping him or her avoid opportunistic illnesses
   c. Reducing sexual and drug-use behaviors that may spread HIV
   d. All of the above

13-16. *Increase in years of life of an HIV-infected person by extending the interval of time between an AIDS diagnosis and death (developmental).* Related to this objective, all of the following are correct except:
   a. From 1996 through 1998, there has been a steady increase in deaths from AIDS.
   b. The number of persons living with AIDS has been increasing.
   c. If declines continue in newly diagnosed AIDS cases in the coming years, an increasing number of persons will be living with HIV infection.
   d. As cases of HIV-infected persons increase it will be important to monitor and treat to people with asymptomatic infection or mild illness.

13-17. *Reduction in new cases of perinatally acquired HIV infection (developmental).* Related to this objective, all of the following are correct except:

   a. Perinatal transmission of HIV accounts for virtually all new HIV infections in children.
   b. The United States has adopted a national policy of universal HIV testing, with patient notification as a routine component of prenatal care.
   c. The risk of perinatal HIV transmission could be reduced by as much as two-thirds with the use of zidovudine therapy.
   d. Counseling and voluntary testing, combined with zidovudine therapy, are highly effective in preventing HIV transmission from mother to unborn child.

FOCUS AREA 14: IMMUNIZATION AND INFECTIOUS DISEASES

This focus area's goal is to prevent disease, disability, and death from infectious diseases, including vaccine-preventable diseases.

Diseases Preventable Through Universal Vaccination

14-1. *Reduction in or elimination of indigenous cases of vaccine-preventable diseases.* All of the following vaccine-preventable diseases are targeted for total elimination except:
   a. Mumps
   b. Rubella
   c. Pertussis
   d. Tetanus

14-2. *Reduction in chronic hepatitis B virus infections in infants and young children (perinatal infections).* The reduction of hepatitis B in infants and young children can best be accomplished by
   a. Screening pregnant women during an early prenatal visit to identify if they are hepatitis B infected
   b. Retesting women at high risk for hepatitis B later in their pregnancy
   c. Administering the hepatitis B vaccine series to infants and young children whose mother is hepatitis B infected
   d. All of the above

14-3.   *Reduction in hepatitis B.* Related to this objective, all repre-
       sent high-risk groups for hepatitis B except:
       a. Adults forty years and older
       b. Injection drug users
       c. Men who have sex with men
       d. Occupationally exposed workers

14-4.   *Reduction in bacterial meningitis in young children.* How
       much of a reduction is targeted for this disease in young chil-
       dren?
       a. 14 percent
       b. 34 percent
       c. 54 percent
       d. 74 percent

14-5.   *Reduction in invasive pneumococcal infections.* Related to
       this objective, what is invasive pneumococcal infection? When
       the bacteria *Streptococcus pneumoniae* are
       a. Acquired as a result of medical treatment while in the hos-
          pital
       b. Isolated from a normally sterile site such as blood, cere-
          brospinal fluid, or pleural fluid
       c. Spread from one anatomic site to another site in the body
       d. Transmitted to humans by arthropods, primarily mosqui-
          toes, ticks, and fleas

Diseases Preventable Through Targeted Vaccination

14-6.   *Reduction in hepatitis A.* Related to this objective, which age
       group has the highest rate of hepatitis A?
       a. Children
       b. Adolescents
       c. Adults
       d. Older adults

14-7.   *Reduction in meningococcal disease.* Related to this objec-
       tive, which of the following is correct?
       a. There is only one strain of meningococcal bacteria.
       b. The current vaccine for meningococcal disease in young
          children is highly effective and has a long duration of pro-
          tection.

206 *Epidemiology for Health Promotion/Disease Prevention Professionals*

c. College students have recently become a high-risk group for certain kinds of meningococcal disease.
d. There are no plans for developing new vaccines for meningococcal disease.

14-8. *Reduction in Lyme disease.* How much of a reduction in Lyme disease is being targeted?
   a. 2 percent
   b. 22 percent
   c. 44 percent
   d. 64 percent

Infectious Diseases and Emerging Antimicrobial Resistance

14-9. *Reduction in hepatitis C.* Related to this objective, which of the following is correct about hepatitis C?
   a. Hepatitis C is the most prevalent chronic bloodborne viral infection in the U.S. population.
   b. Hepatitis C virus is commonly transmitted through sharing of equipment between injection drug users.
   c. Hepatitis C infects persons of all ages, but more so young adults aged twenty to thirty-nine years.
   d. All of the above are correct.

14-10. *Increase in the proportion of persons with chronic hepatitis C infection identified by state and local health departments.* Related to this objective, identification of hepatitis C infected persons allows for
   a. Counseling to prevent further disease transmission
   b. Vaccination to cure the disease
   c. Evaluation for likely kidney complications
   d. All of the above

14-11. *Reduction in tuberculosis.* What is the targeted rate of tuberculosis in the U.S. population?
   a. 1 new case per 100,000 population
   b. 10 new cases per 100,000 population
   c. 100 new cases per 100,000 population
   d. 1,000 new cases per 100,000 population

14-12. *Increase in the proportion of all tuberculosis patients who complete curative therapy within twelve months.* As of 1996,

what percentage of patients completed their therapy within twelve months?
a. 34 percent
b. 54 percent
c. 74 percent
d. 94 percent

14-13. *Increase in the proportion of contacts and other high-risk persons with latent tuberculosis infection who complete a course of treatment.* What is the targeted proportion of these high-risk persons completing treatment?
a. 25 percent
b. 45 percent
c. 65 percent
d. 85 percent

14-14. *Reduction in the average time for a laboratory to confirm and report tuberculosis cases.* As of 1997, what was the average length of time for a laboratory to confirm and report a tuberculosis case?
a. One day
b. Twenty-one days
c. Forty-one days
d. Sixty-one days

14-15. *Increase in the proportion of international travelers who receive recommended preventive services when traveling in areas of risk for select infectious diseases: hepatitis A, malaria, and typhoid (developmental).* Related to this objective, which of the following is correct?
a. The number of international travelers from the United States has increased an average of 3 percent a year for the past decade.
b. Hepatitis A, malaria, and typhoid account for a large proportion of illness and disability for international travelers.
c. Before embarking, some travelers go to a travel clinic, some visit primary care providers, and some receive no pretravel care.
d. All of the above are correct.

14-16. *Reduction in invasive early onset group B streptococcal disease.* Related to this objective, all of the following are correct about group B streptococcus except:
   a. It is a bacterium normally found in the intestines and genital area of the body.
   b. It is harmful to the adult person carrying the germ.
   c. About one in five pregnant women has the bacterium and is capable of transmitting it to the newborn.
   d. It can cause a dangerous infection in the blood, spinal fluid, and lungs of babies born to women having the bacteria.

14-17. *Reduction in hospitalizations caused by peptic ulcer disease in the United States.* Related to this objective, which is most likely to cause peptic ulcers?
   a. Stress
   b. *H. pylori* bacteria
   c. Spicy foods
   d. Excess stomach acid

14-18. *Reduction in the number of courses of antibiotics for ear infections for young children.* How much of a reduction in the number of antibiotic courses for children's ear infections is targeted?
   a. 19 percent
   b. 39 percent
   c. 59 percent
   d. 79 percent

14-19. *Reduction in the number of courses of antibiotics prescribed for the sole diagnosis of the common cold.* How much of a reduction in the number of antibiotic courses for the common cold is targeted?
   a. 10 percent
   b. 30 percent
   c. 50 percent
   d. 70 percent

14-20. *Reduction in hospital-acquired infections in intensive care unit patients.* Related to this objective, which of the following is correct?
   a. Hospital-acquired infections are a leading cause of illness and death in the United States.

    b. Of the 36 million patients admitted annually to U.S. hospitals, about 2 million will acquire an infection from the hospital setting.

    c. About 25 percent of all annual hospital-acquired infections occur in intensive care patients resulting in about 90,000 deaths.

    d. All of the above are correct.

14-21. *Reduction in antimicrobial use among intensive care unit patients.* How much of a reduction in antimicrobial use for these patients is being targeted?

    a. 20 percent

    b. 40 percent

    c. 60 percent

    d. 80 percent

Vaccination Coverage and Strategies

14-22. *Achievement and maintenance of effective vaccination coverage levels for universally recommended vaccines among young children.* What percentage of young children needs to be vaccinated to prevent circulation of viruses and bacteria-causing vaccine-preventable diseases in the general population?

    a. 30 percent

    b. 50 percent

    c. 70 percent

    d. 90 percent

14-23. *Maintenance of vaccination coverage levels for children in licensed day care facilities and children in kindergarten through the first grade.* As of 1998, what percentage of children either entering school or day care facilities has been vaccinated?

    a. 35 percent

    b. 55 percent

    c. 75 percent

    d. 95 percent

14-24. *Increase in the proportion of young children and adolescents who receive all vaccines that have been recommended for universal administration for at least five years.* Related to this objective, which vaccine likely will not be recommended by the year 2010?

a. Polio
b. Measles, mumps, and rubella
c. Diphtheria, pertussis, and tetanus
d. Hepatitis B

14-25. *Increase in the proportion of providers who have measured the vaccination coverage levels among children in their practice population within the past two years.* As of 1997, what percentage of private providers has measured child patients' vaccination coverage?

a. 6 percent
b. 26 percent
c. 46 percent
d. 66 percent

14-26. *Increase in the proportion of children who participate in fully operational population-based immunization registries.* As of 1999, what proportion of children were participating in such a registry?

a. 12 percent
b. 32 percent
c. 52 percent
d. 72 percent

14-27. *Increase in the routine vaccination coverage levels for adolescents.* What is the targeted proportion of adolescents who have adequate vaccination coverage?

a. 30 percent
b. 50 percent
c. 70 percent
d. 90 percent

14-28. *Increase in the hepatitis B vaccine coverage among high-risk groups.* As of 1995, what was the hepatitis B vaccine coverage for occupationally exposed workers?

a. 31 percent
b. 51 percent
c. 71 percent
d. 91 percent

14-29. *Increase in the proportion of adults who are vaccinated annually against influenza and are ever vaccinated against pneumococcal disease.* What is the target proportion of adults ever vaccinated against these two infectious diseases?
   a. 30 percent
   b. 50 percent
   c. 70 percent
   d. 90 percent

Vaccine Safety

14-30. *Reduction in vaccine-associated adverse events.* Related to this objective, which is a vaccine-associated adverse event?
   a. Vaccine-associated paralytic polio
   b. Pertussis vaccine-related seizures
   c. Pertussis vaccine-related febrile seizures
   d. All of the above

14-31. *Increase in the number of persons under active surveillance for vaccine safety via large linked databases.* Related to this objective, all of the following are correct except:
   a. A high standard of safety is expected of vaccines since they are recommended for millions of healthy people, including infants.
   b. Vaccine safety monitoring to identify and minimize vaccine-related reactions is necessary to help ensure safety because no vaccine is completely safe.
   c. Knowledge of vaccine safety is essential to assess accurately the risks and benefits in formulating vaccine use recommendations.
   d. A majority of adverse events show adequate evidence to determine if the vaccine was the cause of the event.

TEST ANSWERS

Focus Area 13

13-1.   (d) All of the above. Effective antiretroviral therapies for HIV-infected persons means a delayed progression to AIDS. Therefore, AIDS incidence is not a time-sensitive indicator of HIV incidence patterns. This should be kept in mind when relying on the baseline incidence rate of 19.5 cases of AIDS per 100,000 and the target rate of 1.0 new case per 100,000 persons. Data are estimated; adjusted for delays in reporting.*

13-2.   (b) 25 percent improvement. In 1998, an estimated 17,847 AIDS cases were diagnosed among men having sex with men. This was a decline from previous years and attributed to prevention efforts such as effective antiretroviral therapies. The target is 13,385 new cases per year. Even with the decline, males having sex with males remains a population at risk for HIV infection. Prevention efforts must promote behavioral risk reduction especially among at-risk youth.

13-3.   (b) 25 percent improvement. In 1998, an estimated 12,099 new cases were diagnosed among thirteen years and older males (8,432) and females (3,667) who injected drugs. This was a decline from previous years and attributed to prevention efforts such as effective antiretroviral therapies. Still, the target is to reduce to 9,075 new cases each year in this at-risk group. Measures should include: preventing the start of the drug-injecting practice, reaching out to this at-risk group through treatment, encouraging safer injecting practices, and promoting safer sexual behavior in this at-risk group.

13-4.   (c) Prevention programs should focus on reaching only those persons who identify themselves as either homosexual or bisexual. This is incorrect because prevention should also focus on those not identifying themselves as either homosexual or bisexual. Besides this, the programming should be directed at both adolescent and adult males as well as those who are or are not HIV infected. Certain racial and ethnic groups, re-

---

*Ages adjusted to the year 2000 standard population.

gardless of whether individuals practice same-gender sex or inject drugs, are at greater risk for AIDS. This is because their proportional share of total AIDS cases exceeds their representation in the overall U.S. population.

13-5.   (d) All of the above are true. Recent advances in HIV treatment have slowed the progression of HIV disease for infected persons on treatment and have contributed to a decline in AIDS incidence. These advances in treatment have diminished the ability of AIDS surveillance data to represent trends in HIV incidence or to represent the impact of the epidemic on the health care system. Now that HIV case surveillance has been implemented nationwide, the Centers for Disease Control and Prevention (CDC) will be able to report baseline data and progress toward the objective of "reducing the annual incidence of HIV infection."

13-6.   (c) 50 percent. Although data pertaining to sexually active adult males are developmental, as of 1995, 23 percent of sexually active adult females aged eighteen to forty-four years reported using condoms and the target for improvement is 50 percent. Correct use of latex condoms is highly effective in preventing HIV transmission and offer a high level protection if one of the partners is HIV infected.

13-7.   (a) Serostatus is the result of a blood test for the antibodies, that the immune system creates to fight specific diseases. Seronegative indicates that a person's blood lacks antibodies, whereas seropostive indicates the presence of antibodies to infections, such as HIV.

13-8.   (c) 58 percent. The target is for 70 percent of substance abuse treatment facilities offering HIV/AIDS education, counseling, and support. This would represent an improvement of 12 percent.

13-9.   (d) All of the above are true. The significance is that incarcerated persons represent a particular high-risk population for HIV infection, yet unlike other high risk groups (homeless, runaway youth, mentally ill) their confinement makes them easier to reach.

13-10. (a) All state prison systems are required to provide HIV testing to all inmates before discharge. This is incorrect. Actually it is the federal prison and not the state prison system that is required to perform testing. This objective focuses on the state prison systems' potential for providing access to treatment and care for persons infected with HIV.

13-11. (c) 55 percent. The target is to increase the proportion of adults aged twenty-five to forty-four years with TB being tested for HIV to 85 percent. Testing is important. There is a rapid rate of progression from infection with TB bacteria to active TB disease among HIV-positive persons. Coinfection with both TB and HIV is estimated to be as high as 25 percent. The symptoms of TB might mask the symptoms of HIV-related diseases and AIDS, thus delaying early detection and necessary care.

13-12. (d) All of the above are correct. Considering that a person with one STD is at risk for having another, it makes sense that a good opportunity to screen for STDs or make available the hepatitis B vaccine would be at sites offering HIV counseling and testing. This would allow health care providers to reach high-risk persons who might not otherwise seek STD screening or immunization services.

13-13. (a) HAART. HAART stands for highly active antiretroviral therapy and represents an aggressive anti-HIV treatment, usually including a combination of drugs called protease inhibitors and reverse transcriptase inhibitors whose purpose is to reduce viral load infection to undetectable levels. A pandemic is an epidemic over a large area or country. CD4+ cells are t-lymphocytes (T cells) that perform a disease-fighting function. Universal infection control precautions are guidelines and procedures to protect health care workers from exposure to infection from blood and other body fluids.

13-14. (d) All of the above are correct. Between 1996 and 1997 there was a 44 percent decline in deaths attributed to HIV infection, which coincides with the advent of new combination drug therapies for this disease. Therapies such as HAART appear to help delay HIV infection progression.

13-15. (d) All of the above. For the HIV-infected person to benefit from treatment advances, HIV counseling and testing programs must facilitate an early diagnosis of HIV infection. Everyone should have equal access to appropriate care and treatment services necessary for maintaining a healthy life.

13-16. (a) From 1996 through 1998, there has been a steady increase in deaths from AIDS. This is incorrect because there has been a steady decline in deaths from AIDS during this time period. All of the remaining responses are correct.

13-17. (b) The United States has adopted a national policy of universal HIV testing with patient notification as a routine component of prenatal care. Although the Institute of Medicine has recommended guidelines for such a national prenatal health care policy, it will not be pursued until all states extend their surveillance systems to include HIV.

Focus Area 14

14-1. (c) Pertussis. Although this disease will be reduced among children due to increasing vaccination coverage it will not be eliminated because the pathogen circulates among older-age persons and the present vaccine is not 100 percent effective.

14-2. (d) All of the above. A large majority of hepatitis B infections in infants and children can be prevented through screenings and vaccination. This objective has targeted a 76 percent reduction in such infections—from 1,682 to 400 per year.

14-3. (a) Adults forty years and older. This is not a high-risk group for hepatitis although its annual incidence rate of 15 per 100,000 has been targeted for reduction to 3.8 per 100,000 persons. For the high-risk groups, a 75 percent reduction in cases is targeted. For one other high-risk group, heterosexually active adults, a 92 percent reduction in cases is targeted.

14-4. (b) 34 percent. The target is reducing new cases of bacterial meningitis in children ages one through twenty-three months from 13 to 8.6 per 100,000. This age group has a higher rate of meningitis than do older children. Vaccines for bacterial meningitis are in various stages of development.

14-5. (b) Isolated from a normally sterile site such as blood, cerebrospinal fluid, or pleural fluid. A hospital-acquired infection occurs as a result of medical treatment while in the hospital. A distant infection spreads from one anatomic site to another site in the body. A vectorborne disease is transmitted to humans by arthropods. Invasive pneumococcal infections can be reduced in two ways. First, the proportion of invasive pneumococcal infections due to drug-resistant strains can be lowered through judicious prescribing of antibiotics. Second, decreasing invasive pneumococcal infections in general can be achieved through the development of effective vaccines.

14-6.   (a) Children. Children have the highest rate of hepatitis A and are a primary source for new infections in the community. A vaccination strategy is under development designed to produce high levels of immunity in children.

14-7.   (c) College students have recently become a high-risk group for certain kinds of meningococcal disease. There are at least three strains or kinds of meningococcal disease: B, C, and Y. A vaccine is available for B, but it is not highly effective with young children, nor does it have long duration in persons of any age. Currently, new vaccines are being developed to address high-risk groups such as college students.

14-8.   (c) 44 percent. As of 1992 to 1996, the baseline was 17.4 new cases of Lyme disease per 100,000 persons and the target is a reduction to 9.7 new cases per 100,000 persons in endemic states. It is important to reduce Lyme disease cases because delayed diagnosis and treatment can result in health complications costing between $2,228 to $6,724 per patient in the first year.

14-9.   (d) All of the above are correct. Hepatitis C virus is the most common chronic bloodborne viral infection in the United States and is usually transmitted through large or repeated percutaneous exposures to blood. Affecting persons of all ages, most new cases occur in twenty to thirty-nine year olds with the highest proportion among whites. However, the highest rates of new cases are among other nonwhite racial and ethnic groups.

14-10.   (a) Counseling to prevent further disease transmission. Although the annual number of new cases of hepatitis C has been in decline, those with the disease are chronically infected and able to transmit the disease to others. The infected person requires counseling about his or her chronic infected state and how to minimize health complications from the disease. Although there is no vaccine either to prevent or to cure hepatitis C, antiviral medications have some effectiveness in treating the infection. Because the disease can cause complications in the liver (and not the kidneys), the infected person should be vaccinated against other strains of hepatitis to prevent additional liver damage.

14-11. (a) 1 new case per 100,000 population. As of 1998, the base line rate was 6.8 new cases per 100,000. Tuberculosis (TB) rates increased in the early 1990s, then decreased in the latter part of the decade. However, there have been outbreaks. There is a concern about antibiotic-resistant strains of TB. In order to reach this objective, improved testing laboratories, strengthened surveillance systems, and intensified therapy compliance programs are needed.

14-12. (c) 74 percent. The targeted improvement is 90 percent. Completion of curative therapy within twelve months is the main goal of TB control programs. Incompletion means patient relapse into illness and becoming contagious again. Given the reality of drug-resistant TB, it might be necessary for some patients to be placed on special drug regimens requiring longer than twelve months of treatment.

14-13. (d) 85 percent. As of 1997, the baseline was 62 percent of tuberculosis contacts and other high-risk persons who started and completed treatment for latent TB infection. Latent infection refers to the state of being infected with the organism *Mycobacterium tuberculosis* without showing signs or symptoms of active TB disease. Increasing the proportion to 85 percent represents a 27 percent improvement.

14-14. (b) About twenty-one days. In 1996, it required about twenty-one days for a laboratory to confirm and report 75 percent of TB cases. The target is for a reduction to two days, which represents a 90 percent reduction in time for testing results. Presently, there is commercial technology capable of detecting TB bacilli within forty-eight hours of receipt, but there are considerations related to the laboratory testing (i.e., sensitivity, costs, quality control, and qualified personnel) that must be addressed before widespread application to public health laboratories is undertaken.

14-15. (d) All of the above are correct. An example of a recommended preventive service for international travelers would be identifying risk areas for malaria and receiving an antimalarial prophylaxis medication.

14-16. (b) It is harmful to adult persons carrying the germ. This is incorrect because it is generally harmless to the adult (e.g., a pregnant woman) who carries the bacterium. Group B streptococcus disease is considered an early onset disease because if transmitted to the newborn, the onset of illness usually takes place within seven days of age.

14-17. (b) *H. pylori* bacteria. Peptic ulcer disease affects up to 25 million persons in the United States and is responsible for about 6,500 annual deaths. Although first believed to be caused by stress, spicy foods, and excess stomach acid, it is now known that at least 90 percent of cases are due to *H. pylori* bacterial infection. Peptic ulcers can be successfully treated though antibiotic regimens.

14-18. (a) 19 percent. During 1996-1997, the two-year average number of antibiotics courses for otitis media ear infections was 108 per 100 children under age five. The two-year average target is a reduction to 88 antibiotic courses per 100 children under five. Reduction is possible by recognizing that certain cases of otitis media do not require antibiotic treatment, and through the use of the recently CDC-approved pneumococcal conjugate vaccine.

14-19. (c) 50 percent. The common cold does not require antibiotic treatment; this should be accepted by both caregivers and patients.

14-20. (d) All of the above are correct. The numbers are correct on persons admitted annually to the hospital, those acquiring an infection in this setting, and how many of these infections are in intensive care patients. Hospital-acquired infections have increased by 36 percent over the past twenty years, probably because a higher number of older (and sicker) patients are being admitted to intensive care units, and these units depend on specialized care equipment, the operation and maintenance of which present challenges to insuring infection control.

14-21. (a) 20 percent. As of 1995, 150 daily doses of antimicrobials were administered per 1,000 patient days in the intensive care unit. The target is to reduce this to 120 daily doses per 1,000 patient days. It is critical to address this matter. Excessive or inappropriate use of antimicrobials, which occurs more so in

intensive care units, encourages antimicrobial-resistant pathogens. These pathogens would then become virtually untreatable. Not only would the health of intensive care patients be compromised, antimicrobial resistance could spread into the community and cause a public health disaster.

14-22. (d) 90 percent. Maintenance of at least 90 percent vaccination coverage in the early childhood population is the best way to prevent the spread of vaccine-preventable childhood diseases and to control these diseases in adulthood (e.g., measles, mumps, rubella, tetanus, diphtheria, pertussis, *Haemophilus influenzae* type b, polio, varicella, and hepatitis B).

14-23. (d) 95 percent. Actually, it is more than 95 percent. This was the target for 2000 and it was successfully achieved. Therefore, efforts are under way to maintain this high percentage.

14-24. (a) Polio. Because of successful worldwide eradication efforts, it is likely that the polio vaccine will not be recommended for children by 2010. Even so, vaccination records that include polio inoculation will still be monitored.

14-25. (a) 6 percent. The target is for 90 percent of private providers to assess their child patients' vaccination coverage. About 66 percent of public providers assess this coverage and their target is also 90 percent. State immunization programs are working with private providers on increasing these kinds of assessments. Also, managed care plans are requiring providers to collect these data.

14-26. (b) 32 percent. About one-third of children under age six participate in a population-based immunization registry, and the target for this age group is an increase to 95 percent. The population-based immunization registry will be a cornerstone of the nation's immunization system by 2010. The registry protects confidential information, enrolls children at birth, allows providers access to vaccination histories, recommends needed vaccinations, notifies when vaccinations are due, profiles the region in terms of coverage, and produces individual records of coverage.

14-27. (d) 90 percent. This is the same target of immunization coverage for children. As of 1997, baseline vaccination coverages for adolescents were hepatitis B 48 percent; measles, mumps, and rubella, 89 percent; DPT, 93 percent; and varicella, 45 percent. Considering that 79 percent of children and adolescents visit a health care provider annually, the physician and other health care professionals are in a strategic position to review and ensure adequate vaccination coverage.

14-28. (c) 71 percent. Persons working in public safety positions who have exposure to blood or body fluids are considered a high-risk group for hepatitis B. The target is for 98 percent of these workers to be vaccinated for hepatitis B.

14-29. (d) 90 percent. Again, this percentage of coverage is consistent with vaccination targets for children and adolescents. Vaccination is an effective strategy to reduce illness and deaths due to pneumococcal disease and influenza. However, current levels of coverage among adults vary widely according age, risk, and racial and ethnic groups.*

14-30. (d) All of the above. The target is total elimination of vaccine-associated paralytic polio by using only the intravenous polio vaccine. The target is a 50 percent reduction in pertussis vaccine-related seizures, especially febrile seizures, through newly developed pertussis vaccines.

14-31. (d) A majority of adverse events show adequate evidence to determine if the vaccine was the cause of the event. The CDC, in conjunction with HMOs, has linked existing databases of some 6 million medical records to study vaccine safety, conduct surveillance of adverse reactions, conduct trials, evaluate vaccine economics, and assess vaccine coverage. The target is to have 13 million records comprising these databases.

---

*Ages adjusted to the year 2000 standard population.

Chapter 8

Investigations

INVESTIGATIVE METHOD

Recall the definition of epidemiology: the study of the occurrence and distribution, cause and control, and treatment and prevention of disease and other morbid conditions. The cause and control of diseases are within the purview of an epidemiological **investigation,** which is a professional response to a greater-than-expected occurrence of disease, known as an **outbreak** or **epidemic.** Epidemiologists tend to refer to infectious disease outbreaks rather than noninfectious or chronic disease epidemics. In this way, we can be more specific in the type of outbreak we are examining, for example, if it occurs within a health care setting, it is called a **nosocomial** disease outbreak. The investigation has a twofold purpose: (1) to determine the cause of the outbreak and, in doing so, (2) to control the outbreak. By fulfilling this purpose, epidemiologists can help prevent further occurrence of the disease or morbid condition.

The concept of "disease detective" emerges clearly during an epidemiological investigation of disease and other morbid conditions. A dramatic example is the legionellosis outbreak of 1976. In Philadelphia, over 100 attendees of the American Legion National Convention were struck down by this virulent respiratory disease. To solve the mystery, disease detectives had to answer a number of questions: Why were the cases primarily middle-age to late-age males? Why were family members spared from this severe infection? Why were most but not all cases associated with lodging at the Bellevue-Stratford Hotel? After months of investigative methodology, the epidemiologists were able to determine the reservoir for legionellosis bacteria was the air conditioning system of the hotel housing the legionnaires, most of whom were adult males. Other hotel visitors, some of whom merely walked by the revolving front door, were also infected. Since it was a common source and not a propagated exposure, the cases did not infect their family members (Stolley and Lasky, 1995).

Before describing an epidemiological investigation, it is worth noting that many diseases do not cooperate with a step-by-step procedure of inquiry. Take syphilis, for example, a bacterial disease primarily transmitted through close physical contact. It became a matter of concern and study in fifteenth-century Europe. Recall that Fracastoro used case studies on syphilis to develop the germ theory (see Chapter 2). This was an amazing accomplishment given the mysterious aspects of this disease. It has a complicated and extended disease process—three clinical stages segmented by two incubation periods. Fracastoro and later epidemiological investigators remarked about the inconsistency of disease manifestation. At least one-quarter of cases do not display characteristic signs and symptoms. Investigators were also stymied by the origin of syphilis, asking: Why had so many cases of this virulent bacterial disease appeared during the 1600s? Some posit that Columbus's contact with Caribbean cultures during the latter 1400s was the source of exposure with subsequent incidence rates of syphilis increasing steadily during following centuries. Other investigators collected evidence and asserted that any culture with a history of **yaws,** a bacterial infection similar to syphilis but requiring venereal contact, could have been the source of this disease. Hence, the early "globalization" efforts of the fifteenth and sixteenth centuries exposed uninfected populations to source populations of the disease (Cartright and Biddiss, 2000).

Many of the infectious diseases requiring a mosquito vector for transmission have baffled epidemiological investigators over the years as well. Malaria is a good example. Each year, this protozoan disease is responsible for more deaths than any other disease, condition, or event, including war. Decade after decade investigators searched, followed the trail of the disease, weighed clues as to its origin, and experimented with possible treatments and cures. It was not until 1902 that the *Anopheles* mosquito was ascertained as the vector.

In another more current example, recent cases of arbovirus (arthropod-borne disease) infection were reported in metropolitan areas of the northeastern United States. During summer 1999, the outbreak first struck bird flocks in New York State. Human cases followed. First considered an "alien virus" of unknown or undetermined origin, it was later assumed to be viral encephalitis. By midautumn of that year, epidemiologists deduced that it was West Nile virus (Moore, 2001). Since then, surveillance efforts to identify West Nile virus-infected birds and to alert the public have intensified in northeast and mid-Atlantic states.

The steps for conducting an investigation of a foodborne outbreak, for example, have been presented by Lilienfeld and Stolley (1994). In order to identify the disease being investigated, epidemiologists must be able to

1. define what a case is;
2. ascertain cases;
3. determine a common event among cases;
4. define the population present at the common event;
5. develop a questionnaire to assess consumption of food items at the common event;
6. administer the questionnaire to all those present at the common event;
7. calculate food-specific attack rates to determine which food item was contaminated;
8. investigate the preparation of the contaminated food item, including medical examination of all food handlers involved in such preparation; and
9. take appropriate public health action to stop the possibility of such outbreaks in the future (e.g., slaughtering of infected flocks producing contaminated eggs).

PROBLEM SOLVING DURING INFECTIOUS DISEASE OUTBREAKS

Epidemiologists, when investigating an infectious disease outbreak, undertake an investigation that typically follows five problem-solving steps. Those steps are:

1. *Determine the problem.* The problem is determined by establishing the existence of an outbreak. While monitoring surveillance data, epidemiologists in local public health departments respond to reported cases of disease. Cases are defined through

diagnosis. A specific biological agent is presumed responsible for infectious disease cases, and investigators conjecture the necessary and sufficiency factors to the disease occurrence. Epidemiologists confer with medical and other health professionals involved in diagnosis, clinical testing, laboratory studies, and environmental health measurements. Criteria for defining individual cases are established. Cases are then placed in categories of confirmed, probable, suspected, and missing. Sometimes, this step in an investigation is referred to as performing **case studies,** because the epidemiologists examine, verify, and classify cases of disease during an outbreak.

2. *Study the problem.* In an investigation, epidemiologists examine and describe the distribution of cases in terms of person, place, and time characteristics. Regarding person characteristics, the distribution of cases is studied according to demographic features such as age, gender, ethnicity, and occupation. Interactions with family and associates are also considered. Regarding place characteristics, epidemiologists like to use spot mapping techniques within which the geographic location of each case is recorded as a dot on a map. Place characteristics, such as climate and typography, work and school sites, and proximity to the suspected source of the etiological agent, are also considered. Regarding time characteristics, **secular** (or long-term) and cyclical trends in disease distribution are considered. The epidemiologists create an epidemic curve. Usually, the public is alerted at this stage, and the professional community is told about the seriousness of the outbreak and of the ongoing investigation.

3. *Suggest a solution to the problem.* In other words, epidemiologists generate a **hypothesis** and set forth a tentative and testable explanation about how the outbreak happened.

4. *Test the solution.* Needed data to test the hypothesis are gathered and analyzed. Attack rates and relative risk ratios are calculated. Data can also be inserted into two-by-two epidemiological tables to determine relationships between exposure to agents or risk factors and the occurrence of disease cases. Risks are determined. It is through these calculations that epidemiologists attempt to figure out the etiological source and the means of agent transmission (e.g., vehicles or vectors) to the infected cases.

5. *Evaluate the solution.* This means making a decision regarding how the outbreak happened. During decision making, the investigators are careful to minimize **bias,** which is the error caused by systematically favoring some findings over others. The decision is not based on the calculations in step four only, but is also based on passing the findings through the principle of causality. Once assured of bias minimization, epidemiologists present recommendations about preventing further outbreaks. In these recommendations, epidemiologists identify susceptible groups in the population who are at risk of exposure to the agent, given specified place and time characteristics.

$$\text{Attack rate} = \frac{\#\,\text{cases in specified time}}{\text{persons exposed to agent}} \times 10^{(n)}$$

$$\text{Relative risk} = \frac{\text{incidence rate of exposed}}{\text{incidence rate of nonexposed}}$$

The chief type of disease outbreak that launches epidemiological investigations is foodborne disease. It is for this reason that an examination of foodborne diseases is covered in the next section (Timmreck, 1998).

Foodborne Diseases

A disease that relies on food as a vehicle of transmission is a **foodborne disease.** There are three major kinds of foodborne diseases: poisoning, infection, and contamination or intoxication. Each is generally characterized by **gastroenteritis,** an inflammation of the gastrointestinal tract, with symptoms such as nausea, vomiting, and anorexia, and can be accompanied by fever, abdominal discomfort, and diarrhea. Some foodborne diseases can affect the nervous and excretory systems as well. This is probably due to the presence of an enterotoxin, the poisonous products from bacteria infesting the gastrointestinal tract. Foodborne diseases are primarily treated through fluid replacement and supportive care. Foodborne diseases caused by toxic chemical agents from the environment would be more likely to affect liver, kidneys, and the nervous system rather than produce gastrointestinal discomfort (Stone et al., 1996).

Food infection occurs when a host consumes a microorganism and then proceeds through a disease process as a result of the agent incubating and growing in number inside. Common infectious bacteria capable of causing food infection are salmonella, campyloacter, shigella, and listeria. In fact, *Salmonella typhi* and campylobacter, which have an affinity for meat and dairy products, are believed responsible for 80 percent of all reported cases of foodborne disease. Common viral infections include hepatitis A, and Norwalk virus (and other agents causing gastroenteritis). Protozoan infections include giardiasis and amoebic dysentery, while metazoan infections include trichinosis.

Food poisoning occurs when a host consumes a microorganism and then proceeds through a disease process as a result of toxins or poisons produced by the agent. Common infectious bacteria capable of causing food poisoning are clostridium, staphylococcus, and *Escherichia coli* (*E. coli*).

Food contamination (or intoxication) occurs when a host consumes a hazardous substance and then proceeds through a disease process as a result of the exposure. It should be mentioned that food contamination could also refer to presence of a biological agent in or on food. For the purpose of clarity, though, this text will regard the contaminant as a chemical agent. Pesticides, herbicides, and fungicides contain hazardous substances such as chlorinated hydrocarbons, organophosphates, and mercury. Less likely would be contamination during food preparation from cookware and vessels (e.g., cadmium or lead). Of course, there are a range of food additives and preservatives considered harmless when consumed on a short-term bases, yet on a long-term basis are suspected in causing a cumulative toxic effect. Some food sources might contain naturally occurring toxic substances and might be consumed accidentally (e.g., mushrooms, fish, and shellfish).

When comparing the three kinds of foodborne diseases, it is worth noting that poisonings generally have shorter incubation periods and clinical stages than do food infections and contaminations. Transmission of foodborne diseases from source to food occurs at one or more points during the **food cycle**: production, processing, or preparation.

During food production there are several opportunities for agent exposure and infestation. Shigella is transmitted directly from its environmental source, through the consumption of sewage-contaminated water. It can also be transmitted indirectly when an infected person contaminates food or water during its preparation. Listeria bacteria may pose a risk for illness if soil and manure used as fertilizers contaminate vegetables. Hepatitis A can infect shellfish prior to processing.

Of course, hazardous substances can contaminate agricultural crops as well as livestock. During processing, bacteria such as salmonella, campylobacter, and *E. coli* reside in animal intestines and can infect the meat, especially poultry and beef products if not properly washed and processed. These bacteria are also found in unpasteurized dairy products.

During preparation, clostridium might be inadvertently bottled or canned and allowed to produce its toxin. Within anaerobic conditions, clostridium botulism can produce a neurotoxin that results in a high rate of mortality among its consumers. Food handlers might act as carriers of staphylococcus, perhaps through pustules on their hands or face, and inadvertently transmit the bacteria to food. Sometimes food preparers **cross-contaminate,** which is the indirect transmission of a biological agent to a host via one fomite to another. An example would be neglecting to clean a previously used cutting board and thus exposing other food to agents residing on the fomite.

INVESTIGATING NONINFECTIOUS DISEASE EPIDEMICS

Similar to the preceding section on infectious disease investigation, epidemiologists follow the same five steps of problem solving to determine the cause of noninfectious disease epidemics and make attempts to control them.

1. *Determine the problem.* In an investigation the problem is determined by establishing the existence of an epidemic. Relying on surveillance data, epidemiologists in local public health departments respond to reported cases of disease and define cases through diagnosis. Physical, chemical, behavioral, social, or genetic agents are presumed responsible for noninfectious disease cases. Investigators conjecture the necessary and sufficiency factors to the disease occurrence. Epidemiologists work with

medical and other health promotion and disease professionals involved in diagnosis, clinical testing, laboratory studies, and environmental health measurements to establish criteria for defining individual cases. Cases are categorized in terms of confirmed, probable, suspected, and missing. As we have learned, this step in an investigation involves case studies which are especially preferred in the investigation of a noninfectious disease epidemic.

2. *Study the problem.* In such investigations, epidemiologists examine and describe the distribution of cases in terms of person, place, and time characteristics. Regarding person characteristics, the distribution of cases is studied according to demographic features such as age, gender, ethnicity, and occupation. Interactions with family and associates are also considered. Regarding place characteristics, epidemiologists like to use spot mapping techniques. Place characteristics such as climate and typography, work and school sites, and proximity to suspect source of etiological agent are considered. Place characteristics probably play more of a role in noninfectious disease epidemics than in infectious disease outbreaks. Regarding time characteristics, secular (or long-term) and cyclic trends in disease distribution are considered. An epidemic curve is created. Usually at this step of the investigation epidemiologists alert the public and the professional community to the seriousness of the epidemic and the ongoing investigation.

3. *Suggest a solution to the problem.* Epidemiologists generate a hypothesis about what has caused the epidemic and set forth a tentative and testable explanation.

4. *Test the solution.* Needed data to test the hypothesis are gathered and analyzed. Attack rates and ratios are calculated. Data are inserted into two-by-two epidemiological tables; risks are determined. It is through these calculations that epidemiologists attempt to figure out the etiological source and the means of host exposure, either point or nonpoint, to the suspected agent.

5. *Evaluate the solution.* This means making a decision regarding how the epidemic happened. During decision making, the investigators are careful to minimize bias, which is the error caused by systematically favoring some findings over others. The decision is not based on the calculations in step four only, but is also

based on passing the findings through the principle of causality. Once assured of bias minimization, recommendations about preventing further epidemics are presented. In these recommendations, epidemiologists identify susceptible groups in the population who are at risk of exposure to the agent given specified place and time characteristics.

Investigating Injuries in High School and College Sports, 1982-1997

Investigators have been able to draw the connection between certain kinds of sports-related practices and the incidence of athlete injury. The results of these investigations have prompted recommendations and regulations regarding game rules. For example, "spearing" in football has been prohibited. In swimming, there are specifications regarding water depth and the racing dive. These regulations are based on epidemiological data on deaths and catastrophic injuries, and are meant to promote the safety of young athletes. There are other examples: anchoring movable soccer goals to prevent tipping, improving preparation of high school wrestling coaches (i.e., adhering to athlete weight management guidelines), prohibiting pushing or checking from behind in ice hockey, wearing protective helmets for baseball batting-practice pitchers, and instituting barriers around the discus circle in track and field (Cantu and Mueler, 1999, pp. 1-6).

This relates to Healthy People 2010 Objective 15-31: *(developmental) Increase in the proportion of public and private schools that require use of appropriate head, face, eye, and mouth protection for students participating in school-sponsored physical activities* (Healthy People 2010, 2000, 15-34). (See Chapter 8 activities for more information.)

Let us examine an example of a noninfectious condition investigation that involved the carbon monoxide poisoning deaths of several campers in Georgia. **Carbon monoxide** (CO) is a colorless, odorless gas produced as a result of incomplete burning of carbon-containing fuels. Carbon monoxide reduces the blood's ability to carry oxygen, and as an agent, causes the highest number of fatal, unintentional poisonings in the nation. The highest mortality incidence involving CO occurs within homes or automobiles during the cold-weather months. In 1999, however, two deadly CO outbreaks occurred outdoors among six campers in Georgia. In one outbreak, on March 14, a man with three children and a pet dog were discovered dead in their zipped-up ten-by-fourteen-feet two-room tent. A propane gas stove was burning inside the tent upon discovery. The investigators deduced that the stove was brought into the tent to provide warmth. A postmortem examination revealed high levels of CO in each victim's bloodstream. The following week, at a different campsite, a man and his young son were found dead in practically the same circumstances, although this time a charcoal-burning grill had been brought inside their zipped-up tent to provide warmth. Again, CO concentrations in the bloodstream were high, indicating lethal CO poisoning (VDH, 1999).

Investigating Childhood Suffocation

Investigations of childhood (fourteen years and younger) suffocation reveal that a majority occur in the home. Most fatal incidents occur in children four years and younger with a chief explanation being the ingestion of toys or toy parts. Many cases of sudden infant death syndrome (SIDS) are found in potentially suffocating environments, such as when infants are placed in unsafe sleeping positions (e.g., on their stomachs, with their noses and mouths covered by soft bedding)(Willinger, Hoffman, and Hartford, 1994).

This relates to Healthy People 2010 Objective 16: *Reduction in deaths from sudden infant death syndrome* (Healthy People 2010, 2000, 16-16). (See Chapter 8 activities for more information.)

INVESTIGATING CHRONIC DISEASES

Investigating chronic diseases has the same twofold purpose of controlling the epidemic as well as preventing further occurrence. The difference lies in the nature of chronic diseases when compared to infectious diseases. Recall from Chapter 4 that chronic diseases characteristically have multiple risk factors including long latency, long disease process, and difficulty treating to the point of full recovery. Given these distinctions from infectious disease, the following problem-solving steps could be followed:

1. *Determine the problem.* This means confirming cases of chronic disease in a population through surveillance systems. The criteria for identifying individual cases should be consistent with ICD-10 codes. Incidence and prevalence rates of the chronic disease are calculated.

2. *Study the problem.* Knowing rates of occurrence, the epidemiologist tries to explain the distribution of cases through person, place, and time characteristics. For instance, risks of being diagnosed with a chronic disease might vary according to age, gender, and personal lifestyle. It is worth noting that most leading causes of death are chronic in nature and that they share similar risk factors.

3. *Suggest a solution.* Generate a hypothesis, meaning, epidemiologists set forth a tentative and testable explanation about how this epidemic of chronic disease happened.

4. *Test the solution.* Needed data to test the hypothesis are gathered and analyzed through prospective, prevalence, and retrospective epidemiological studies (studied in Chapters 9 through 12).

5. *Evaluate the solution.* Make a decision regarding the hypothesis. Validate the results of the study by minimizing bias and assessing causality. Epidemiologists also recommend disease control and future prevention measures. This involves identifying susceptible populations that are at increased risk of exposure to the risks (or agents) of chronic disease.

SUMMARY

Epidemiologists act as "disease detectives," answering crucial questions related to disease outbreaks and epidemics. An epidemiological investigation is designed to determine what caused the outbreak, how to control it, and how to prevent further occurrence. Epidemiologists follow a five-step problem-solving protocol, which can be applied to infectious and noninfectious diseases, as well as chronic and morbid conditions. Epidemiological investigations are well suited for addressing foodborne diseases such as food infection, poisoning, and contamination. Investigations can also be directed at morbid conditions such as unintentional injuries and deaths from toxic substances. Investigations can also be used to better understand chronic diseases, although these conditions pose challenges (i.e., multiple risk factors, long latency, long disease process, and difficulty in treating to the point of full recovery) to the investigative method.

REVIEW QUESTIONS

1. What is an epidemiological investigation? Can you identify and present in correct order the five problem-solving steps to conducting an investigation? Can you explain what takes place during each problem-solving step?
2. Do you know the definitions of the important terms in bold print within this chapter?
3. Can you explain how an epidemiological investigation takes place for infectious versus noninfectious diseases? For chronic diseases? Could you present an example of each kind of investigation?
4. What is a case study?
5. What is a foodborne disease? Can you identify and describe common foodborne diseases?
6. Do you know the answers to the following chapter activity questions based on objectives from Healthy People 2010 focus areas 15 and 16?

WEB SITE RESOURCES

Center of Complex Infectious Diseases
<http://www.ccid.org/>

Centers for Disease Control, Epi Info Software Program
<http://www.cdc.gov/epiinfo/>

Global Infectious Disease and Epidemiology Network
<http://www.cyinfo.com/>

REFERENCES

Cantu, R.C. and Mueler, R.O. (1999). Fatalities and catastrophic injuries in high school and college sports, 1982-1997: Lessons for improving safety. *The Physician and Sportsmedicine,* 27(8): 1-6.

Cartright, F.F. and Biddiss, M. (2000). *Disease and history.* London, England: Sutton Publishing.

Healthy People 2010 (2000). *Healthy People 2010: Objectives for improving health*. Washington, DC: Office of Disease Prevention and Health Promotion, U.S. Department of Health and Human Services.

Lilienfeld, D.E. and Stolley, P.D. (1994). *Foundations of epidemiology* (Second edition). New York: Oxford Press.

Moore, P. (2001). *Killer germs and rogue diseases of the 21st century*. London, England: Carlton Books.

Stolley, P.D. and Lasky, T. (1995). *Investigating disease patterns*. New York: Scientific American Library.

Stone, D.B., Armstrong, W.R., Macrina, D.M., and Pankau, J.W. (1996). *Introduction to epidemiology*. Madison, WI: Brown and Benchmark.

Timmreck, T.C. (1998). *An introduction to epidemiology* (Second edition). Sudbury, MA: Jones and Bartlett Publishers.

VDH (1999). *Health alert: accidental carbon monoxide deaths*. Richmond, VA: Virginia Department of Health, Office of Epidemiology.

Willinger, M., Hoffman, H.J., and Hartford, R.B. (1994). Infant sleep position and risk for sudden infant death syndrome: Report of meetings held January 13 and 14, 1994, National Institutes of Health, Bethesda, MD. *Pediatrics,* 93(5): 814-819.

Purpose: (1) to acquaint the reader with Healthy People 2010 targets for improvement and (2) present examples of epidemiology as the underlying science to health promotion and disease prevention.

Directions: Check out your knowledge of these Healthy People 2010 focus areas by taking the following tests (answers follow in a separate section).

FOCUS AREA 15:
INJURY AND VIOLENCE PREVENTION

This focus area's goal is to reduce injuries, disabilities, and deaths due to unintentional injuries and violence.

Injury Prevention

15-1. *Reduction in hospitalization for nonfatal head injuries.* If the 1998 baseline rate was 60.6 hospitalizations for nonfatal head injuries per 100,000 population, which of the following represents a targeted 26 percent reduction?
a. Five hospitalizations per 100,000 population
b. Twenty-five hospitalizations per 100,000 population
c. Forty-five hospitalizations per 100,000 population
d. Sixty-four hospitalizations per 100,000 population

15-2. *Reduction in hospitalizations for nonfatal spinal cord injuries.* Related to this objective, all of the following are correct except:
a. The physical and emotional toll associated with head and spinal cord injuries can be significant for the survivors and their families.

b. Persons with existing disabilities from head and spinal cord injuries are at lower risk for further secondary disabilities.

c. Prevention efforts should target motor vehicle crashes, falls, firearm injury, diving, and water safety.

d. Among pedalcyclists killed, most died from head injuries.

15-3. *Reduction in firearm-related deaths.* Related to this objective, which education level is associated with the highest rate of firearm-related deaths?
a. Less than high school
b. High school graduate
c. At least some college
d. Postbaccalaureate

15-4. *Reduction in the proportion of persons living in homes with firearms that are loaded and unlocked.* As of 1998, what proportion of persons lived in homes with loaded, unlocked firearms?
a. 19 percent
b. 39 percent
c. 59 percent
d. 79 percent

15-5. *Reduction in nonfatal firearm-related injuries.* Related to this objective, efforts to promote proper storage of firearms in homes can help reduce the risk of:
a. Assaultive shootings
b. Intentional self-inflicted shootings
c. Unintentional shootings
d. All of the above

15-6. *Extension of state-level child fatality review of deaths due to external causes for children aged fourteen years and under (developmental).* As of 1997, what percentage of injuries occurring to children was violent in nature?
a. 13 percent
b. 33 percent
c. 53 percent
d. 73 percent

15-7. *Reduction in nonfatal poisonings.* As of 1996, which type of poisoning had the highest rate of occurrence in the U.S. population?
   a. Assaultive
   b. Attempted homicide
   c. Intentional suicide attempt
   d. Unintentional poisoning

15-8. *Reduction in deaths caused by poisonings.* Related to this objective, all of the following are correct except:
   a. Children are at significantly greater risk from poisoning death and exposure than adults.
   b. Children are more likely to ingest potentially harmful chemicals.
   c. Persons aged four years and under accounted for nearly half of all children's deaths caused by poisoning.
   d. Approximately 90 percent of all poison exposures in children occurred outside a residence, such as at school.

15-9. *Reduction in deaths caused by suffocation.* Related to this objective, which of the following is correct?
   a. A majority of persons dying from suffocation are children.
   b. Most children dying from suffocation are over the age of four.
   c. A majority of childhood suffocations occur in the home.
   d. Sudden infant death syndrome is an unexplained phenomenon in which infants die for no apparent reason.

15-10. *Increase in the number of states and in the District of Columbia with statewide emergency department surveillance systems that collect data on external causes of injury.* As of 1998, how many states had statewide emergency department surveillance systems that collected data on external causes of injury?
   a. Two states
   b. Twelve states
   c. Twenty-two states
   d. Thirty-two states

15-11. *Increase in the number of states and the District of Columbia that collect data on external causes of injury through hospital discharge data systems.* As of 1998, how many states had collected data on external causes of injury through hospital discharge data systems?

a. Three states
b. Thirteen states
c. Twenty-three states
d. Thirty-three states

15-12. *Reduction in hospital emergency department visits caused by injuries.* Related to this objective, which of the following is correct?

a. Emergency department patient records are an important source of public health surveillance.
b. Emergency departments are well positioned to provide data on cause and severity of injuries.
c. Access to injury data collected by emergency departments can help with the development of population-based public health interventions.
d. All of the above are correct.

Unintentional Injury Prevention

15-13. *Reduction in deaths caused by unintentional injuries.* Which population has the highest rate of deaths from unintentional injuries?

a. American Indian or Alaska Native males
b. Black or African-American males
c. Hispanic males
d. White males

15-14. *Reduction in nonfatal unintentional injuries (developmental).* Related to this objective, what is an unintentional injury?

a. Fatal injury intentionally caused to one human being by another
b. A type of injury that occurs without purposeful intent
c. Actual or threatened physical or sexual violence or psychological and emotional abuse by an intimate partner
d. A characteristic that has been demonstrated statistically to be associated with a particular injury

15-15. *Reduction in deaths caused by motor vehicle crashes.* How much of a reduction is being targeted?
a. 1 percent
b. 21 percent
c. 41 percent
d. 61 percent

15-16. *Reduction in pedestrian deaths on public roads.* How much of a reduction is being targeted?
a. 10 percent
b. 30 percent
c. 50 percent
d. 70 percent

15-17. *Reduction in nonfatal injuries caused by motor vehicle crashes.* How much of a reduction is being targeted?
a. 1 percent
b. 21 percent
c. 41 percent
d. 61 percent

15-18. *Reduction in nonfatal pedestrian injuries on public roads.* How much of a reduction is being targeted?
a. 8 percent
b. 28 percent
c. 48 percent
d. 68 percent

15-19. *Increase in use of safety belts.* As of 1998, what percent of the total population used seatbelts?
a. 29 percent
b. 49 percent
c. 69 percent
d. 89 percent

15-20. *Increase in use of child restraints.* As of 1998, what percent of motor vehicle occupants ages four years and under used child restraints?
a. 32 percent
b. 52 percent
c. 72 percent
d. 92 percent

15-21. *Increase in the proportion of motorcyclists using helmets.* As of 1998, what percent of motorcyclists used helmets?
   a. 27 percent
   b. 47 percent
   c. 67 percent
   d. 87 percent

15-22. *Increase in the number of states and the District of Columbia that have adopted a graduated driver licensing model law.* Related to this objective, which of the following is correct?
   a. Graduated licensing allows a young driver to gain driving experience at incremental levels.
   b. Graduated licensing is a system for phasing in on-road driving.
   c. Graduated licensing allows beginning drivers to obtain their initial experience under lower risk conditions.
   d. All of the above are correct.

15-23. *Increase in use of helmets by bicyclists (developmental).* Bicycle helmets reduce the risk of bicycle-related head injury by how much?
   a. 25 percent
   b. 45 percent
   c. 65 percent
   d. 85 percent

15-24. *Increase in the number of states and the District of Columbia with laws requiring bicycle helmets for bicycle riders.* Which of the following is correct?
   a. There are states having bicycle helmet laws that apply to riders of all ages.
   b. Most states have helmet laws that apply to young bicyclists under age eighteen.
   c. Several localities have ordinances that require some or all bicyclists to wear helmets.
   d. All of the above are correct.

15-25. *Reduction in residential fire deaths.* Related to this objective, all of the following are correct except:
   a. Residential fires are the second leading cause of unintentional injury death among children.

b. Compared to the total population, children ages four years and under have a fire death rate more than twice the national average.

c. Children are disproportionately affected because they react more effectively to residential fires than adults.

d. Children generally sustain more severe burns at lower temperatures than adults do.

15-26. *Increase in functioning residential smoke alarms.* As of 1998, what percentage of residences had functioning smoke alarms on every floor?
a. 28 percent
b. 48 percent
c. 68 percent
d. 88 percent

15-27. *Reduction in deaths from falls.* Related to this objective, all of the following are correct except:
a. Falls have become the leading cause of injury deaths among adults ages sixty-five years and older.
b. Falls are the most common cause of injuries and hospital admissions for trauma among elderly persons.
c. For persons ages sixty-five years and older, 60 percent of fatal falls occur in public places.
d. For all ages combined, alcohol use has been implicated in 35 to 63 percent of deaths from falls.

15-28. *Reduction in hip fractures among older adults.* Related to this objective, all of the following are correct except:
a. The most serious fall-related injury is hip fracture.
b. 75 to 80 percent of all hip fractures are sustained by males.
c. Half of all elderly adults hospitalized for hip fracture cannot return home or live independently after the fracture.
d. Some factors contributing to falls are difficulties in gait and balance, disabilities, medications, as well as environmental hazards.

15-29. *Reduction in drownings.* Related to this objective, all of the following are correct except:
a. Drownings represent about half of deaths from unintentional injuries.

    b. Drowning is the second leading cause of injury-related death for persons between ages one and nineteen years.

    c. Males' drowning rates are almost two to four times greater than rates for females.

    d. African-American children are twice as likely to drown as white children.

15-30. *Reduction in hospital emergency department visits for nonfatal dog bite injuries.* Related to this objective, all of the following are correct except:

    a. Each year, at least 500,000 (and probably much higher) persons in United States are bitten by dogs.

    b. Half of all people are believed to have been bitten by a dog during their adulthood.

    c. Children are likely to be bitten in the head, face, or neck.

    d. Effective prevention strategies are needed to reduce the painful and costly burden of dog bites.

15-31. *Increase in the proportion of public and private schools that require use of appropriate head, face, eye, and mouth protection for students participating in school-sponsored physical activities (developmental).* Related to this objective, which of the following is correct?

    a. Trauma to the head, face, eyes, and mouth occurs frequently during school-sponsored physical activities.

    b. Schools with recreation and sports programs can reduce traumas by requiring students to use appropriate protective gear.

    c. To ensure injury protection in school sports, it must be accepted that most injuries are predictable and preventable.

    d. All of the above are correct.

Violence and Abuse Prevention

15-32. *Reduction in homicides.* As of 1998, which age group experienced the highest homicide rate?

    a. Persons under one year

    b. Persons aged one to nine years

    c. Persons aged ten to fourteen years

    d. Persons aged fifteen to thirty-four years

15-33. *Reduction in maltreatment and maltreatment fatalities of children.* How much of an improvement is targeted in reducing maltreatment and its fatalities in children?
a. 20 percent improvement
b. 40 percent improvement
c. 60 percent improvement
d. 80 percent improvement

15-34. *Reduction in the rate of physical assault by current or former intimate partners.* Related to this objective, which of the following is correct?
a. Both females and males experience family and intimate violence and sexual assault.
b. Perpetrators can be the same or opposite sex.
c. Male victimization of females is more common in intimate partner violence and sexual assault.
d. All of the above are correct.

15-35. *Reduction in the annual rate of rape or attempted rape.* Related to this objective, which of the following is correct?
a. Survey data on rape, attempted rape, or sexual assault tend to be accurate (e.g., 1 million U.S. females have been victims of forcible rape at some time in their lives).
b. Rape takes place in heterosexual but not homosexual relationships.
c. Rape is best defined as physically forced sexual intercourse.
d. None of the above is correct.

15-36. *Reduction in sexual assault other than rape.* Related to this objective, which of the following is correct?
a. Teen dating violence is a concern that may stem from childhood abuse or other experiences with violence.
b. Battering in teen relationships is very different from interpersonal violence (IPV) that occurs between adults.
c. The issue of teen dating violence requires national attention and prevention efforts that need to continue focusing on adolescent violence within the larger context of family violence.
d. All of the above are correct.

15-37. *Reduction in physical assaults.* Related to this objective, all of the following are correct except:
   a. Physical assault victimization among adolescents took place less as often as compared to the general population.
   b. Assaults were significantly higher among males.
   c. Assaults were higher for those with lower household incomes.
   d. As of 1998, total assaults for blacks, whites, Hispanics, and non-Hispanics were similar.

15-38. *Reduction in physical fighting among adolescents.* In 1999, what percent of adolescents in grades nine through twelve engaged in physical fighting in the previous twelve months?
   a. 16 percent
   b. 36 percent
   c. 56 percent
   d. 76 percent

15-39. *Reduction in weapon carrying by adolescents on school property.* In 1999, what percent of adolescents in grades nine through twelve carried weapons on school property during the past thirty days?
   a. 6.9 percent
   b. 26.9 percent
   c. 46.9 percent
   d. 66.9 percent

FOCUS AREA 16:
MATERNAL, INFANT, AND CHILD HEALTH

This focus area's goal is to improve the health and well-being of women, infants, children, and families.

Fetal, Infant, Child, and Adolescent Deaths

16-1. *Reduction in fetal and infant deaths.* Related to the objective, after the first month of life what is the leading cause of death in infants?

a. Respiratory distress
b. Sudden infant death syndrome
c. Birth defects
d. Disorders related to short gestation

16-2. *Reduction in the rate of child deaths.* How much of a reduction is targeted for child deaths in the one to four year age range?
a. 27 percent
b. 47 percent
c. 67 percent
d. 87 percent

16-3. *Reduction in deaths of adolescents and young adults.* Related to this objective, the leading cause of death for younger and older adolescents and young adults is:
a. Congenital disease
b. Motor vehicle crashes
c. HIV
d. Homicide

Maternal Deaths and Illnesses

16-4. *Reduction in maternal deaths.* Related to this objective, which of the following is correct?
a. A large number of maternal deaths take place each year.
b. Most maternal deaths are not preventable.
c. Ectopic pregnancy is the leading cause of maternal death in the first trimester.
d. Maternal mortality ratios are equivalent among the races.

16-5. *Reduction in maternal illness and complications due to pregnancy.* How much of a reduction is targeted in complications during labor and delivery?
a. 5 percent
b. 25 percent
c. 45 percent
d. 65 percent

Prenatal Care

16-6. *Increase in the proportion of pregnant women who receive early and adequate prenatal care.* As of 1997, what proportion of pregnant women received first trimester prenatal care?
   a. 23 percent
   b. 43 percent
   c. 63 percent
   d. 83 percent

16-7. *Increase in the proportion of pregnant women who attend a series of prepared childbirth classes (developmental).* Related to this objective, all of the following are correct except:
   a. Prepared childbirth classes should begin in the first trimester of pregnancy.
   b. Prepared childbirth classes should be conducted by a certified childbirth educator.
   c. Prepared childbirth classes help women relieve anxiety and manage pain, making delivery a more positive experience.
   d. Minimally, prepared childbirth classes comprise information on labor and birth, exercises, self-help and support, and preference for care during labor and birth.

Obstetrical Care

16-8. *Increase in the proportion of very low birth weight (VLBW) infants born at level III hospitals or subspecialty perinatal centers.* Related to this objective, what is a level III hospital?
   a. A "medical home"
   b. A birthing center
   c. A medical facility equipped to care for very small infants
   d. An emergency department

16-9. *Reduction in cesarean births among low-risk (full term, singleton, vertex presentation) women.* As of 1998, what percentage of live births by women having their first child were cesarean births?
   a. 18 percent
   b. 38 percent
   c. 58 percent
   d. 78 percent

Risk Factors

16-10. *Reduction in low birth weight (LBW) and very low birth weight (VLBW)*. Related to the objective, all of the following are correct except:
   a. Low birth weight is a risk factor to neonatal death.
   b. Neonatal death is best addressed through improvements in care rather than by reducing the rate of very low birth weight babies.
   c. Low birth weight babies are at greater risk for long-term developmental and neurologic disabilities.
   d. Maternal smoking accounts for 20 to 30 percent of all low birth weight births in the United States.

16-11. *Reduction in preterm births*. Related to this objective, which of the following is correct?
   a. About two-thirds of low birth weight babies, and 98 percent of very low birth weight babies, are born preterm.
   b. The leading cause of neonatal deaths that are not associated with birth defects is preterm birth.
   c. Infancy survival rates increase in correlation with gestational age, even among very preterm infants.
   d. All of the above are correct.

16-12. *Increase in the proportion of mothers who achieve a recommended weight gain during their pregnancies (developmental)*. What is the recommended weight gain for mothers who have a normal prepregnancy body mass index?
   a. 15 to 25 pounds
   b. 25 to 35 pounds
   c. 28 to 40 pounds
   d. 30 to 42 pounds

6-13. *Increase in the percentage of healthy full-term infants who are put down to sleep on their backs*. As of 1996, what percentage of these infants was put down to sleep properly?
   a. 15 percent
   b. 35 percent
   c. 55 percent
   d. 75 percent

Developmental Disabilities and Neural Tube Defects

16-14. *Reduction in the occurrence of developmental disabilities.* As of 1994, what percentage of children have disabilities?
a. 2 percent
b. 12 percent
c. 22 percent
d. 32 percent

16-15. *Reduction in the occurrence of spina bifida and other neural tube defects (NTDs).* How much of a reduction is targeted in the occurrence of these neural tube defects?
a. 10 percent
b. 30 percent
c. 50 percent
d. 70 percent

16-16. *Increase in the proportion of pregnancies begun with an optimum folic acid level.* Related to this objective, which of the following is correct?
a. Neural tube defects including spina bifida occur when the fetal neural tube fails to close fully during first trimester of development.
b. About half of pregnancies with neural tube defects could be prevented through adequate folic acid consumption by the mother from one month before through the first trimester of pregnancy.
c. Women of childbearing age should consume 400 µg of folic acid daily.
d. All of the above are correct.

Prenatal Substance Exposure

16-17. *Increase in abstinence from alcohol, cigarettes, and illicit drugs among pregnant women.* As of 1998, approximately what percentage of pregnant women abstained from smoking cigarettes and from drinking alcohol?
a. 26 percent
b. 46 percent
c. 66 percent
d. 86 percent

16-18. *Reduction in the occurrence of fetal alcohol syndrome (FAS) (developmental)*. Related to this objective, all of the following are correct except:

a. FAS can be consistently diagnosed at birth.

b. FAS is one of the leading preventable causes of mental retardation.

c. FAS is a leading cause of birth defects.

d. Because of the risk of FAS, a safe level of alcohol consumption during pregnancy has not been identified.

Breast-Feeding, Newborn Screening, and Service Systems

16-19. *Increase in the proportion of mothers who breast-feed their babies*. Related to this objective, all of the following are correct except:

a. Breast-feeding is recommended for the first six months of infancy.

b. Human breast milk presents the most complete form of nutrition for infants.

c. Women who test positive for HIV should not breast-feed to help prevent transmission of the virus to their infants.

d. Breast-feeding rates have decreased over the years especially in early infancy.

16-20. *Assurance of appropriate newborn bloodspot screening, follow-up testing, and referral to services (developmental)*. Which of the following is correct?

a. Newborn screening programs have only started in the past ten years with the test for phenylketonuria.

b. All states perform newborn screenings for the same birth defects and disorders.

c. Diagnostic testing should be provided to newborns who screen positive, followed by treatment and referral to appropriate interventions.

d. After screening and diagnosis for phenylketonuria and congenital hypothyroidism, all states report cases.

16-21. *Reduction in hospitalization for life-threatening sepsis among children aged four years and under with sickling hemoglobinopathies (developmental)*. Related to this objective, all of the following are correct except:

a. Sepsis is a severe bacterial infection.
b. Sickle-cell disease is an example of hemoglobinopathy.
c. Children with sickle-cell disease are more susceptible to severe bacterial infections such as meningitis, pneumonia, and septicemia.
d. Sickle-cell disease is the leading cause of death in children.

16-22. *Increase in the proportion of children with special health care needs who have access to a medical home (developmental)*. Related to this objective, what is a "medical home"?

a. Medical care for infants and children that is accessible, continuous, comprehensive, family centered, coordinated, and compassionate
b. Medical care for infants and children for which all prepaid and indemnity health insurance plans will pay for expenses
c. Medical care for infants and children that is culturally appropriate and linguistically competent
d. All of the above

16-23. *Increase in the proportion of territories and states that have service systems for children with special health care needs.* As of 1997, what portion of territories and states had such service systems that meet federal (Title V) standards?

a. 15.7 percent
b. 25.7 percent
c. 45.7 percent
d. 65.7 percent

TEST ANSWERS

Focus Area 15

15-1. (c) Forty-five hospitalizations per 100,000 population. This is determined through simple mathematical calculation in which 60.6 is multiplied by .26 and the product (15.8) is subtracted from 60.6. Aside from the "mechanics" of this item, males and blacks are two groups having higher rates of nonfatal head injuries requiring hospitalization.*

15-2. (b) Persons with existing disabilities from head and spinal cord injuries are at lower risk for further secondary disabilities. This is incorrect because persons with existing disabilities from head and spinal cord injuries are at high risk for further secondary disabilities. The 1998 baseline rate was 4.5 hospitalizations for nonfatal spinal cord injuries per 100,000 population, and the target is a reduction to 2.6 hospitalizations for nonfatal spinal cord injuries per 100,000 population.

15-3. (a) Less than high school. Among adults aged twenty-five to sixty-four years, those with less than high school experience had a 21.4 deaths per 100,000 population followed by high school graduate (17.7) and at least some college (7.0). No data are available on postbaccalaureate. This is compelling evidence of the risk reduction influence of formal education. Overall, the 1998 baseline of 11.3 firearm-related deaths per 100,000 population has a targeted reduction to 4.1 deaths per 100,000 population.

15-4. (a) 19 percent. The target is for persons living in homes with firearms that are loaded and unlocked to be reduced to 16 percent.

15-5. (d) All of the above. It is worth adding that for every firearm-related fatality reported at hospital emergency departments, there are twice as many nonfatal firearm-related injuries being treated. As of 1997, there were 24.0 nonfatal firearm-related injuries per 100,000 population and the target for improvement is 8.6 injuries per 100,000 population.

15-6. (b) 33 percent. Of the nearly 19,000 children aged nineteen years who were injury cases, under one-third were victims of

---

*Ages adjusted to the year 2000 standard population.

violence while the remaining two-thirds were victims of unintentional injury. Following California's lead, states are now
forming multidisciplinary teams of reviewers who examine
the deaths of youth, present explanations for the fatalities,
and offer recommendations for prevention.

15-7.   (d) Unintentional poisoning. With a rate of 268.0 per
100,000, unintentional poisoning ranks highest followed by
intentional suicide attempt (63.0), and assaultive or attempted
homicide (6.0). Overall, the 1997 baseline rate of nonfatal
poisonings was 348.4 per 100,000 and the targeted rate is a
reduction to 292.

15-8.   (d) Approximately 90 percent of all poison exposures in children occurred outside a residence, such as at school. This is
incorrect because 90 percent of these exposures do take place
in a residence (home or elsewhere). In trying to reduce fatal
poisonings from 6.8 deaths per 100,000 (1998) to 1.5 deaths
per 100,000, it is important to target children who are at a
noticeably higher risk.

15-9.   (c) A majority of childhood suffocations occur in the home.
All the other responses are incorrect. In 1997, of the 10,650
persons dying from suffocation, 934 were children ages fourteen years and under. Most fatal childhood suffocations occur
in children four years and younger, with a chief explanation
being the ingestion of toys or toy parts. Many cases of sudden
infant death syndrome are found in potentially suffocating
environments, such as when infants are placed in unsafe
sleeping positions (i.e., on their stomachs, with their noses
and mouths covered by soft bedding).

15-10.   (b) Twelve states. The target is for all states and the District of
Columbia to have such a system.

15-11.   (c) Twenty-three states. The target is for all states and the
District of Columbia to have such systems.

15-12.   (d) All of the above are correct. As of 1997, the baseline was
131 hospital emergency department visits per 1,000 population were caused by injury, and the target is a reduction to 126
hospital emergency department visits per 1,000 population.

15-13.   (a) American Indian or Alaskan Native males. In 1998, this
population had 83.6 deaths from unintentional injuries per
100,000. The other populations had rates in this order: black

or African-American males, 60.8; white males, 48.7; and Hispanic males, 46.2. The overall baseline rate of deaths from unintentional injuries is 35.0 deaths per 100,000 population in 1998, and the target is a reduction to 17.5 deaths per 100,000 population.

15-14. (b) A type of injury that occurs without purposeful intent. As of 1998, the baseline rate from unintentional injuries was 35.0 deaths per 100,000 population. The target rate is a reduction to 17.5 deaths per 100,000 population.

15-15. (c) 41 percent. As of 1998, the baseline rate was 15.6 deaths per 100,000 population and the target is a reduction to 9.2 deaths per 100,000. This represents about a 41 percent reduction.

15-16. (c) 50 percent. As of 1998, the baseline rate was 1.9 pedestrian deaths per 100,000 population and the target is to reduce that number to 1.0 pedestrian death per 100,000.

15-17. (b) 21 percent. As of 1998, the baseline rate was 1,181 nonfatal injuries per 100,000 population caused by motor vehicle crashes and the target is to lower that to 933 nonfatal injuries per 100,000 population.

15-18. (b) 28 percent. As of 1998, the baseline rate was twenty-six nonfatal pedestrian injuries per 100,000 population occurred on public roads and the target is nineteen nonfatal injuries per 100,000 population.

15-19. (c) 69 percent. The target is to increase to 90 percent of the total population using seatbelts.

15-20. (d) 92 percent. Although this might seem an encouraging percent, the target is for 100 percent of motor vehicle occupants aged four years and under using child restraints.

15-21. (c) 67 percent. The target is to increase to 79 percent of motorcycle operators and passengers using helmets.

15-22. (d) All of the above are correct. As of 1999, twenty-three states had a graduated driver licensing model law. The model law was drawn up by the National Committee on Uniform Traffic Laws and Ordinances and calls for a minimum of six months in the learner stage and a minimum of six months in the intermediate license stage with night driving restrictions. Applicants for intermediate and full licenses cannot have any safety belt or zero-tolerance violations and must be conviction free during the mandatory holding periods.

15-23. (d) 85 percent. Persons of all ages should wear helmets. In fact, more bicycle deaths occur with older bicyclists.

15-24. (c) Several localities have ordinances that require some or all bicyclists to wear helmets. There are no states having bicycle helmet laws applying to riders of all ages. Only fifteen states have laws applying to young bicyclists under age eighteen years.

15-25. (c) Children are disproportionately affected because they react more effectively to residential fires than adults. This is incorrect because children react less effectively than adults do. All of the other responses are correct. The target is for less than one person dying from residential fires per 100,000 population.

15-26. (d) 88 percent. The target is for 100 percent of residences having functioning smoke alarms.

15-27. (c) For persons ages sixty-five years and older, 60 percent of fatal falls occur in public places. This is incorrect since most fatal falls for older adults take place in the home. For the overall population, the target is 3.0 deaths from falls per 100,000 population.

15-28. (b) 75 to 80 percent of all hip fractures are sustained by males. This is incorrect because it is females having more hip fractures. All of the other responses are correct. The targets are to reduce hip fracture from falls by 20 percent in older adult males and 60 percent in older adult females.

15-29. (a) Drownings represent about half of deaths from unintentional injuries. This is incorrect because motor vehicle crashes actually represent that number. However, drowning is one of the major causes of death from unintentional injuries. In 1998, the baseline rate was 1.6 drownings per 100,000 population and the target is to reduce this to less than one drowning per 100,000 population.

15-30. (b) Half of all people are believed to have been bitten by a dog during their adulthood. This is incorrect because it is actually during childhood that people are more likely to have been bitten. Prevention strategies should focus on children and include persons of older ages in terms of better surveillance, identifying high-risk situations, and addressing high-risk dogs. The baseline rate in 1997 was 151.4 hospital emergency department visits per 100,000 population, which were for non-fatal dog bite injuries; the target is to reduce this to 114 visits per 100,000.

15-31. (d) All of the above are correct. Injuries from school-sponsored physical activities are preventable especially when schools require appropriate protective gear.

15-32. (d) Persons aged fifteen to thirty-four years. This group's rate was 13.0 homicides per 100,000 persons. Persons under one year of age had the next higher rate at 8.1. Homicide is the second leading cause of death in fifteen- to twenty-four-year-olds and the leading cause of death in black Americans in this age group. Overall, the baseline rate in 1998 was 6.5 homicides per 100,000 population, and the target rate is a reduction to 3.0 homicides per 100,000 population.

15-33. (a) 20 percent improvement. The baseline rate in 1998 was 12.9 child victims of maltreatment per 1,000 children under age eighteen. The target rate is 13.3 child victims of maltreatment per 1,000 children under age eighteen years.

15-34. (d) All of the above are correct. As of 1998, the baseline rate was 4.4 physical assaults per 1,000 persons aged twelve years and older by current or former intimate partners. The target rate is a reduction to 3.3 physical assaults per 1,000 persons aged twelve years and older.

15-35. (d) None of the above is correct. Survey data are on rape, attempted rape, and sexual assault are estimates of a serious problem that tends to be underreported. Rape includes psychological coercion as well as physical force. Rape occurs regardless of a person's sexual orientation. As of 1998, the baseline rate was 0.8 rapes or attempted rapes per 1,000 persons aged twelve years and older. The target is to reduce this to 0.7 rapes or attempted rapes per 1,000 persons aged twelve years and older.

15-36. (d) All of the above are correct. As of 1998, the baseline rate was 0.6 sexual assaults other than rape per 1,000 persons aged twelve years and older. The target is 0.4 sexual assaults other than rape per 1,000 persons aged twelve years and older.

15-37. (a) Physical assault victimization among adolescents took place less as often as compared to the general population. This is incorrect because physical assault takes place twice as much among adolescents compared to the overall population. All other responses are correct. As of 1998, the baseline rate was 31.1 physical assaults per 1,000 persons aged twelve years and older. The target rate is 13.6 physical assaults per 1,000 persons aged twelve years and older.

15-38. (b) 36 percent. The target is to decrease to 32 percent of adolescents in grades nine through twelve engaging in physical fighting in the previous twelve months.

15-39. (a) 6.9 percent. The target is to reduce to 4.9 percent of adolescents in grades nine through twelve carrying weapons on school property during the past thirty days.

Focus Area 16

16-1. (b) Sudden infant death syndrome. After the first month of life, SIDS is the leading cause of infant death, accounting for about one-third of all infant deaths during this period.

16-2. (b) 47 percent. The baseline death rate in 1998 was 34.6 per 100,000 children aged one to four. The target rate is 18.6 per 100,000 age-specific population.

16-3. (b) Motor vehicle crashes. The deaths of young adolescents, older adolescents, and young adults are more likely due to external causes such as unintentional injuries sustained through motor vehicle crashes. The targeted reductions in age-specific death rates are: younger adolescents (24 percent), older adolescents (44 percent), and young adults (49 percent).

16-4. (c) Ectopic pregnancy is the leading cause of maternal death in the first trimester. A total of 327 maternal deaths were reported in 1997, and even though the number is small, the significance is that a large proportion of these deaths were preventable. Also, these deaths have a significant impact on the families of the fatalities. African-American women consistently have maternal mortality ratios three to four times that of white women.

16-5. (b) 25 percent. The baseline rate in 1998 was 31.2 maternal complications during hospitalized labor and delivery per 100 deliveries. The target rate is a reduction to twenty-four complications per 100 deliveries.

16-6.   (d) 83 percent. Although a noticeable majority of pregnant women start prenatal care during the first trimester, the target is for 100 percent to do so. Prenatal care involves risk assessment, treatment for medical conditions or risk reduction, and education.

16-7.   (a) Prepared childbirth classes should begin in the first trimester of pregnancy. This is incorrect because these classes are recommended for the third trimester so that information learned will be used relatively soon after presentation.

16-8.   (c) A medical facility equipped to care for very small infants. In 1996-1997, 73 percent of very low birth weight infants were born at level III hospitals or subspecialty perinatal centers. The target is for 90 percent of these infants to be born in such facilities.

16-9.   (a) 18 percent. Cesarean births have been declining in pregnant women having either first or latter children. Still, the target is to reduce cesarean sections to 15 percent of live births in low-risk women.

16-10.   (b) Neonatal death is best addressed through improvements in care rather than by reducing the rate of very low birth weight babies. This is incorrect because some experts believe that little more in the advances of care for very low birth weight infants can be done to reduce neonatal death rates. The focus should be on preventing very low birth weight infants by addressing risk factors such as reducing maternal tobacco smoking. As of 1998, about 8 percent of babies born had low birth weight, and a little over 1 percent had very low birth weight. The target to reduce to 5 percent and less than 1 percent respectively.

16-11.   (d) All of the above are correct. As of 1998, the percent of live births that were preterm was 11.6, and the target is 7.6 percent.

16-12.   (b) 25 to 35 pounds. It is recommended that a graduated level of weight gain take place during pregnancy, one that is based on a woman's prepregnancy body mass index. A woman with normal BMI should gain 25 to 35 pounds during pregnancy.

Those with a below-normal BMI should gain 28 to 40 pounds. Overweight women should gain 15 to 25 pounds.

16-13. (b) 35 percent. The target is for 70 percent of healthy full-term infants to be put down to sleep on their backs. A nonprone sleeping position (i.e., sleeping on the side or back rather than on stomach) greatly decreases the risk of sudden infant death syndrome among healthy full-term infants

16-14. (b) 12 percent. A disability is considered a limitation in one or more functional areas, and 12 percent of persons under age eighteen years meet this criterion.

16-15. (c) 50 percent. As of 1996, there were six new cases of spina bifida or another NTD per 10,000 live births. The target is to reduce to three new cases per 10,000 live births.

16-16. (d) All of the above are correct. The baseline in 1991-1994 was 21 percent of nonpregnant women, ages fifteen to forty-four years old consumed at least 400 µg of folic acid daily. The target is for 80 percent of this population to consume adequate daily amounts of this nutrient.

16-17. (d) 86 percent. This is correct for both cigarette smoking and for alcohol drinking. Ninety percent abstained from binge drinking and 98 percent from illicit drugs. The abstinence targets are: alcohol, 94 percent; binge drinking, 100 percent; cigarette smoking, 99 percent; and illicit drugs, 100 percent.

16-18. (a) FAS can be consistently diagnosed at birth. Despite having characteristic signs and symptoms, FAS diagnosis is difficult to perform consistently because of the difficulty in evaluating the newborn's nervous system, lack of training by health care providers, and the human factor of minimizing alcohol's contribution to the evident birth defect. Estimates of FAS incidence are 0.2 to 1.0 per 1,000 live births with alcohol-related birth disorders occurring three to four times greater.

16-19. (d) Breast-feeding rates have decreased over the years especially in early infancy. This is incorrect because breast-feeding rates have actually increased over the years, particularly in early infancy. However, breast-feeding rates among women of all races decrease substantially by five to six months postpartum, even though a minimum of six months is recommended.

16-20. (c) Diagnostic testing should be provided to newborns who screen positive, followed by treatment and referral to appropriate interventions. This response is correct while the other responses are incorrect. Newborn screening (NBS) programs began as early as the 1960s. Although all states screen for phenylketonuria and hypothyroidism, screening tests vary considerably state to state. Even though screening takes place, reporting might not.

16-21. (d) Sickle-cell disease is the leading cause of death in children. This is incorrect because injuries actually are the leading cause of death in this age group. However, sickle-cell disease does place children at greater risk for some of the leading causes of death: meningitis, pneumonia, and septicemia. That is why these children are prescribed a regimen of penicillin to prevent bacterial disease, although this practice might also encourage antimicrobial-resistant bacteria.

16-22. (d) All of the above. The concept of a "medical home" is in response to the historically inappropriate, inadequate, or inefficient services available to children (and families) with special health care needs.

16-23. (a) 15.7 percent. If this is the baseline, then the target is for 100 percent of territories and states meeting Title V for service systems for children with special health care needs. These services would include health services (e.g., health education, primary care, and therapeutics), early interventive services (e.g., educational and vocational support), and transitional services (i.e., school to work).

Chapter 9

Prevalence Studies

THE NATURE OF STUDIES

An epidemiological **study** is made up of research on the distribution and cause of disease as well as interventions that treat and prevent disease. The study relies on a **research design** that lays out predetermined procedures and methods that researchers utilize during a study. A study can be descriptive, analytic, or experimental. An epidemiological study of a descriptive nature focuses on the distribution of disease and other health-affecting conditions. A **descriptive** study is concerned with and designed to describe existing distributions of variables without regard to causal or other hypotheses. Examples would include a community health survey used to determine the health status of the people in a community, or perhaps analyses of cancer registry data to measure risks. A small-scale descriptive study is seen during the investigation of an outbreak. Recall how epidemiologists study the problem—the distribution of disease cases according to person, place, and time characteristics. Other efforts at descriptive research are seen when epidemiologists conduct surveys to determine the nature of the population affected by a particular disease, also noting person, place, and time characteristics.

An epidemiological study can also be of an **analytic** nature. An analytic study focuses on risk factors and causes of disease. An analytic study can follow disease occurrence and distribution for years to determine variations in morbidity and mortality. Whereas an epidemiologist attempts to uncover the cause of an outbreak, analytic studies take a step further by trying to establish causal relationships between agents, factors, and diseases of all kinds.

Last, an epidemiological study can be of an **experimental** or **trial** nature. This kind of study determines the effectiveness of interventions meant to treat or prevent disease. It can take the shape of a **clinical**

trial, meaning the subjects are individual persons, or a **community,** meaning a group of persons. The results are applied to preventive health services. A trial usually involves the administration of a test regimen to evaluate its efficacy and safety. A trial should have treatment and control groups, although this is not always the arrangement. Random selection of subjects and random assignment to either of these groups are also normal occurrences. In a nutshell, trials focus on the intervention rather than the disease. This will be discussed more in Chapter 12.

Types of Studies

Given their general nature, an easy way to categorize epidemiological studies is according to when the disease occurs (see Figure 9.1). If studying a disease that is *presently occurring,* it is likely that a **prevalence study** will be conducted. This chapter examines the prevalence study in great detail. A prevalence study could also be called a cross-sectional study, or disease frequency survey. It examines the relationships between disease and its agents, or person, place, and time characteristics. Note that disease prevalence, rather than incidence, is normally recorded in a cross-sectional study. The temporal sequence of cause and effect cannot necessarily be determined in a cross-sectional study.

A study that begins *after* a disease has occurred is called a **retrospective study.** A primary example is the case control study, which is covered in Chapter 10. Its research design tests an etiological hypothesis about disease resulting from exposure to risk factor(s). The essential feature of the case control study is that some of the persons un-

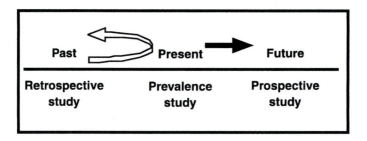

FIGURE 9.1. Type of study based on when disease occurs (*Source:* Adapted from Timmreck, 1998, p. 259)

der study have the disease and are matched in terms of person, place, and time characteristics with persons who do not have the disease.

If the study begins *before* a disease has occurred, it is known as a **prospective study,** although it can also be called a concurrent, follow-up, incidence, or longitudinal study. These variations study subjects who might have already started a disease process. A cohort study is another kind of prospective study that examines a group of persons exposed to factors who are followed over time and tracked for the incidence of disease. The cohort study will be examined in Chapter 11.

Prevalence of Food Allergy

Food allergy affects between 6 and 7 million Americans, and 90 percent of allergic reactions are caused by peanuts, tree nuts, milk, eggs, wheat, soy, fish, and shellfish. Severe allergic reactions called **anaphylaxis** (same as for bee stings, medications, and latex) cause about 30,000 visits to emergency departments each year, and kill 100 to 200 people in the United States, often within thirty minutes after onset. There is no cure. Only strict avoidance of the offending allergen will prevent a reaction. When a severe reaction does occur, the medication of choice is epinephrine (adrenaline). The medication must be administered promptly after the onset of a reaction and be followed up soon after by treatment at a medical facility (Sampson, 1998).

This relates to Healthy People 2010 Objective 17-1: *Increase in the proportion of health organizations that are linked in an integrated system that monitors and reports adverse events* (Healthy People 2010, 2000, 17-13). (See Chapter 9 activities for more information.)

WHAT IS PREVALENCE?

Prevalence was introduced in Chapter 7 when studying morbidity rates. **Prevalence** is the number of instances of a given disease or condition in a given population during a designated time period. Essentially, it refers to existing cases that started before but then extended into the reporting year, as well as any case during the time period studied. Prevalence is usually expressed as a rate and is calculated using existing cases during a specified time. If no reference is made to the time period, then epidemiologists will use the simple expression prevalence. Prevalence is similar to **incidence,** since both refer to the instance of a case, but incidence equates to new cases or new events, not existing ones. For example, diabetes is a significant health problem in the United States. According to the American Diabetes Association (1996), 10.5 million persons have been diagnosed with diabetes while 5.5 million are estimated to have the disease but remain undiagnosed. This represents prevalence. In a given year there are about 800,000 new cases of diabetes, which amounts to 2,200 per day. This represents incidence. The relationship between prevalence and incidence can best be described as the former being the existing quantity in a container, and the latter being the new contribution to the volume (Gordis, 1996).

Measuring prevalence is important to health promotion and disease prevention activity. In keeping with the example of diabetes, epidemiologists have noticed that the annual prevalence rate has been increasing each year over the past two decades, especially within Latino and Hispanic racial and ethnic groups (Flegal et al., 1991; Vinicor, 1994). Considering that diabetes ranks seventh as a leading cause of death in the adult population, and given its implications with cardiovascular disease, kidney disease, blindness, and amputation, it is critical that communities with higher prevalence be addressed through preventive health services.

Most times, prevalence rates for specific diseases and other morbid conditions are calculated during a cross-sectional or prevalence study. Epidemiologists can calculate annual, period, point, and even lifetime prevalence rates from data procured in studies.

Problem Solving Within the Prevalence Study

Prevalence studies attempt to take a snapshot of the present health status of a population. Commonly, surveys are conducted to better understand the affected population in terms of host characteristics such as age, gender, ethnicity, occupation, etc. They ascertain the population's existing characteristics as well as its experiences with disease. They are descriptive in nature because they focus on the distribution of disease and other health-affecting conditions. Although a prevalence study is not designed to infer causality, researchers can examine the data to ascertain possible risk relationships between population characteristics and the disease. One of the chief distinctions of the prevalence study is its reliance on surveys in addition to other data collection techniques. The surveys are examined for validity and reliability, and then administered preferably to representative samples of the population (Coggon, Rose, and Barker, 1997). Given the descriptive nature of prevalence research, the five problem-solving steps, similar to conducting an investigation, can also be used when performing a prevalence study.

1. *Determine the problem.* Relying on surveillance systems at the local, state, or national levels, epidemiologists attempt to ascertain a population's characteristics as well as its experiences with disease. Epidemiologists need to define the characteristic as well as disease cases in order to note existence in the population. For example, different criteria might be recognized for the disease by different professional associations. So, epidemiologists have to use a commonly accepted set of diagnostic signs and symptoms (known as ICD-10) for catagorizing diseases. Also at this step, the researchers will conjecture the necessary and sufficiency factors for disease occurrence.

2. *Study the problem.* Relying on surveillance data, epidemiologists examine existing cases and attempt to describe the distribution in terms of person, place, and time characteristics. Regarding person, the distribution of cases is studied according to demographic features such as age, gender, ethnicity, occupation, and so forth. Regarding place characteristics, questions are posed regarding the geographic location of each case and are entered as individual dots on a map. Place characteristics such as climate and typography, and work and school sites are also considered. Subjects might be queried on sociocultural place characteristics such as rating the degree of stress experienced during commuting, proximity to available preventive health services, or availability of linguistically and culturally appropriate health-related literature. Regarding time characteristics, secular and cyclic trends in disease occurrence are noted. This would be procured by asking subjects to identify when their disease cases were diagnosed and for how long they have experienced the disease process.

3. *Suggest a solution to the problem.* Epidemiologists generate a hypothesis, a tentative and testable explanation about existing cases of disease. The explanation is presented in terms of associations between one or more independent variables and a de-

pendent variable. For instance, subjects with one or more person, place, or time characteristics identified as factors are more likely to be a disease case.

4. *Test the solution.* This step requires analyzing collected data with the intent of either supporting or not supporting the hypothesis generated in step three. Given the nature of a prevalence study, statistical analysis will most likely be descriptive. Cross-sectional sampling, however, is preferred. That is, the proportions of person characteristics in the sample are similar to the proportions of person characteristics in the population. Relying on the preset definitions of a disease case as well as person, place, and time characteristics, researchers can determine the prevalence of a disease along with related population characteristics. At this step, various rates and ratios can be calculated, including incidence, prevalence, and standard morbidity or mortality ratios. Risk calculations can also be performed, such as absolute risk, attributable risk, and relative risk. Although data analysis results can be used readily to accept or not accept the hypothesis, the epidemiologist usually waits until the next step to make the final decision.

5. *Evaluate the solution.* In preparing for the decision, epidemiologists should first ensure the minimization of bias, which is error caused by systematically favoring some findings over others. A common source of error is the intentional or inadvertent misrepresentation by subjects (e.g., they might not want to report a person characteristic such as age or race, or they might not know they are a case of disease). Error can also occur on the part of the researcher who might not ask questions relevant to the study, or who might prompt subjects to respond in a desired way. Another error could be caused by subject self-selection. The study is only as good as the sample or respondents who choose to participate, and it is highly unlikely that 100 percent of the originally selected subjects will respond. Therefore, it would be prudent for researchers to further examine why some persons decide not to participate since they also represent an important source of information.

Satisfied with their steps at solving the problem, epidemiologists make a decision regarding the prevalence of the disease as well as the variables that are associated with this prevalence. Epidemiologists also recommend disease control and future prevention measures. They identify susceptible populations—persons with particular characteristics and who are likely exposed to the risk factors of the disease. Bear in mind that a prevalence study can present associations or relationships between variables but is limited in establishing causal or directional relationships between variables.

Prevalence of Mental Disorders

Mental disorders are health conditions characterized by alterations in thinking, mood, or behavior, or some combination thereof. Mental disorders spawn a host of problems that may include personal distress, impaired functioning and disability, pain, or death. These disorders can be the result of family history, genetics, or other biological, environmental, social, or behavioral factors that occur alone or in combination. They can occur across the life span and can affect persons of all racial and ethnic groups, both genders, and all educational and socioeconomic groups. In the United States, about 22 percent of persons aged eighteen to sixty-four years have a diagnosable mental disorder. Younger persons have the same prevalence. Extreme mental disorders exist in about 5 percent of the population. An estimated 25 percent of persons over sixty-five experience specific mental disorders, such as depression, anxiety, substance abuse, dementia, and Alzheimer's disease (Friedman, Katz-Levey, and Manderschied, 1996).

This relates to Healthy People 2010 Objective 18-6: *Increasing the number of persons seen in primary health care who receive mental health screening and assessment* (Healthy People 2010, 2000, 18-17). (See Chapter 9 activities for more information.)

Risk Calculations

Risk calculations rely primarily on incidence data but can also be performed in prevalence studies. This is true as long as it is understood that cases are measured during the time period of the study. Three common risk calculations used during prevalence studies follow.

- **Absolute risk:** the number of cases of disease occurring in a given time period divided by the population exposed to the risk, with its quotient multiplied by 100 (essentially, it is an incidence rate in an exposed population). Absolute risk would not be a primary risk calculation during a prevalence study because it relies on incidence data. Many times it is presented as a secondary risk calculation, providing supporting evidence of the presence of the disease in relation to specified person, place, and time characteristics. In this case, epidemiologists use the following statement: "The absolute risk for 'such and such' disease was 'so many' cases per 100,000 population occurring during that year."

- **Attributable risk:** portion of disease occurrence that appears to be explained by exposure to a particular factor. The simple calculation is to subtract the incidence rate of those not exposed from those exposed, although there are more strenuous ways to calculate attributable risk. Attributable risk is reported in a statement such as: "Of the number of cases of 'such and such' disease, a certain percentage is associated with exposure to 'such and such' factor."

- **Relative risk:** a ratio in which the incidence rate of those exposed to a factor is divided by the incidence rate of those not exposed to the same factor is called a relative risk ratio. This calculation allows epidemiologists to say: "Persons exposed to 'such and such' factor are 'so many times more (or less) likely' to develop 'such and such' disease." If the resulting quotient is equal to one, then the risk from exposure is the same as the risk of nonexposure. A quotient greater than one means the risk of disease is that much greater for those exposed. It is customary for relative risk (and its estimate, odds ratio, which is studied in Chapter 10) to be subjected to a nonparametric statistical test called a chi square. This would provide more support that the calculated risk was due to the factor, and not the probability of chance (Stone et al., 1996).

Descriptive Statistics

Think of a **descriptive statistic** as a numerical value resulting from a calculation that represents a person, place, or time characteristic. Common descriptive statistics are frequency and correlation. Descriptive statistics differ from inferential statistics in that the former represents the group whereas the latter represents the population. Another distinction rests on the four levels of measurement: nominal, ordinal, interval, and ratio. Descriptive statistics are derived from nominally and ordinally measured characteristics. Inferential statistics rely on interval and ratio levels of measurement.

In the following example (see Table 9.1), the variable of gender is measured nominally, that is, the subject is either female or male. There is no order as to how these variable levels are scored. On the other hand, physical activity appears to be measured at the ordinal level, and there is increasing value in scoring from not active through ≥3 days weekly. Therefore, the descriptive statistic of frequency has been calculated and presented in percentage format.

The table of results from the National College Health Risk Behavior Survey does not present clear examples of interval and ratio measurement levels. Had the researchers posed the following item, it would be an interval measurement:

> If you have used alcohol, when did this take place?
> a. Past 30 days
> b. Past 31 to 60 days
> c. Past 61 to 90 days
> d. Past 91 to 120 days

The possible responses to this question could be scored not only in order but with an equal interval (30 days) between the values. Therefore, it would be scored on the interval measurement level. If the survey questionnaire had posed the following item to respondents:

> How many alcoholic beverage servings have you had in the past 30 days? _____

the responses could range from 0 to however many servings. Therefore, the possible responses would have a zero starting point and increase incrementally in order and in equal interval value. This would be an example of scoring at the ratio measurement level.

The term **biostatistics** is meant as the application of statistics to biological or medical problems. It encompasses both descriptive and inferential statistics. Sound biostatistics during prevalence studies require valid and reliable measurement instruments, i.e. the survey questionnaire. Representative sampling of the population usually occurs through a cross-sectional method. In addition, there needs to be a minimization of bias during data collection, and, of course, the appropriate use of descriptive statistical analyses for nominal- and ordinal-scaled variables and inferential statistics for interval- and ratio-scaled variables.

TABLE 9.1. Percentage of substance use by level of physical activity and gender, National College Health Risk Behavior Survey (N = 4,838)

	Not Active	Physically Active ≥2 days weekly	Physically Active ≥3 days weekly
Alcohol use past 30 days			
Females	62.1	66.0	68.6
Males	64.6	72.1	70.1
≥5 drinks consumed past 30 days			
Females	29.6	31.3	39.7
Males	36.8	47.9	50.7
Cigarettes ever tried			
Females	68.2	66.5	67.4
Males	67.5	71.6	66.0
Cigarettes used past 30 days			
Females	29.2	28.2	25.6
Males	32.7	26.0	24.2
Cigarettes regularly smoked—ever			
Females	22.9	21.1	17.5
Males	24.5	22.2	15.0
Smokeless tobacco used past 30 days			
Females	.2	.8	1.0
Males	9.0	13.4	14.2
Marijuana used past 30 days			
Females	17.8	13.6	12.3
Males	14.8	20.8	18.3
Cocaine used past 30 days			
Females	1.4	.5	.0
Males	1.9	.3	.9
Volatile inhalants used ever			
Females	9.6	7.7	6.4
Males	13.4	11.6	10.1

Source: CDC, 1995.

In addition to tables, the results of prevalence studies are commonly presented as charts and figures. Most statistical analysis software has chart generation capabilities. Epidemiologists also use spreadsheet software in population data analysis, where subject records are entered as rows, and variables of measurement are arranged in columns. Each cell or coordinate represents a subject's response to a particular item from the prevalence survey. After data have been entered, descriptive statistics and limited inferential statistical calculations can be performed. Charts and graphs, such as pie, column, line, bar, or scatter, are an easy few steps away once this point is reached.

Prevalence Data from Surveillance Systems

Prevalence studies are usually dependent upon surveillance systems that are operated at local, state, and national levels as studied in Chapter 8. Here again are some common surveillance systems:

- National Employer Health Insurance Survey
- National Health Care Survey
  —Ambulatory Health Care Data (NAMCS/NHAMCS)
  —Hospital Discharge and Ambulatory Surgery Data
  —National Home and Hospice Care Survey
  —National Nursing Home Survey
- National Health Interview Survey
- National Health and Nutrition Examination Survey
- National Immunization Survey
- National Maternal and Infant Health Survey
- National Mortality Followback Survey
- National Survey of Family Growth
- National Vital Statistics System

A good example of collecting prevalence and incidence data is provided by the National Institutes of Health (NIH) in its Consensus Development Panel on Rehabilitation of Persons with Traumatic Brain Injury (TBI). The findings report that amateur athletes in football, soccer, and other contact sports often sustain mild head injuries that consequently affect their written and verbal test-taking abilities. Each year, approximately 300,000 amateur athletes, including those at interscholastic and intercollegiate levels, will endure the incidence of **traumatic brain injury (TBI).** TBI is a syndrome of signs and symptoms such as headaches, sleep disturbances, and inability to concentrate that indicate a range of neurological damage from mild—impaired written and verbal test-taking abilities—to severe—long-term disability and death. Whereas medical professionals can readily diagnose concussion, the prevalence on neurological damage might be overlooked. Signs and symptoms such as complaints of headaches, sleep disturbances, and inability to concentrate appear, which may be caused by mild brain injuries. About 5 percent of all injuries in high-school athletes could be classified as mild traumatic brain injuries. Most of the injuries were found in players participating in football, 63.4 percent; wrestling, 10.5 percent; girls' soccer, 6.2 percent; and boys' soccer, 5.7 percent. Clinical interviews and tests of college football players revealed the prevalence of neuropsychological disorders among athletes with existing learning disabilities and among those who also had a history of two or more prior concussions. Further, it appears that athletes might continue playing even though they have long-term neuropsychological damage. Players should be monitored closely after head injuries and sidelined until they no longer experience headaches or other symptoms. This does not mean, however, that young athletes should abandon sports (Collins, 1999).

SUMMARY

In this chapter we examined the various kinds of epidemiological studies. These studies are of a descriptive, analytic, or experimental (trial) nature. We can categorize studies according to disease occurrence. Categories include presently occurring—prevalence study, after occurrence—retrospective, and before occurrence—prospective. Focusing on the prevalence study, this chapter brought to light the five problem-solving steps with examples of actual prevalence studies.

REVIEW QUESTIONS

1. What is an epidemiological study? Can you distinguish the three types of studies?

2. Do you know the definitions of the important terms in bold print throughout this chapter?
3. Studies can be categorized according to time of disease occurrence—which study is conducted before, during, and after disease occurrence?
4. Can you explain the difference between descriptive and inferential statistics? Which levels of measurement are used in each kind? Could you present examples?
5. What is a prevalence study? What is its relationship to surveillance systems?
6. Can you distinguish incidence from prevalence? Could you explain this difference when using the example of traumatic brain injuries in athletes?
7. If given an example of a prevalence study, could you identify the five problem-solving steps?
8. Do you know the answers to the following chapter activities questions based on objectives from Healthy People 2010 focus areas 17 and 18?

WEB SITE RESOURCES

The Center for Health and Health Care in Schools
<http://www.healthinschools.org/home.asp>

U.S. Department of Agriculture, Agricultural Research Service, Continuing Survey of Food Intakes by Individuals and 1994-1996 Diet and Health Knowledge Survey
<http://www.barc.usda.gov/bhnrc/foodsurvey/home.htm>

REFERENCES

American Diabetes Association (1996). *Diabetes 1996: Vital statistics.* Alexandria, VA: American Diabetes Association.

CDC. (1995). Substance use by level of physical activity and gender, National College Health Risk Behavior Survey. Atlanta, GA: U.S. Centers for Disease Control and Prevention.

Coggon, D., Rose, G., and Barker, D.J.P. (1997). Epidemiology for the uninitiated. BMJ Publishing Group. Available online: <http://www.bmj.com/epidem/epid.html>.

Collins, D. (1999). Neuropsychological outcomes of TBI in athletes. *Journal of the American Medical Association,* 282: 964-980.

Flegal, K., Ezzati, T., and Harris, M. (1991). Prevalence of diabetes in Mexican Americans, Cubans and Puerto Ricans from the Hispanic Health and Nutrition Examination Survey, 1982-1984. *Diabetes Care,* 14: 628-638.

Friedman, R.M., Katz-Levey, J.W., and Manderschied, R.W. (1996). Prevalence of serious emotional disturbance in children and adolescents. In Manderscheid, R.W. and Sonnen-Schein, M.A., (Eds.), *Mental Health, United States, 1996* (pp. 71-78). Rockville, MD: Center for Mental Health Services (CMHS).

Gordis, L. (1996). *Epidemiology.* Philadelphia, PA: W.B. Saunders.

Healthy People 2010 (2000). *Healthy People 2010: Objectives for improving health.* Washington, DC: Office of Disease Prevention and Health Promotion, U.S. Department of Health and Human Services.

Sampson, H.A. (1998). Fatal food-induced anaphylaxis. *Allergy,* 53(Suppl. 46): 125-130.

Stone, D.B., Armstrong, W.R., Macrina, D.M., and Pankau, J.W. (1996). *Introduction to epidemiology.* Madison, WI: Brown and Benchmark.

Timmreck, T.C. (1998). *An introduction to epidemiology* (Second edition). Boston, MA: Jones and Bartlett Publishers.

Vinicor, F. (1994). Is diabetes a public health disorder? *Diabetes Care* 17(S1): 22-27.

Purpose: (1) to acquaint the reader with Healthy People 2010 targets for improvement and (2) present examples of epidemiology as the underlying science to health promotion and disease prevention.

Directions: Check out your knowledge of these Healthy People 2010 focus areas by taking the following tests (answers follow in a separate section).

FOCUS AREA 17: MEDICAL PRODUCT SAFETY

This focus area's goal is to ensure the safe and effective use of medical products.

17-1. *Increase in the proportion of health organizations that are linked in an integrated system that monitors and reports adverse events (developmental).* Such an integrated system would be helpful in:
   a. Monitoring suspected associations between drug exposures and adverse events
   b. Securing answers to specific drug safety questions
   c. Providing exposure data on new molecular entities that have been approved within the past five years in the United States
   d. All of the above

17-2. *Increase in the use of linked, automated systems to share information (developmental).* How could prescribers and pharmacists use these linked, automated systems?
   a. To review a patient's medical record regarding pharmaceutical history, allergies and contraindications to medications, drug sensitivities, etc.

b. To process prescription claims and payments, measure the quality of health care, perform cost analyses, provide drug information, etc.

c. To provide warnings about dosing errors and potential adverse events among medications dispensed by different sources to individual patients.

d. All of the above are correct.

17-3. *Increase in the proportion of primary care providers, pharmacists, and other health care professionals who routinely review with their patients aged sixty-five years and older, and patients with chronic illnesses or disabilities, all new prescribed and over-the-counter medicines (developmental).* Related to the objective, all of the following are correct except:

a. Although persons sixty-five years and older make up about 15 percent of the population, they consume about 33 percent of all retail prescriptions.

b. Persons sixty-five years and older purchase at least 40 percent of all over-the-counter medications.

c. Persons sixty-five years and older are more likely to suffer from multiple chronic diseases with each disease requiring a specific medication.

d. Persons sixty-five years and older routinely visit a single physician who is familiar with all medications that have been recently prescribed.

17-4. *Increase in the proportion of patients receiving information that meets guidelines for usefulness when their new prescriptions are dispensed (developmental).* As of 1992, what proportion of patients received prescriptive information within these guidelines?

a. 14 percent
b. 34 percent
c. 54 percent
d. 74 percent

17-5. *Increase in the proportion of patients who receive verbal counseling from prescribers and pharmacists on the appropriate use and potential risks of medications.* As of 1995,

what percent of patients received this counseling from pre-scribers and pharmacists?
a. From prescribers, 14 percent; and from pharmacists, 32 percent
b. From prescribers, 34 percent; and from pharmacists, 52 percent
c. From prescribers, 54 percent; and from pharmacists, 72 percent
d. From prescribers, 74 percent; and from pharmacists, 92 percent

17-6. *Increase in the proportion of persons who donate blood, and in so doing ensure an adequate supply of safe blood.* How much of an improvement is targeted in increasing the proportion of persons donating blood?
a. 20 percent improvement
b. 40 percent improvement
c. 60 percent improvement
d. 80 percent improvement

FOCUS AREA 18:
MENTAL HEALTH AND MENTAL DISORDERS

This focus area's goal is to improve mental health and ensure access to appropriate, quality mental health services.

Mental Health Status Improvement

18-1. *Reduction in the suicide rate.* Related to this objective, all of the following are correct except:
a. As of 1996, suicide was the ninth leading cause of death in the United States.
b. At least 90 percent of all people who kill themselves have a mental disorder or a substance abuse disorder, or a combination of disorders.
c. Suicide is easy to predict and prevent once the risk factors are known.
d. Risk factors include prior suicide attempt(s), stressful life events, and access to lethal suicide methods.

18-2.   *Reduction in the rate of suicide attempts by adolescents.* Related to this objective, which of the following is correct?
   a. Suicide is the third leading cause of death for persons between ages fifteen and twenty-four.
   b. Suicide occurs most frequently as a consequence of a mental disorder.
   c. Suicide prevention involves reducing access to lethal methods and recognition and treatment of mental and substance abuse disorders.
   d. All of the above are correct.

18-3.   *Reduction in the proportion of homeless adults who have serious mental illness (SMI).* As of 1996, what was the proportion of homeless adults having such an illness?
   a. 5 percent
   b. 15 percent
   c. 25 percent
   d. 35 percent

18-4.   *Increase in the proportion of persons with serious mental illness (SMI) who are employed.* What is the targeted proportion of persons with serious mental illness being employed?
   a. 11 percent
   b. 31 percent
   c. 51 percent
   d. 71 percent

18-5.   *Reduction in the relapse rates for persons with eating disorders including anorexia nervosa and bulimia nervosa (developmental).* What is the relapse rate for persons with eating disorders?
   a. As high as 10 percent within year of treatment
   b. As high as 30 percent within year of treatment
   c. As high as 50 percent within year of treatment
   d. As high as 70 percent within year of treatment

Treatment Expansion

18-6.   *Increase in the number of persons seen in primary health care who receive mental health screening and assessment (developmental)*. Related to this objective, all of the following are correct except:

 a. Each year, about 6 percent of adult persons use the general medical sector (physicians, nurses, etc.) for mental health care.

 b. Each year, adult persons make about four mental health visits to the general medical sector.

 c. Each year, adult persons make about fourteen visits to the specialty medical sector.

 d. The general medical sector has only recently been identified as the initial point of contact for many adults with mental disorders.

18-7. *Increase in the proportion of children with mental health problems who receive treatment (developmental)*. Related to this objective, all of the following are correct except:

 a. For many youth eighteen years and younger, lifelong mental disorders are not likely to start until after adolescence.

 b. In any given year, 20 percent of persons between age nine and seventeen have been diagnosed with a mental disorder.

 c. Mental, behavioral, and emotional disorders in youth can lead to school failure, substance use, violence, or suicide.

 d. About 5 percent of youth are extremely impaired by mental, behavioral, and emotional disorders.

18-8. *Increase in the proportion of juvenile justice facilities that screen new admissions for mental health problems (developmental)*. Related to this objective, which of the following is correct?

 a. Over 100,000 youth are placed in juvenile justice facilities annually.

 b. Within the juvenile justice system, the proportion of youth with mental disorders is considerably higher than in the general population.

 c. Suicide, self-injurious behavior, and other disorders are significant among youths in the juvenile justice system.

 d. Within the juvenile justice system, screening activities such as interviewing parents or caregivers should be conducted by qualified mental health personnel.

18-9. *Increase in the proportion of adults with mental disorders who receive treatment.* Related to this objective, which of the following is correct?
   a. Today's mental health treatments are of limited effectiveness.
   b. There is no "one size fits all" treatment; rather, there is a variety of treatment options available for most disorders.
   c. There exists today a limited array of treatment settings.
   d. A person has limited options in selecting a setting for mental health treatment and may have to settle for one that is neither covered by health insurance nor best for his or her kind of mental condition.

18-10. *Increase in the proportion of persons with co-occurring substance abuse and mental disorders who receive treatment for both disorders (developmental).* Related to this objective, what percentage of the U.S. adult population (eighteen to sixty-four year olds) had a diagnosis of a co-occurring mental and addictive disorder in the past year?
   a. 9 percent
   b. 19 percent
   c. 29 percent
   d. 39 percent

18-11. *Increase in the proportion of local governments with community-based jail diversion programs for adults with serious mental illness (SMI) (developmental).* What proportion of the jail population has a serious mental illness?
   a. 7 percent
   b. 17 percent
   c. 27 percent
   d. 37 percent

18-12. *Increase in the number of states and the District of Columbia that track consumers' satisfaction with the mental health services they receive.* In 1999, how many states tracked consumers' satisfaction?
   a. Six states
   b. Sixteen states
   c. Twenty-six states
   d. Thirty-six states

18-13. *Increase in the number of states, territories, and the District of Columbia with an operational mental health plan that addresses cultural competence (developmental).* Related to this objective, which of the following is correct?

    a. Health care providers need to understand the differences in how various populations in the United States perceive mental health and mental illness.

    b. Select populations use mental health services differently in terms of how they seek it, present their symptoms, and participate in the care they receive.

    c. Select populations may not seek mental health services in the formal system, may drop out of care, or may seek care at much later stages of illness.

    d. All of the above are correct.

18-14. *Increase in the number of states, territories, and the District of Columbia with an operational mental health plan that addresses mental health crisis interventions, ongoing screening, and treatment services for elderly persons.* Related to this objective, what percentage of adults sixty-five years and older experience specific mental disorders, such as depression, anxiety, substance abuse, and dementia, that are not part of normal aging?

    a. 5 percent

    b. 15 percent

    c. 25 percent

    d. 35 percent

282 Epidemiology for Health Promotion/Disease Prevention Professionals

TEST ANSWERS

Focus Area 17

17-1.   (d) All of the above. There is a complex benefit-risk balance to using medical care products. Several parties are involved: manufacturers, federal authorities, health care providers, consumers, etc. This elaborate benefit-risk system lacks the integration needed to ensure optimal public health and safety. Therefore, an integrated data information system is needed.

17-2.   (d) All of the above. In addition, these linked, automated systems can prevent prescribing, dispensing, and administration errors.

17-3.   (d) Persons sixty-five years and older routinely visit a single physician who is familiar with all medications that have been recently prescribed. This is incorrect because most older adults actually visit multiple physicians, each of whom may be unaware of other medicines that have been prescribed.

17-4.   (a) 14 percent. A 1992 survey conducted by the FDA of the amount of information received by consumers found that 14 percent of people received information about prescription drugs from prescribers, and 32 percent from pharmacists.

17-5.   (a) From prescribers, 14 percent; and from pharmacists, 32 percent. The target is 95 percent from both prescribers and from pharmacists.

17-6.   (c) 60 percent improvement. The baseline proportion was 5 percent of the total population donated blood in 1994. The target is 8 percent of the total population. Educational efforts toward encouraging increasing donation should center on the safety of the procedure and the benefits to recipients, such as cancer patients.

Focus Area 18

18-1.   (c) Suicide is easy to predict and prevent once the risk factors are known. This is incorrect since it is difficult to predict, and the best that can be done preventively is to focus on the risk factors. As of 1998, the baseline rate was 11.3 suicides per

100,000 population. The target is 5.0 suicides per 100,000 population.*

18-2.   (d) All of the above are correct. As of 1999, the twelve-month average was 2.6 percent of adolescents in grades nine through twelve attempted suicide and the target is a reduction to 1.0 percent of adolescents in grades nine through twelve attempting suicide.

18-3.   (c) 25 percent. The baseline was 25 percent of homeless adults aged eighteen years and older with a serious mental illness, and the targeted reduction is 19 percent. A serious mental illness is a diagnosable mental disorder found in persons aged eighteen years and older that is so long lasting and severe that it seriously interferes with a person's ability to take part in major life activities.

18-4.   (c) 51 percent. As of 1994, 43 percent of persons aged eighteen years and older with severe mental illness were employed. Recovering from a severe mental illness involves independent living and maintenance of employment. Employment offers personal as well as economic benefits that factor into a person's ability to manage his or her life.

18-5.   (c) As high as 50 percent within year of treatment. Anorexia nervosa is characterized by extreme and often life-threatening weight loss. About 30 to 50 percent of patients relapse within a year of treatment. Cognitive-behavioral therapy seems effective in reducing relapse rates. Bulimia nervosa is characterized by binge eating and then purging. Relapse rates can be as high as 50 percent within a year of treatment. However, there are effective short-term treatments.

18-6.   (d) The general medical sector has been identified only recently as the initial point of contact for many adults with mental disorders. This is incorrect because the general medical sector has long been identified as the first point of contact for many adults with mental disorders. The significance is that providers in the general medical sector represent the only source of mental health services for many adult persons. Therefore, the providers play a key role in the early detection of and intervention for mental health problems.

---

*Ages adjusted to the year 2000 standard population.

18-7.   (a) For many children aged eighteen years and younger, life-long mental disorders may start in childhood or adolescence. This is incorrect since lifelong mental disorders may in fact begin in childhood or adolescence. Effective services for youth, especially those with severe mental illness, require a collaboration of support from families, social services, health services, mental health services, juvenile justice, and the schools.

18-8.   (d) Within the juvenile justice system, screening activities such as interviewing parents or caregivers should be conducted by qualified mental health personnel. Given the numbers of youth entering the justice system, and the kinds of mental conditions they present, proper screening will ensure that youths possessing a treatable mental health problem are identified and receive appropriate treatment.

18-9.   (b) There is no "one size fits all" treatment; rather, there is a variety of treatment options available for most disorders. This is correct, but the other responses are incorrect. Modern treatments for mental disorders are highly effective. There is a diverse array of treatment settings from which a person can choose based on preference, insurance coverage, type of treatment needed, and other factors.

18-10.   (b) 19 percent. In addition, 22 percent of the population had a diagnosis of mental disorder alone.

18-11.   (a) 7 percent. Each year, about 700,000 persons with a serious mental illness are incarcerated in jails. Their proportion exceeds the proportion in the general population. To those arrested for nonviolent crimes, they would probably benefit more from a divergent program or a community-based mental health treatment program.

18-12.   (d) Thirty-six states. The target is to increase this number to all fifty states and the District of Columbia with regard to a system for tracking consumer satisfaction with the mental health services they receive in public and private sectors.

18-13.   (d) All of the above are correct. Considering select population differences in seeking and participating in treatment, a community-based mental health service system needs a plan that centers on cultural relevance, responsiveness, and accessibility.

18-14. (c) 25 percent. Although a majority of persons aged sixty-five years and older cope well with the changes associated with aging and maintain their mental health, about 25 percent develop mental conditions. One disorder, Alzheimer's disease, is responsible for most cases of dementia and is a leading cause of nursing home placements.

Chapter 10

Retrospective Studies

Epidemiologists look back to factors from the past that can perhaps help explain present time diseases and other morbid conditions. They are directed to the past since it holds clues to present causes of morbidity and mortality. Hippocrates was actually the first epidemiologist to conduct retrospective studies; he insisted on close observation of the disease experience with attention to preceding environmental conditions that may have disturbed the body's humoural balance. Retrospective studies began appearing in the professional literature about 1920, when epidemiologists explored the relationship between breast cancer and prior reproductive factors. By the mid-twentieth century, retrospective study design became the preferred method of cancer researchers.

Retrospective studies can be population based, that is, cases are limited to a geographic area; hospital based, in which cases are admitted patients; or group based, in which cases represent a local outbreak or epidemic (Schlesselman, 1982). Retrospective studies are popularly conducted and their results have immediate applications to professionals in health promotion and disease prevention. There are two major kinds of retrospective studies: the case study and the case control study (Gordis, 1996) (see Figure 10.1).

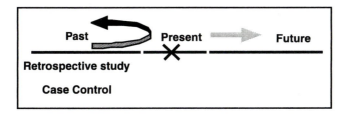

FIGURE 10.1. The case control study (*Source:* Adapted from Timmreck, 1998, p. 259)

CASE STUDY

The **case study,** sometimes called the case-based study or the case history study by clinicians, starts with the identification and sampling of persons with a disease or condition. The intent is to study what preceding factors could explain the occurrence of disease in these cases. In addition, the case study sometimes samples the exposed population and makes comparisons between those with the disease and those without the disease—again, to try to determine the causative factors to the disease.

Mantel and Haenzel (1959) were among the first researchers to prompt medical clinicians to use implicit control groups during a case history study. For example, clinicians were encouraged to compare their diagnoses of specified disease cases with their diagnoses of patients having other diseases. The recollection of signs of symptoms and comparisons made between patient groups assisted the clinician in his or her decision making. Mantel and Haenzel are also credited with devising chi square statistical tests that are used to calculate health risk during a retrospective study. The chi square test is a nonparametric statistic used to determine significant differences in the number of disease cases when comparing persons exposed versus those not exposed to an agent or risk factor.

The case study is customarily performed during the investigation of an epidemic or outbreak. Recall the problem-solving steps of an epidemiological investigation. During the first step, epidemiologists examine, verify, and classify cases of disease. This is essentially a case study. However, a case study can easily be conducted independent from epidemiological responses to epidemics or outbreaks.

CASE CONTROL STUDY

Case control studies are analytic in nature. They attempt to determine the agents or risk factors of disease. These studies are also retrospective since they begin after the occurrence of disease. The design utilizes two groups. The **cases** are persons with the disease or health-affecting condition, whereas the **controls** are those without the disease. Being retrospective, the investigators will look back in time to determine possible agents or risk factors responsible for the disease.

Case control studies are the "next generation" beyond case studies because controls are added. Case control studies are used for diseases that generate a low number of cases. The design allows for a prompt response to disease. This is especially important when the need to know the cause(s) is imminent. By having a matched control, the researchers can better test hypotheses—suspected agents or risk factors. The case control study is relatively inexpensive to conduct in comparison with other analytic efforts such as the cohort study, which will be discussed in Chapter 11.

Case Control Study of Food Intake and Prostate Cancer Risk

There is established epidemiological evidence linking high fruit and vegetable intakes with decreased risks of many cancers. Epidemiologists have wondered if this would hold true for prostate cancer. In a case control study of men under sixty-five years of age from Seattle, Washington, cases represented 628 persons newly diagnosed with prostate cancer. The cases were matched by age with 602 controls—persons from the same geographic place but without prostate cancer. Self-administered food-frequency questionnaires were used to assess diet over the preceding three- to five-year period. Daily nutrient intake was determined using dietary recall software, which was recently updated with analytic values for carotenoids. Risk calculations were performed on analyzed data. No associations were found between fruit intake and prostate cancer risk. However, persons who consumed twenty-eight or more servings of vegetables per week were at a decreased risk of developing prostate cancer. The calculated risk was 0.65. This result means that a person eating less than twenty-eight servings of vegetables was 35 percent more likely to become a prostate cancer case. Accordingly, persons who consumed three or more servings of cruciferous ("crunchy") vegetables per week were at less of a risk for the same cancer. The risk was 0.59. On the flip side, persons who consumed fewer than fourteen servings of vegetables per week were at a higher risk for prostate cancer, as were those who consumed less than one portion of cruciferous vegetables per week (Cohen, Kristal, and Sanford, 2000).

This relates to Healthy People 2010 Objective 19-6: *Increase in the proportion of persons aged two years and older who consume at least three daily servings of vegetables, with at least one-third being dark green or orange vegetables* (Healthy People 2010, 2000, 19-19). (See Chapter 10 activities for more information.)

One unique use of the case control study method is during clinical trials, when a tested intervention or treatment inadvertently yields adverse reactions in the subjects (more on this in Chapter 12). The re-

searchers would then try to determine the cause(s) of the adverse reactions by matching affected cases with nonaffected controls.

Proposed steps for understanding how case control studies are
conducted have been presented by professionals at George Washington University's School of Public Health and Health Services. In abbreviated format, the steps are:

1. *Study design:* Deciding on the question to be answered by the
   study and the study hypothesis, and determining the size of the
   case and control groups.
2. *Assignment:* Setting criteria for whom the subjects are, from
   which population they will be drawn, the method of assignment
   to either case or control groups, and who is aware of the assignment.
3. *Assessment:* Determining the results of the study in case and
   control groups and ensuring validity and reliability of the results.
4. *Analysis:* Comparing results between case and control groups
   with consideration for proper comparison, necessary age-ad-
   justment, appropriate statistical analysis, and minimization of
   error.
5. *Interpretation:* Drawing conclusions about the meaning of differences between the case and control groups while making sure
   results are valid and reliable, and that the differences are significant enough to be clinically useful.
6. *Extrapolation:* Drawing conclusions from the study for possible
   application to persons of other populations experiencing similar
   risk factors to disease (GWU, 1999).

Problem Solving Within the Case Control Study

Given the features of a case control study, it is time to look at the
five problem-solving steps within the study. Although these steps are
similar to those within a prevalence study (see Chapter 9), aspects of
each step are unique to the case control study.

1. *Determine the problem.* During this step, the researchers are notified about the occurrence of a disease, and identify and con-

firm cases of the disease. This calls for a suitable case definition. During this and subsequent steps, the researchers want to
minimize bias (further discussed in step five). For example, it is
advisable to use incident (new) cases rather than prevalent (existing) cases. The main reason is that it is easier to determine the
possible risk factors or causes with new cases. Hence, cases of
disease are confirmed through medical evaluations, interviews,
records, and clinical tests.

2. *Study the problem.* Epidemiologists examine and describe the
distribution of cases, which are examined according person,
place, and time characteristics. This is important for two reasons.
First, a representative sample of cases should be matched with a
representative sample of controls according to person, place, and
time characteristics. Second, the distribution of cases will furnish
indicators or clues to the suspected risk factors or causes.

3. *Suggest a solution.* The researchers generate a hypothesis, an
explanation, for the risk factors/cause of the disease. They will
attempt to establish a valid and reliable relationship between
risk/cause and the disease.

4. *Test the solution.* During this step, the researchers need to match
the selected cases with selected controls and then collect and analyze data pertaining to the independent/dependent variable relationship. Cases are matched with their controls on similar person (demographics), place (life situations), and time (period of
exposure) characteristics. Whereas the cases should be representative of persons who have the disease, controls should be
representative of the population that is at risk for developing the
disease but who have not begun a disease process. Ideally, the
matching should be stratified according to levels within the demographic variables. Minimally, a one to four case to control ratio is used. Data collection can be performed through self-administered questionnaires or interviews. While collecting data
on exposure to suspected risks/causes, epidemiologists have
come to realize the potential for bias (addressed in step five). A
two-by-two epidemiological table is constructed. Thereafter, an
odds ratio is calculated, which is a calculation of risk that is
more appropriate for case-control studies because the incidence

of morbidity/mortality in persons without the disease has been controlled (is zero) (see Figure 10.2). Therefore, it would be meaningless to use the standard relative risk calculation. If the risk is 1.0 or greater, the researchers will subject the odds ratio calculation to a chi square test, a nonparametric inferential statistical analysis. If there is significant difference, this allows researchers to report that "'such and such' cause makes the person 'so many times' more likely to develop 'such and such' disease." Separate analyses (tabling) can be performed on levels of causes as well as levels of disease. The aggregate of chi square testing on these various tables is handled through what are known as Mantel/Haentzel and Cochran chi squares tests (Lilienfeld and Stolley, 1994, pp. 239-240).

5. *Evaluate the solution.* Given the results of risk calculation and statistical analysis, the researchers make a decision regarding the risk factors/cause of the disease. Essentially, they accept or reject the hypothesis. Recall the necessity to minimize **bias,** which is the error caused by systematically favoring some findings over others. Minimizing bias increases the likelihood that the best solution will be employed, as opposed to the favored solution.

	Disease Cases	Controls
Factor present (exposed)	# a	# b
Factor absent (nonexposed)	# c	# d

$$\text{odds ratio} = \frac{a \times d}{b \times c}$$

FIGURE 10.2. The odds ratio calculation as an estimate of relative risk (*Source: Adapted from Timmreck, 1998, p. 374*)

Epidemiologists should have been careful during the preceding steps to address the following potential sources of bias:

- During step one, epidemiologists must be careful about misclassification of cases. Given the nature of case control studies, it is difficult to derive a representative group of subjects with the disease. In an effort to secure the representative sample, the chance of misclassification increases. Therefore, epidemiologists confirm that cases meet the ICD-10 classification based on physician diagnosis.
- During step two, epidemiologists must be careful not to confuse the independent variables with the dependent variable. Cases represent the **dependent variable** (DV) and are under the influence of one or more independent variables. An **independent variable** (IV) has an actual or assumed directional relationship with a dependent variable so that change in the IV influences change in the DV.
- During step three, epidemiologists try to minimize unauthentic relationships between agents, risk factors, and diseases, known **spurious relationships.**
- During step four, data gathering should be standardized for cases and controls; however, the researchers will likely have prior knowledge of who is a case and who is a control, and this might influence data gathering (e.g., during an interview of a case the researcher might prompt the subject for a desired response). Cases usually have better personal recall of their exposure to suspect risk factors/causes than do controls. The validity of such information will depend in part on the subject matter. People may be able to remember quite well where they lived in the past or what jobs they held. On the other hand, long-term recall of dietary habits is probably less reliable.

The best way for epidemiologists to avoid the aforementioned bias would be to rely on the principles of causation or the "five Ps" (Chapter 3). In brief, the agent/risk is always **p**resent when the disease/condition occurs. The agent/risk consistently **p**recedes the disease/condition. There is a **p**ropensity in the relationship: increase the agent/

risk and there is a corresponding increase in the disease/condition. The agent/risk relationship to disease/condition appears in other **per-sons**. In other words, the agent/risk factor-disease relationship is demonstrable in diverse populations of susceptible hosts. The agent/risk relationship to disease/condition appears in be consistent despite **p**lace. Once the epidemiologists are satisfied with their evaluation, it is time to apply the findings to preventive health services.

Case Control Study of Back Injury in Municipal Workers

A case control study was undertaken to identify factors associated with acute low back injury among municipal employees of a large city. For each of 200 injured case patients, two co-worker controls were randomly selected, the first matched on gender, job, and department, while the second matched on gender and job classification only. In-person interviews were conducted to collect data on demographics, work history, work characteristics, work injuries, back pain, psychosocial and work organization, health behaviors, and anthropometric and ergonomic factors related to the job. Psychosocial work organization variables were also examined. Of all factors studied, high job strain was the most important in explaining back injury. The odds ratio risk calculation was 2.12, so workers exposed to high job strain were over twice as likely to experience lower back pain. Other significant factors that contributed to increased risk of lower back pain and injury were workers' body mass index, odds ratio risk calculation 1.54; and work movements involving twisting, extended, reaching, and stooping, odds ratio risk calculation 1.42. Results suggested that increasing workers' control over their jobs reduced levels of job strain. Ergonomic strategies and work-site health promotion may help reduce other risk factors (Myers et al., 1999).

This relates to Healthy People 2010 Objective 20-9: *Increase in the proportion of work sites employing fifty or more persons that provide programs to prevent or reduce employee stress* (Healthy People 2010, 2000, 20-15). (See Chapter 10 activities for more information.)

SUMMARY

This chapter dealt with retrospective studies, among which are the case study and the case control study. Both are analytic in nature with case studies used in clinical practice, and case control studies in epidemiological practice. The retrospective study is conducted after disease occurrence. In case studies there are selected efforts at matching cases with controls. The idea behind the case control study is to match cases with controls to determine the causes or risk factors to disease. The case control study is widely used, considering its cost effectiveness and convenience. We can use the five problem-solving steps to understand how a case control study is conducted. Since this kind of study attempts to determine causality, epidemiologists rely on risk calculations, most notably, the odds ratio.

REVIEW QUESTIONS

1. What is a case control study and how does it differ from a case study? When is it conducted in terms of disease occurrence?
2. Do you know the definitions of the important terms in bold print in this chapter?
3. Can you describe the five problem-solving steps in conducting a case control study? Could you identify these steps if given case control study examples?
4. Are you familiar with the odds ratio risk calculation? Could you perform this calculation?
5. What are sources of bias in a case control study, and how do epidemiologists minimize bias?
6. Can you explain how a case control study was used to determine the risk factors of prostate cancer? Back injury?
7. Do you know the answers to the following chapter activity questions based on objectives from Healthy People 2010 focus areas 19 and 20?

WEB SITE RESOURCES

Case Control and Other Epidemiological Studies at WebMD
<http://webmd.lycos.com/>

Residential Radon and Lung Cancer Case-Control Study, Center for Health Effects of Environmental Contamination,
University of Iowa
<http://www.cheec.uiowa.edu/misc/radon.html>

REFERENCES

Cohen J.H, Kristal, A.R., and Stanford, J.L. (2000). Fruit and vegetable intakes and prostate cancer risk. *Journal of the National Cancer Institute* 92(1): 61-68.

Gordis, L. (1996). *Epidemiology*. Philadelphia, PA: W.B. Saunders.

GWU. (1999). George Washington University School of Public Health and Health Services, Evaluating the Health Research Literature: The Uniform Framework for Case Control Studies. Accessed online: <http://learn.gwumc.edu/sphhs/sstt/casecontrol.htm>.

Healthy People 2010 (2000). *Healthy People 2010: Objectives for improving health*. Washington, DC: Office of Disease Prevention and Health Promotion, U.S. Department of Health and Human Services.

Lilienfeld, D.E. and Stolley, P.D. (1994). *Foundations of epidemiology* (Second edition). New York: Oxford Press.

Mantel, N. and Haenzel, W. (1959). Statistical aspects of the analysis of data from retrospective studies of disease. *Journal of National Cancer Institute* 22: 719-748.

Myers, A.H., Baker, S.P., Li, G., Smith, G.S., Wiker, S., Liang, K., and Johnson, J.V. (1999). Back injury in municipal workers: A case-control study. *American Journal of Public Health* 89: 1036-1041.

Schlesselman, J.J. (1982). *Case-control studies*. New York: Oxford Press.

Timmreck, T.C. (1998). *An introduction to epidemiology* (Second edition). Boston, MA: Jones and Bartlett Publishers.

Purpose: (1) to acquaint the reader with Healthy People 2010 targets for improvement and (2) present examples of epidemiology as the underlying science to health promotion and disease prevention.

Directions: Check out your knowledge of these Healthy People 2010 focus areas by taking the following tests (answers follow in a separate section).

FOCUS AREA 19:
NUTRITION AND WEIGHT MANAGEMENT

This focus area's goal is to promote health and reduce chronic disease associated with diet and weight.

Weight Status and Growth

19-1. *Increase in the proportion of adults who are at a healthy weight.* As of 1988-1994, what proportion of adults were at healthy weight?
a. 22 percent
b. 42 percent
c. 62 percent
d. 82 percent

19-2. *Reduction in the proportion of adults who are obese.* As of 1988-1994, what proportion of adults were obese?
a. 23 percent
b. 43 percent
c. 63 percent
d. 83 percent

19-3.   *Reduction in the proportion of children and adolescents who are overweight or obese.* As of 1988-1994, what proportion of youth eleven to nineteen years old were obese?
a. 11 percent
b. 33 percent
c. 53 percent
d. 73 percent

19-4.   *Reduction in growth retardation among low-income children under age five years.* Related to this objective, how is growth retardation determined in a population of children age five years and younger?
a. When body mass indexes do not meet certain standards
b. When greater than 5 percent of the group does not meet the fifth percentile of expected height for that age group
c. When families spend at least 40 percent of the food budget on away-from-home foods purchased at food service outlets
d. When a child's height and weight do not meet expected standards

Food and Nutrient Consumption

19-5.   *Increase in the proportion of persons aged two years and older who consume at least two daily servings of fruit.* What is the targeted proportion of persons two years and older consuming at least two servings of fruit daily?
a. 25 percent
b. 50 percent
c. 75 percent
d. 100 percent

19-6.   *Increase in the proportion of persons aged two years and older who consume at least three daily servings of vegetables, with at least one-third being dark green or orange vegetables.* What is the targeted proportion of persons two years and older consuming at least three servings of vegetables, one being of dark green leafy, daily?
a. 35 percent
b. 55 percent
c. 75 percent
d. 95 percent

19-7. *Increase in the proportion of persons aged two years and older who consume at least six daily servings of grain products, with at least three being whole grains.* What is the targeted proportion of persons two years and older consuming at least six servings of grains (three being whole grains) daily?
a. 35 percent
b. 55 percent
c. 75 percent
d. 95 percent

19-8. *Increase in the proportion of persons aged two years and older who consume less than 10 percent of calories from saturated fat.* What is the targeted proportion of persons two years and older consuming less than 10 percent of daily calories from saturated fat?
a. 35 percent
b. 55 percent
c. 75 percent
d. 95 percent

19-9. *Increase in the proportion of persons aged two years and older who consume no more than 30 percent of calories from total fat.* What is the targeted proportion of persons two years and older consuming no more than 30 percent of daily calories from total fat?
a. 35 percent
b. 55 percent
c. 75 percent
d. 95 percent

19-10. *Increase in the proportion of persons aged two years and older who consume 2,400 mg or less of sodium daily.* What is the targeted proportion of persons two years and older consuming 2,400 mg or less of sodium daily?
a. 25 percent
b. 45 percent
c. 65 percent
d. 85 percent

19-11. *Increase in the proportion of persons aged two years and older who meet dietary recommendations for calcium.* What is the targeted proportion of persons two years and older who meet dietary recommendations for calcium?
   a. 35 percent
   b. 55 percent
   c. 75 percent
   d. 95 percent

Iron Deficiency and Anemia

19-12. *Reduction in iron deficiency among young children and females of childbearing age.* As of 1988-1994, what percentage of nonpregnant females ages twelve to forty-nine years had iron deficiency?
   a. 11 percent
   b. 31 percent
   c. 51 percent
   d. 71 percent

19-13. *Reduction in anemia among low-income pregnant females in their third trimester.* As of 1996, what percent of these females had anemia in their third trimester?
   a. 9 percent
   b. 29 percent
   c. 49 percent
   d. 69 percent

19-14. *Reduction in iron deficiency among pregnant females (developmental).* Related to this objective, which of the following is correct?
   a. Only one-fourth of all females ages twelve to forty-nine years consume sufficient dietary iron.
   b. Iron deficiency among females of childbearing age may be prevented by periodic anemia screening and appropriate treatment, and by dietary counseling.
   c. Iron-rich foods are whole grain and enriched breads; lean meats; turkey dark meat; shellfish; spinach; and cooked dry beans, peas, and lentils.
   d. All of the above are correct.

Schools, Work Sites, and Nutrition Counseling

19-15. *Increase in the proportion of children and adolescents aged six to nineteen years whose intake of meals and snacks at school contributes to good overall dietary quality (developmental).* Related to this objective, the U.S. Department of Agriculture requires schools to plan menus that meet the 1995 Dietary Guidelines for Americans, but this applies only to:
   a. Foods served through the school lunch program
   b. Foods sold in school snack bars
   c. Foods sold in school stores
   d. Food sold in school vending machines

19-16. *Increase in the proportion of work sites that offer nutrition or weight management classes or counseling.* During 1988-1999, what percentage of work sites with fifty or more employees offered nutrition/weight management education?
   a. 15 percent
   b. 35 percent
   c. 55 percent
   d. 75 percent

19-17. *Increase in the proportion of physician office visits made by patients with a diagnosis of cardiovascular disease, diabetes, or hyperlipidemia that include counseling or education related to diet and nutrition.* As of 1997, what proportion of physician office visits for nutrition-related diseases involved professionally offered nutrition education and counseling?
   a. 22 percent
   b. 42 percent
   c. 62 percent
   d. 82 percent

Food Security

19-18. *Increase in food security among U.S. households, and in so doing reduce hunger.* Related to this objective, what is food security?
   a. Access by all people at all times to enough food for an active, healthy life.

b. The set of processes by which nutrients and other food components are taken in by the body and used.

c. A pattern of behavior that is relatively inactive, such as a lifestyle characterized by a lot of sitting.

d. Limited or uncertain availability of nutritionally adequate and safe foods or limited and uncertain ability to acquire acceptable foods in socially acceptable ways.

FOCUS AREA 20:
OCCUPATIONAL SAFETY AND HEALTH

This focus area's goal is to promote the health and safety of people at work through prevention and early intervention.

20-1.   *Reduction in deaths from work-related injuries.* Related to this objective, what has been the general trend in deaths from work-related injuries since 1980?
a. Death rates have been increasing.
b. Death rates have been decreasing.
c. Death rates have been stabilizing.
d. Deaths have been practically nonexistent.

20-2.   *Reduction in work-related injuries resulting in medical treatment, lost time from work, or restricted work activity.* How much of a reduction is targeted in these work-related injuries?
a. 10 percent
b. 30 percent
c. 50 percent
d. 70 percent

20-3.   *Reduction in the rate of injury and illness cases involving days away from work due to overexertion or repetitive motion.* How much of a reduction is targeted in injuries from overexertion or repetitive motion?
a. 10 percent
b. 30 percent
c. 50 percent
d. 70 percent

20-4. *Reduction in pneumoconiosis deaths.* Related to this objective, what is pneumoconiosis?
a. A major category of lung disease caused by breathing in certain types of occupational dusts.
b. Hearing loss caused by repeated exposures to sounds at various loudness levels over an extended period of time.
c. An immediate hypersensitivity reaction to one or more natural rubber latex proteins that can result in a wide spectrum of signs and symptoms.
d. A musculoskeletal disorder due to repetitive motion, forceful exertions, or constrained or extreme postures.

20-5. *Reduction in deaths from work-related homicides.* Related to this objective, how many workers die each week as a result of workplace homicides in the United States?
a. 1
b. 20
c. 40
d. 60

20-6. *Reduction in work-related assaults.* How much of a reduction is targeted in work-related assaults?
a. 9 percent
b. 29 percent
c. 49 percent
d. 69 percent

20-7. *Reduction in the number of persons who have elevated blood lead concentrations from work exposures.* How much of a reduction is targeted in elevated blood lead concentrations from work exposures?
a. 25 percent reduction
b. 50 percent reduction
c. 75 percent reduction
d. 100 percent reduction (total elimination)

20-8. *Reduction in occupational skin diseases or disorders among full-time workers.* Related to this objective, occupational skin diseases represent what percent of all reported occupational illnesses?
a. 13.5 percent

b. 33.5 percent
c. 53.5 percent
d. 73.5 percent

20-9.   *Increase in the proportion of work sites employing fifty or more persons that provide programs to prevent or reduce employee stress.* What proportion of work sites employing fifty or more persons are targeted for offering stress management programs?
a. 25 percent
b. 50 percent
c. 75 percent
d. 100 percent

20-10. *Reduction in occupational needlestick injuries among health care workers.* Related to this objective, all of the following are correct except:
a. Needlestick injuries pose the greatest risk of occupational transmission of bloodborne bacteria.
b. Needlestick injuries occur mostly among nursing staff, however laboratory staff, physicians, housekeepers, and other health care workers are also at risk.
c. A 30 percent reduction in needlestick injuries is feasible by using present technologies and adopting changes in techniques (e.g., not trying to cap a used hypodermic needle).
d. Over a half a million occupational needlestick exposures to blood occur annually to health care workers.

20-11. *Reduction in new cases of work-related, noise-induced hearing loss (developmental).* Related to this objective, which of the following are correct? Noise-induced hearing loss is:
a. Caused by repeated exposures to sounds at various loudness levels over an extended period of time
b. The cumulation of many temporary hearing losses, all of which is permanent hearing loss
c. Insidious, often unnoticed by the sufferer until listening and communication are impaired
d. All of the above

TEST ANSWERS

Focus Area 19

19-1. (b) 42 percent. Relying on body mass index (BMI), healthy weight for adults twenty years and older is between 18.5 to 25. While the relation of BMI to body fat differs by age and gender, it is used when comparing persons across racial and ethnic groups. The target is to increase the proportion of healthy weight adults to 60 percent of the adult population.*

19-2. (a) 23 percent. Relying on body mass index (BMI), obesity for adults twenty years and older is a BMI of 30 or greater. A shortcoming to the BMI is that is does not offer information on body fat distribution which is an indicator of health risk. The target is to decrease the proportion of obese adults to 15 percent of the adult population.

19-3. (a) 11 percent. Relying on body mass index (BMI), obesity for youth eleven to nineteen years old is defined as at or above the gender- and age-specific ninety-fifth percentile of BMI based on the revised CDC Growth Charts for the United States. This method of setting an obesity standard is necessary because measures of body fat and body weight are difficult to interpret in youth without measures of sexual maturity. The target is to decrease the proportion of obese youth to 5 percent of the youth population.

19-4. (b) When greater than 5 percent of the group does not meet the fifth percentile of expected height for that age group. It is to be expected that 5 percent of healthy children are below the fifth percentile of height for age due to normal biologic variation. But when the proportion of children not meeting the fifth percentile exceeds 5 percent, this is an indication that some children in that group are not meeting full growth potential. In some select groups of low-income children, as much as 15 percent of that group does not meet the fifth percentile of expected height. The baseline in 1997 was 8 percent of low-income children under age 5 years were growth retarded. The target is to decrease this to 5 percent of low-

---

*Ages adjusted to the year 2000 standard population.

income children falling below the fifth percentile of expected growth.

19-5. (c) 75 percent. As of 1994-1996, only 28 percent of persons two years and older were eating two servings of fruit daily.

19-6. (b) 55 percent. As of 1994-1996, only 3 percent of persons two years and older were eating at least three servings of vegetables (one being of dark green leafy) daily. Although the average consumption was five servings, only 7-10 percent of the vegetable servings comprised dark green or deep yellow/ orange vegetables. Only 5 to 6 percent of the servings included legumes such as beans and peas.

19-7. (b) 55 percent. As of 1994-1996, only 7 percent of persons two years and older were eating at least six servings of grains, three being whole grains, daily. Although the average consumption was about seven servings, only about 14 to 15 percent of the servings included whole grains such as those found in bread.

19-8. (c) 75 percent. As of 1994-1996, only 36 percent of persons two years and older were eating less than 10 percent of daily calories from saturated fat. Although the role of fat in the diet is complicated because different types of fatty acids have different health effects, it is a fact that the U.S. population consumes too much fat, within which too much is from saturated fatty acids.

19-9. (c) 75 percent. As of 1994-1996, only 33 percent of persons two years and older were eating no more than 30 percent of daily calories from total fat. The target can be achieved by consuming most calories from plant foods (grains, fruits, vegetables) that have little added fat.

19-10. (c) 65 percent. As of 1988-1994, only 21 percent of persons aged two years and older consumed 2,400 mg or less of sodium daily from foods, dietary supplements, tap water, and table salt. Salt should not be added at the table since both home foods and away-from-home foods provide excessive amounts of sodium.

19-11. (c) 75 percent. As of 1988-1994, only 46 percent of persons aged two years and older were at or above approximated mean calcium requirements. This was based on consideration of calcium from foods, dietary supplements, and antacids.

Daily recommended consumption for ascending age groups are children ages one to three, 500 mg; children ages four to eight, 800 mg; adolescents ages nine to eighteen, 1,300 mg; adults ages nineteen to fifty, 1,000 mg; and adults ages fifty-one and older, 1,200 mg.

19-12. (a) 11 percent. The target is to reduce the number of non-pregnant females (ages twelve to forty-nine) with iron deficiency to 7 percent. Iron deficiency ranges from depleted iron stores without functional or health impairment to iron deficiency with anemia, which affects the functioning of several organ systems.

19-13. (b) 29 percent. The target is to reduce to 20 percent of low-income pregnant females in their third trimester being anemic. Being anemic is defined as having a hemoglobin count that is <11.0 g/dL. This can be prevented through daily intake of at least 15 mg of iron.

19-14. (d) All of the above are correct. Besides eating iron-rich foods, persons at risk for iron deficiency can take iron supplements especially during pregnancy. Certain foods also enhance iron absorption in the body, such as orange juice and other citrus products whereas there are foods to avoid, such as coffee and tea, since they inhibit iron absorption.

19-15. (a) Foods served through the school lunch program. Improving the quality of students' dietary intake in school settings is important because, for many children, meals and snacks consumed at school make a major contribution to their total daily consumption of food and nutrients.

19-16. (c) 55 percent. Work sites can offer nutrition and weight management instruction and counseling either on site or through their health plans (e.g., education materials offered to members of an HMO). The target is to increase this education to 85 percent of work sites with fifty or more employees.

19-17. (b) 42 percent. The target is to provide nutrition education and counseling during 75 percent of physician office visits that involve patients with a diagnosis of either cardiovascular disease, diabetes, or elevated cholesterol. Primary care providers are well positioned in the health care system to provide preventive services, including nutrition screening and assessment, referral, and counseling.

19-18. (a) Access by all people at all times to enough food for an active, healthy life. It includes at a minimum (1) the ready availability of nutritionally adequate and safe foods and (2) an assured ability to acquire acceptable foods in socially acceptable ways. In 1995, 88 percent of U.S. households were food secure, and the target is for 94 percent of households to be food secure.

Focus Area 20

20-1. (b) Deaths have been decreasing. However, in recent years there has been a stabilization of about 4.3 deaths per 100,000 workers each year. The target is to reduce death rates in most occupations by as much as 30 percent.

20-2. (b) 30 percent. As of 1997, the baseline rate of work-related injuries resulting in lost time from work, medical treatment, or restricted work activity was 6.6 cases per 100 full-time workers. This amounted to about 6.1 million workers. The target is a reduction to 4.3 cases per 100 full-time workers. Clearly, this is a major health and business concern, and prevention efforts are needed to reduce the tremendous burden of these injuries on individual workers as well as society.

20-3. (c) 50 percent. As of 1997, the baseline rate was 675 injuries per 100,000 full-time workers due to overexertion or repetitive motion. The target is 338 injuries per 100,000 full-time workers. About 32 percent of occupational injuries and illnesses resulting in days away from work involved overexertion (e.g., lifting) or repetitive motion (e.g., key entry).

20-4. (a) A major category of lung disease caused by breathing in certain types of occupational dusts. The dust deposited in the lung can result in inflammation and scarring, with associated respiratory symptoms, reduced lung function, and disability. A number of types of dust (for example, asbestos, silica, or coal mine dust) are known to cause pneumoconiosis. In 1997, there were 2,928 pneumoconiosis deaths among persons aged 15 years and older. The target is a reduction to no more than 1,900 deaths per year.

20-5. (b) 20. An average of twenty workers die weekly from workplace homicides. As of 1998, the baseline was 0.5 deaths per

100,000 workers aged sixteen years and older were work-related homicides. The target is 0.4 deaths per 100,000 workers. At-risk jobs have the following characteristics: interacting with the public, handling exchanges of money, working alone or in small numbers, and working late night or early morning hours. Prevention efforts need to recognize these characteristics and launch workplace violence prevention efforts as a part of a comprehensive occupational safety and health program.

20-6.   (b) 29 percent. Between 1987-1992, the baseline rate was 0.85 assaults per 100 workers aged sixteen years and older. The target is to reduce that occurrence to 0.60 assaults per 100 workers. Reducing the number of workplace assaults as well as homicides will require improved surveillance.

20-7.   (d) 100 percent reduction (total elimination). The baseline rate, as of 1998, was 93 per 1 million persons aged sixteen to sixty-four years with blood lead concentrations of 25 µg/dL or greater. The target is zero per million persons aged sixteen to sixty-four years having blood lead concentrations of 25 µg/dL. Lead exposure most likely takes place in battery manufacturing, nonferrous foundries, radiator repair shops, lead smelters, construction, demolition, and firing ranges. Also at risk are persons working in sheltered workshops, where mentally and physically challenged adults work. Lead from work exposure can be inadvertently brought home and can harm children and spouses. Lead exposures while making pottery and stained glass, or during casting of ammunition and fishing weights, cause additional cases, as do exposures during certain home renovation and remodeling projects.

20-8.   (a) 13.5 percent. Occupational skin diseases or disorders are the most common nontrauma-related occupational illnesses. Examples of such illnesses include dermatitis and allergic reactions to chemical substances at the job site. As of 1997, the baseline rate was sixty-seven new cases of occupational skin diseases or disorders per 100,000 full-time workers aged sixteen years and older. The target is to reduce that number to forty-seven new cases per 100,000 full-time workers.

20-9.   (b) 50 percent. Work-related stress is considered a risk factor in cardiovascular disease, musculoskeletal disorders, and injuries on the job. About one-third of employees report experiencing high stress levels. Work-site programs attempt to help workers cope with stress and/or attempt to alter sources of stress through job redesign. In 1992, the baseline was 37 percent of work sites with fifty or more employees provided work-site stress reduction programs for their employees.

20-10. (a) Needlestick injuries pose the greatest risk of occupational transmission of bloodborne bacteria. This is incorrect because actually, bloodborne viruses such as HIV, hepatitis B, and C, pose the greatest threat to health care workers. The baseline in 1996 was 600,000 occupational needlestick exposures to blood among health care workers. The target is a reduction to 400,000 occupational needlestick exposures annually. Present and newly developed technology, along with safer "sharps" handling practices, can reduce these serious incidents.

20-11. (d) All of the above. The National Institute for Occupational Safety and Health, in partnership with more than 500 outside organizations and individuals, has identified noise-induced hearing loss as one of the top twenty-one research priorities for occupational safety and health.

Chapter 11

Prospective Studies

Epidemiologists prospect during studies—that is, they look into the future for factors that explain the development of disease and other morbid conditions. They make a major commitment in time and resources by following groups of persons for years at a time and monitoring their exposure to risk factors and their incidence of disease and death. The prospective study also goes by names such as concurrent, follow-up, incidence, and longitudinal. There are variations of the prospective study in which large groups of persons are traced for extended periods of time. Some research designs start with a group of cases (those with disease) and follow them through time to study their disease process progression. Other prospective studies will match the cohort, called the study group, with another cohort, deemed the control group. However, the most common prospective study is the **cohort study** within which a group of persons without the disease are assessed periodically for long periods of time to see if there is a factor exposure and disease incidence relationship.

A classic example of a prospective study is the Framingham Heart Study. Beginning in 1948, a same-age group of skilled and semi-skilled males was followed for decades and given annual health assessments to measure each person's exposure to suspected risk factors, as well as to record incidents of cardiovascular-related death. Later, other same-age groups, comprised of both genders, were researched in parallel to the initial study. It is from this classic prospective study that epidemiologists deduced the relationship between serum cholesterol levels (≤ 220 mg/dL) and increased risk of cardiovascular disease. They also confirmed the contributions of high blood pressure, cigarette smoking, and other factors to heart disease (Kannel, Dawber, and McGee, 1980). Based on this and other prospective studies, health promotion and disease prevention professionals now know that all adults twenty years of age and older should have their cholesterol levels checked every five years. If at risky levels, persons are encouraged to make lifestyle changes such as moderating consumption of saturated fat and cholesterol, becoming more physically active, and managing body weight.

COHORT STUDY

A cohort study is a kind of analytic study in which exposed persons in a group are followed over time to observe disease incidence and mortality. A cohort study is prospective because it starts before a disease occurs. This kind of study is also called a longitudinal study, given the forward progress time frame. Essentially, epidemiologists are looking for associations between agent or risk exposure and the incidence of morbidity or mortality.

Prospective Studies and Oral Health

Oral health is an essential and integral component of health throughout life. Poor oral health and untreated oral diseases and conditions can have a significant impact on quality of life. Dental caries is the single most common chronic disease of childhood, occurring five to eight times as frequently as asthma, the second most common chronic disease in children. Prospective studies have been able to demonstrate that despite the reduction in cases of caries in recent years, more than half of all children have caries by the second grade. By the time students finish high school, about 80 percent have caries. Unless arrested early, caries is irreversible. Presently under study is early childhood caries, which affects the primary teeth of infants and young children ages one to six years. Although the exact cause of this condition is not known, factors such as large family size, nutritional status of the mother and the infant, the transfer of infectious organisms from caregiver to infant, and allowing sweetened drinks and pacifiers to remain in sleeping infants' mouths are being considered. Studies have demonstrated that inadequate dental health practices and lack of access to either fluoridated water or topical treatments are factors to dental caries in older children, adolescents, and adults. Future studies will examine how baby boomers will likely have more teeth in their later years than previous generations, however, those teeth will continue to be at risk for dental caries (Ismail and Sohn, 1999).

This relates to Healthy People 2010 Objective 21-1: *Reduction in the proportion of children and adolescents who experience dental caries in their primary or permanent teeth* (Healthy People 2010, 2000, 21-11). (See Chapter 11 activities for more information.)

The cohort study receives its name from the group or cohort that is followed through time. A **cohort** is composed of same-aged persons with varying degrees of exposure to risk. The component of the population that comprises a cohort are those born during a particular period, and are identified by period of birth so that characteristics (e.g., causes of death and numbers still living) can be ascertained as it enters successive time and age periods. The term can be broadened to describe any designated group of persons who are followed or traced over a period of time. Depending on the size and complexity of the cohort study design, a cohort can be made up of subcohorts (subgroups).

Some cohort studies are conducted for years whereas others are for weeks or months, as in an episode of acute occupational exposure to a toxic substance. During such a study, subjects are periodically assessed on risk exposure and health outcomes. It should be mentioned that in a longitudinal study, sometimes a control group is compared to the cohort. However, for the purposes of this text, the cohort study will be considered to have one group—a cohort—in the design.

There are two major kinds of cohort studies (see Figure 11.1). The first and most typical, called a **concurrent prospective,** starts in the present and proceeds into the future. The research design calls for a cohort of subjects to be selected and then periodically assessed for risk exposure and disease occurrence for months or years to follow. The second kind of cohort study is the **nonconcurrent prospective** which begins in the past. The nonconcurrent study is conducted by reconstructing data about persons at a time or times in the past. This method uses existing records about the health or other relevant aspects of a population as it was at some time in the past, and seeks to determine the current (or subsequent) status of population members

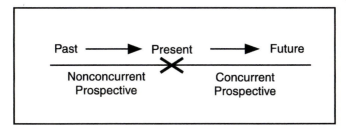

FIGURE 11.1. Cohort studies can be concurrent and nonconcurrent (*Source:* Adapted from Timmreck, 1998, p. 259)

with respect to the condition. Different past exposure levels to risk factor(s) of interest must be identifiable for subsets of the population.

A good example of a concurrent cohort study design took place recently in New York City. Epidemiologists examined the relationship between meat and fat intake and breast cancer. The study started in 1985 and continued to 1991. A cohort of 14,291 women self-reported their dietary intake. During the study, 180 invasive breast cancer cases were diagnosed. There was an evident increase in the relative risk of breast cancer for increasd consumption of red meat, especially meat having a high fat content. According to the study's findings, women who had higher levels of animal source protein which was rich unsaturated fat, were about five times more likely to develop breast cancer than those who consumed lower levels. Other sources of protein (e.g., dairy products, fish, and poultry) did not demonstrate this significant relative risk (NYU, 1999).

An example of a nonconcurrent cohort study took place among shipbuilders, which examined the suspected link between asbestos fiber exposure and lung disease. By the end of the 1950s, public and occupational health surveillance systems noted an increased rate of asbestosis in the United States. **Asbestosis** is a fibrous lung disease caused by prolonged inhalation of asbestos fibers. A type of pneumoconiosis, it is found primarily among workers whose occupations involved asbestos, principally mining, construction, and the manufacture of insulation, fireproofing, cement products, and automobile brakes. The disease is not limited to asbestos workers; it is also known to strike people living near mines, factories, and construction sites. Inhaled asbestos fibers remain in the lungs for years and eventually cause excessive scarring and fibrosis, resulting in a stiffening of the lungs that continues long after exposure ceases. Greater effort is needed to make the stiffened lungs expand during breathing, resulting in shortness of breath and inadequate oxygenation of the blood. Persons with advanced cases of the disease have a chronic dry cough, and the increased cardiac effort needed to expand the lungs may induce a secondary heart disease. An increased incidence of lung cancer and of malignant **mesothelioma,** a rare cancer of the membrane lining of the lungs and abdominal organs, is also associated with asbestos inhalation and asbestosis. There is no effective treatment for asbestosis, and it usually results after at least ten years of asbestos exposure. By contrast, mesothelioma can develop after relatively little exposure to asbestos. The first symptoms do not appear until many years after the initial exposure. Shipyard workers exposed to asbestos during World War II began developing asbestosis in the 1960s and 1970s. Also, it is now known that cigarette smoking seriously aggravates the symptoms of asbestosis. Incidence of asbestosis increased after 1950, probably due to the increasingly widespread industrial use of asbestos. This use declined during the 1970s and had become prohibited in many countries by the 1990s (Mausner and Kramer, 1985).

Another kind of cohort study less in use is the **historical cohort study.** Its design calls for control subjects from whom data were collected at a time preceding that at which the data are gathered on the group being studied. Because of the difference in exposures, etc., use of historical controls can lead to bias in analysis.

Proposed steps for understanding how a cohort study is conducted have been presented by professionals at George Washington University's School of Public Health and Health Services. They follow in abbreviated format.

1. *Study design:* Deciding on the study question and study hypothesis, and determining the size of the study and control groups.
2. *Assignment:* Setting criteria for who is a subject, from which population drawn, method of assignment to either cohort or control (if used), and who is aware of the assignment.
3. *Assessment:* Determining the results of the study in cohort and control groups and ensuring validity and reliability of the results.
4. *Analysis:* Comparing results between cohort and control groups with consideration to proper comparison, necessary age adjustment, appropriate statistical analysis, and minimization of error.
5. *Interpretation:* Drawing conclusions about the meaning of and differences between the cohort and control groups while making sure results are valid and reliable, and that the differences are significant enough to be clinically useful.
6. *Extrapolation:* Drawing conclusions from the study for possible application to persons of other populations experiencing similar risk factors to disease (GWU, 1999).

Problem Solving Within the Cohort Study

Like other analytic studies, there are identifiable problem-solving steps:

1. *Determine the problem.* During this step, the researchers become aware of a health problem, such as a chronic disease, and seek to determine the risk factors/causes of this disease. They must be able to identify and confirm cases of the disease as the study proceeds because, at the start, the cohort members are disease free. This calls for a suitable case definition. During this and subsequent steps, the researchers want to minimize bias (further discussed in step five). For instance, epidemiologists have to account for subjects dropping out during study, which may cause the remaining subjects to be different (e.g., more health conscious) from those who quit.

2. *Study the problem.* Prior to beginning the study, epidemiologists examine and describe the distribution of disease cases in the general population according to person, place, and time characteristics. The distribution of cases will furnish indicators or clues as to the suspected agents or risk factors. These agents or risks should be delineatable, meaning that the researchers should be able to measure risk exposure and then delineate subjects into low and high exposure or risk groups.

3. *Suggest a solution.* The researchers generate a hypothesis, an explanation, for the agent or risk factors to the disease. They will attempt to establish a valid and reliable relationship between the suspected cause(s) and the disease.

4. *Test the solution.* The epidemiologists collect and analyze periodic data on exposure and incidence of disease. Typically, the cohort is assessed annually. Over time, epidemiologists should see a gradient of disease (which is the dependent variable) due to increasing exposure to the risk (the independent variable). In fact, the cohort should be delineatable in terms of exposure to agent/risk. That is, over time, the epidemiologists can distinguish those who are at high and low risk. The delineation between high and low risk cohort members should have an observable association with subsequent incidence of morbidity or mortality. Two-by-two tables are constructed. Relative risk and attributal risk calculations are performed. Any relative risk ratio that is greater than 1.0 is subjected to a chi square test.

5. *Evaluate the solution.* Given the results of risk calculation and statistical analysis, the researchers make a decision regarding the cause(s) of the disease. They essentially accept or reject the hypothesis. Recall the necessity to minimize bias, which is the error caused by systematically favoring some findings over others.

Epidemiologists are careful during these steps to address the following potential sources of bias:

- During step one, epidemiologists try to retain the cohort's original members. Agreed-upon definitions of the risk/cause, as well as the case, are necessary.
- During step two, epidemiologists make sure they can delineate exposure (independent variable) at the start of the study. Likewise, a system of diagnosing the dependent variable is necessary (e.g., screenings).
- During step three, epidemiologists try to minimize unauthentic agent/risk factor-disease relationships, known as spurious relationships.
- During step four, data gathering should be standardized for each member of the cohort. Given the time period of a cohort, the epidemiologists have been guarded against inadvertently influencing the subjects to recall their risk/causal factors under investigation. Also, an ethical issue surfaces. If the epidemiologists diagnose the disease, they are compelled to refer the subjects to available community health resources. The best way for epidemiologists to avoid the aforementioned biases would be to rely on the principles of causation, the "five Ps" (Chapter 3). In brief, the agent/risk is always **p**resent when the disease/condition occurs. The agent/risk consistently **p**recedes the disease/ condition. There is a **p**ropensity in the relationship—increase the agent/risk and a corresponding increase in the disease/condition occurs. The agent/risk relationship to disease/condition appears in other **p**ersons. In other words, the agent/risk factor-disease relationship is demonstrable in diverse populations of susceptible hosts. The agent/risk relationship to disease/condition appears to be consistent despite **p**lace. Once the epidemiologists are satisfied with their evaluation, it is time to apply the findings to preventive health services.

Recreational Physical Activity and the Risk of Cholecystectomy in Women

Physical inactivity appears to be a risk factor to gallstone disease in women, having both a direct and indirect influence along with being overweight. In a prospective study, the recreational physical activity (such as jogging, running, and bicycling) and sedentary behavior (such as spending hours watching television) was examined in relation to the risk of **cholecystectomy,** or gallbladder removal, in a cohort of 60,290 women who were forty to sixty-five years of age in 1986 and had no history of gallstone disease. As part of the Nurses' Health Study, the women reported on questionnaires mailed to them every two years both their activity level and whether they had undergone cholecystectomy. During a ten-year follow-up period (1986 to 1996), 3,257 cases of cholecystectomy were reported. Recreational physical activity was inversely related to the risk of cholecystectomy. In contrast, sedentary behavior was independently related to an increased risk of cholecystectomy. Women who spent less than six hours per week sitting while at work or driving were compared to women who spent forty-one to sixty hours per week sitting. The less active women had a relative risk calculation of 1.42 (42 percent more likely to have had a cholecystectomy). This risk increased for women who spent more than sixty hours per week sitting while at work or driving (relative risk calculation of 2.32). These associations persisted after the researchers controlled for body weight and weight change (Leitzmann et al., 1999).

This relates to Healthy People 2010 Objective 22-1: *Reduction in the proportion of adults who engage in no leisure-time physical activity* (Healthy People 2010, 2000, 22-8). (See Chapter 11 activities for more information.)

SUMMARY

This chapter discussed prospective studies, which look into the future for factors that can explain the development of disease and other morbid conditions. The most common prospective study is the cohort study, of which there are two major kinds: concurrent and nonconcurrent. The concurrent study has its start in the present and progresses into the future, while the nonconcurrent study has its start in the past and also progresses forward into the future. Usually, a cohort study has one group of same-age persons whom the epidemiologists periodically measure for the presence of risk factors as well as incidence of disease. Sometimes a cohort study uses a control group. Either way, the logic is that over time, the ever-increasing presence of risk factors should be associated with increased incidence rates of disease or death. From these data, risk calculations can be made. Similar to other epidemiological studies, the cohort study can be explained using the five steps of problem solving.

REVIEW QUESTIONS

1. What is a prospective study? What is a cohort study? How is a cohort study different from other kinds of epidemiological studies? What does it mean that a cohort study determines if there is a factor exposure/disease incidence relationship?
2. What does it mean that a cohort study can be concurrent and nonconcurrent? Can you distinguish them?
3. What is a historical cohort study?
4. Do you know the definitions of terms in bold print in this chapter?
5. If given an example of a cohort study, could you recognize the five steps of problem solving?
6. Do you know the answers to the following chapter activity questions based on objectives from Healthy People 2010 focus areas 21 and 22?

WEB SITE RESOURCES

The Centre for Longitudinal Studies, Institute of Education, Great Britain, is responsible for two of Britain's birth cohort studies
<http://www.cls.ioe.ac.uk/Cohort/cstudie.html>

Established Populations for Epidemiologic Studies of the Elderly (EPESE), Duke University Center for the Study of Aging and Human Development
<http://www.geri.duke.edu/research/epese.html>

The Framingham Heart Study, American Heart Association
<http://www.americanheart.org/>

George Washington University School of Public Health and Health Services, Evaluating the Health Research Literature: The Uniform Framework for Cohort Studies
<http://learn.gwumc.edu/sphhs/sstt/cohort.htm>

The Henry F. Jackson Foundation for the Advancement of Military Medicine, Millennium Cohort Study
<http://www.millenniumcohort.org/>

Multicenter AIDS Cohort Study (MACS), Johns Hopkins University School of Public Health
<http://www.statepi.jhsph.edu/macs/macs.html>

NYU Women's Health Study, NYU School of Medicine Department of Environmental Medicine
<http://www.med.nyu.edu/Biostat-Epi/homepage.htm>

REFERENCES

GWU (1999). *Evaluating the Health Research Literature: The Uniform Framework for Cohort Studies.* Washington, DC: George Washington University School of Public Health and Health Services, The George Washington University Medical Center. Accessed online: <http://learn.gwumc.edu/sphhs/sstt/cohort.htm>.

Healthy People 2010 (2000). *Healthy People 2010: Objectives for improving health.* Washington, DC: Office of Disease Prevention and Health Promotion, U.S. Department of Health and Human Services.

Ismail, A.I. and Sohn, W.A. (1999). A systematic review of clinical diagnostic criteria of early childhood caries. *Journal of Public Health Dentistry* 59(3): 171-191.

Kannel, W.B., Dawber, T.R., and McGee, D.L. (1980). Perspectives on systolic hypertension, the Framingham Study. *Circulation* 61: 1179-1182.

Leitzmann, M.F., Willett, W.C., Rimm, E.B., Stampfer, M.J., Spiegelman, D., Colditz, G.A., and Giovannucci, E. (1999). Recreational physical activity and the risk of cholecystectomy in women. *New England Journal of Medicine* 341: 777-784.

Mausner, J.S. and Kramer, S. (1985). *Epidemiology: An introductory text.* Philadelphia, PA: W.B. Saunders.

NYU (1999). NYU Women's Health Study, NYU School of Medicine Department of Environmental Medicine. Accessed online: <http://www.med.nyu.edu/Biostat-Epi/homepage.htm>.

Timmreck, T.C. (1998). *An introduction to epidemiology* (Second edition). Boston, MA: Jones and Bartlett Publishers.

Purpose: (1) to acquaint the reader with Healthy People 2010 targets for improvement and (2) present examples of epidemiology as the underlying science to health promotion and disease prevention.

Directions: Check out your knowledge of these Healthy People 2010 focus areas by taking the following tests (answers follow in a separate section).

FOCUS AREA 21: ORAL HEALTH

This focus area's goal is to prevent and control oral and craniofacial diseases, conditions, and injuries, and to improve access to related services.

21-1. *Reduction in the proportion of children and adolescents who experience dental caries in their primary or permanent teeth.* Related to this objective, all of the following are correct except:
   a. Dental caries is the second most common chronic disease of childhood following asthma, which is the first most common.
   b. About half of all children have a dental caries experience by second grade.
   c. About 80 percent of students completing high school have had a dental caries experience.
   d. A dental caries experience can be prevented, but once it develops it is irreversible.

21-2. *Reduction in the proportion of children, adolescents, and adults with untreated dental decay.* What is the targeted proportion of adolescents and adult persons with untreated dental decay?
   a. 15 percent
   b. 35 percent

c. 55 percent
d. 75 percent

21-3. *Increase in the proportion of adults who have never had a permanent tooth extracted because of dental caries or periodontal disease.* As of 1988-1994, what proportion of adults have never had a tooth extraction because of caries or disease?
a. 11 percent
b. 31 percent
c. 51 percent
d. 71 percent

21-4. *Reduction in the proportion of older adults who have had all their natural teeth extracted.* As of 1997, what proportion of older adults have had all natural teeth extracted?
a. 20 percent
b. 40 percent
c. 60 percent
d. 80 percent

21-5. *Reduction in periodontal disease.* Related to this objective, what is periodontal disease?
a. An infectious disease that results in demineralization and ultimately cavitation of the tooth surface if not controlled or remineralized.
b. An inflammatory condition of the gum tissue, which can appear red and swollen and bleeds frequently and easily.
c. A disease caused by bacterial infections and resulting in inflammatory responses and chronic destruction of the soft tissues and bone that support the teeth.
d. A congenital opening or fissure occurring in the lip or palate.

21-6. *Increase in the proportion of oral and pharyngeal cancers detected at the earliest stage.* Related to this objective, all of the following are correct except:
a. Whether a person's oral/pharyngeal cancer was detected during early or late stages of the disease, the five-year survival rate is about the same.

b. The proportion of oral/pharyngeal cancer cases detected during early stage is low, about 35 percent.

c. Only 19 percent of African Americans with oral/pharyngeal cancers are diagnosed during early stage compared to 38 percent of whites.

d. Oral/pharyngeal cancers primarily affect adults over age fifty-five.

21-7. *Increase in the proportion of adults who, in the past twelve months, report having had an examination to detect oral and pharyngeal cancers.* As of 1998, what proportion of adults reported having had an oral/pharyngeal cancer examination within the past year?

a. 13 percent
b. 33 percent
c. 53 percent
d. 73 percent

21-8. *Increase in the proportion of children who have received dental sealants on their molar teeth.* What is the targeted proportion of children receiving molar teeth sealants?

a. 25 percent
b. 50 percent
c. 75 percent
d. 100 percent

21-9. *Increase in the proportion of the U.S. population served by community water systems with optimally fluoridated water.* As of 1992, what percent of community water systems were optimally fluoridated?

a. 22 percent
b. 42 percent
c. 62 percent
d. 82 percent

21-10. *Increase in the proportion of children and adults who use the oral health care system each year.* As of 1996, what proportion of persons visited a the dentist during the previous year?

a. 24 percent
b. 44 percent
c. 64 percent
d. 84 percent

21-11. *Increase in the proportion of long-term care residents who use the oral health care system each year.* What is the targeted proportion of long-term care residents using this system?
   a. 5 percent
   b. 25 percent
   c. 45 percent
   d. 65 percent

21-12. *Increase in the proportion of low-income children and adolescents who received any preventive dental service during the past year.* Related to this objective, which of the following is correct?
   a. As of 1993, only about 20 percent of Medicaid eligible children received any preventive dental services.
   b. Lower-income children have higher caries rates than higher-income children.
   c. Children from low-income households have more unmet dental treatment needs those from higher income households.
   d. All of the above are correct.

21-13. *Increase in the proportion of school-based health centers with an oral health component (developmental).* All of the following are correct except:
   a. A school-based health center is given permission by parents to oversee the provision of health education, preventive services, and treatment services to children.
   b. School-based health centers have been increasing in numbers nationwide.
   c. Many school-based health centers include an oral health component.
   d. School-based oral health preventive services would be fluoride mouth rinses or tablets and dental sealants.

21-14. *Increase in the proportion of local health departments and community-based health centers, including community, migrant, and homeless health centers, that have an oral health component.* As of 1997, what proportion of community-based health programs offer oral health services?
   a. 14 percent
   b. 34 percent

c. 54 percent
d. 74 percent

21-15. *Increase in the number of states and the District of Columbia that have a system for recording and referring infants and children with cleft lips, cleft palates, and other craniofacial anomalies to craniofacial anomaly rehabilitative teams.* Related to this objective, what does craniofacial mean?
a. An unusual condition existing at, and usually before, birth
b. A condition characterized by having one or more natural teeth
c. Pertaining to the head and face
d. A condition characterized by not having any natural teeth

21-16. *Increase in the number of states and the District of Columbia that have an oral and craniofacial health surveillance system.* As of 1999, how many states have such a surveillance system?
a. 0 percent
b. 20 percent
c. 40 percent
d. 60 percent

21-17. *Increase in the number of tribal, state (including the District of Columbia), and local health agencies that serve jurisdictions of 250,000 or more persons that have in place an effective public dental health program directed by a dental professional with public health training (developmental).* Related to this objective, which of the following is correct?
a. Improving the health and quality of life for communities relies on population-based preventive programs and the public and private capacity to provide needed care.
b. The capability to provide services depends on an adequate infrastructure at the tribal, state, and local health department levels.
c. Dental professionals in leadership positions who have public health training are needed in tribal, state, and local health departments to implement necessary oral health programs.
d. All of the above are correct.

FOCUS AREA 22:
PHYSICAL ACTIVITY AND FITNESS

This focus area's goal is to improve health, fitness, and quality of life through daily physical activity.

Physical Activity in Adults

22-1.   *Reduction in the proportion of adults who engage in no leisure-time physical activity.* As of 1997, what proportion of adults engaged in no leisure-time physical activity?
a. 20 percent
b. 40 percent
c. 60 percent
d. 80 percent

22-2.   *Increase in the proportion of adults who engage regularly, preferably daily, in moderate physical activity for at least 30 minutes per interval.* What is considered moderate physical activity?
a. Rhythmic, repetitive physical activities that use large muscle groups at 70 percent or more of maximum heart rate for age
b. Jogging/running, lap swimming, "spinning," aerobic dancing, skating, rowing, jumping rope, cross-country skiing, hiking/backpacking, racquet sports, and competitive group sports
c. Activities that use large muscle groups and are at least equivalent to brisk walking
d. Being relatively inactive and having a characteristic lifestyle which includes a lot of sitting

22-3.   *Increase in the proportion of adults who engage in vigorous physical activity that promotes the development and maintenance of cardiorespiratory fitness three or more days per week for 20 or more minutes per occasion.* What is the targeted proportion of adults to engage in weekly vigorous physical activity?
a. 10 percent
b. 30 percent

    c. 50 percent

    d. 70 percent

Muscular Strength/Endurance and Flexibility

22-4.   *Increase in the proportion of adults who perform physical activities that enhance and maintain muscular strength and endurance.* As of 1998, what proportion of persons do not engage in sufficient muscular strength and endurance activities?

    a. 22 percent

    b. 42 percent

    c. 62 percent

    d. 82 percent

22-5.   *Increase in the proportion of adults who perform physical activities that enhance and maintain flexibility.* Related to this objective, which of the following is correct about flexibility?

    a. Flexibility is improved through stretching exercises such as static stretching, yoga, or T'ai Chi Chuan.

    b. Flexibility can improve the ability to perform tasks of daily living.

    c. Lack of joint flexibility can reduce quality of life and possibly lead to eventual disability.

    d. All of the above are correct.

Physical Activity in Children and Adolescents

22-6.   *Increase in the proportion of adolescents who engage in moderate physical activity for at least 30 minutes on five or more of the previous seven days.* Related to this objective, all of the following are correct except:

    a. The health benefits of moderate and vigorous physical activity are not limited to adults.

    b. Physical activity among children and adolescents is important because of the related health benefits and because a physically active lifestyle adopted early in life may continue into adulthood.

    c. Many children are physically active and their physical activity increases during adolescence.

  d. Even among children aged three to four years, those who were less active tended to remain less active after age three than most of their peers.

22-7. *Increase in the proportion of adolescents who engage in vigorous physical activity that promotes cardiorespiratory fitness three or more days per week for twenty or more minutes per occasion.* As of 1999, what proportion of adolescents engaged in vigorous physical activity?
  a. 5 percent
  b. 25 percent
  c. 45 percent
  d. 65 percent

22-8. *Increase in the proportion of the nation's public and private schools that require daily physical education for all students.* As of 1994, what percent of U.S. middle and secondary schools required daily physical education for students?
  a. Middle, 17 percent; secondary, 2 percent
  b. Middle, 37 percent; secondary, 22 percent
  c. Middle, 57 percent; secondary, 42 percent
  d. Middle, 77 percent; secondary, 62 percent

22-9. *Increase in the proportion of adolescents who participate in daily school physical education.* As of 1999, what proportion of adolescents participated in daily physical education at school?
  a. 9 percent
  b. 29 percent
  c. 49 percent
  d. 69 percent

22-10. *Increase in the proportion of adolescents who spend at least 50 percent of school physical education class time being physically active.* In 1999, what proportion of adolescents were physically active during at least half of the physical education class?
  a. 18 percent
  b. 38 percent
  c. 58 percent
  d. 78 percent

22-11. *Increase in the proportion of adolescents who view television two or fewer hours on a school day.* What is the targeted proportion of adolescents spending two of less hours in front of the television on school days?
a. 25 percent
b. 50 percent
c. 75 percent
d. 100 percent

Access

22-12. *Increase in the proportion of the nation's public and private schools that provide access to their physical activity spaces and facilities for all persons outside of normal school hours— that is, before and after the school day, on weekends, and during summer, and other vacations (developmental).* Related to this objective, which of the following is correct?
a. Participation in regular physical activity depends, in part, on the availability and proximity of community facilities and on environments conducive to physical activity.
b. The use of a physical activity facility generally increases as facility distance from a person's residence increases.
c. People are more likely to use community resources located a few minutes away by biking or walking than a few miles away.
d. All of the above are correct.

22-13. *Increase in the proportion of work sites offering employer-sponsored physical activity and fitness programs.* As of 1998-1999, what proportion of work sites offered these programs?
a. 6 percent
b. 26 percent
c. 46 percent
d. 66 percent

22-14. *Increase in the proportion of trips made by walking.* Related to this objective, all of the following are correct except:
a. People prefer walking travel for over 75 percent of all trips less than 1 mile.

b. The number of walking trips as a percentage of all trips taken (of any distance) has declined over the years.
c. Walking trips made by adults has dropped from 9.3 percent in 1977 to 5.4 percent in 1995.
d. Walking has declined even more so for children.

22-15. *Increase in the proportion of trips made by bicycling.* As of 1995, what proportion of trips of five miles or less (for adults) was made by bicycling?
a. 0.6 percent
b. 10.6 percent
c. 20.6 percent
d. 30.6 percent

TEST ANSWERS

Focus Area 21

21-1.   (a) Dental caries is the second most common chronic disease of childhood following asthma, which is the first most common. This is incorrect. Dental caries is the single most common chronic disease of childhood, occurring five to eight times as frequently as asthma, the second most common chronic disease in children. Between 1988-1994, 18 percent of children aged two to four years had dental caries experiences. The target is to reduce to 11 percent of this age group having a dental caries experience.

21-2.   (a) 15 percent. This is the target for all adolescents and adults, but it is higher for younger persons. As of 1988-1994, the baseline proportions of untreated dental decay were: younger children ages two to four, 16 percent; older children ages six to eight, 29 percent; adolescents age fifteen, 20 percent; and adults ages thirty-five to forty-four, 27 percent. The target for younger children is 9 percent, and for older children it is 21 percent.

21-3.   (b) 31 percent. The target is 42 percent of adults aged thirty-five to forty-four years never having a permanent tooth extracted because of dental caries or periodontal disease. A full dentition is defined as having twenty-eight natural teeth, exclusive of third molars and teeth removed for orthodontic treatment or as a result of trauma. Most persons can keep their teeth for life with optimal personal, professional, and population-based preventive practices.

21-4.   (a) 20 percent. As of 1997, 26 percent of adults aged sixty-five to seventy-four years had lost all their natural teeth. This condition can factor into psychological, social, and physical impairments. Even with dentures, individuals might experience speech, chewing ability, taste perception, and quality of life limitations.

21-5.   (c) A disease caused by bacterial infections and resulting in inflammatory responses and chronic destruction of the soft tissues and bone that support the teeth. Periodontal disease is a broad term encompassing several diseases of the gums and tissues supporting the teeth. Dental caries is the demineralization and cavitation of the teeth. Gingivitis is an inflammation of the gum causing swelling, reddening, and bleeding. Cleft lip or palate is a condition at birth in which the lip or palate has an opening or fissure.

21-6.   (a) Whether a person's oral/pharyngeal cancer was detected during early or late stages of the disease, the five-year survival rate is about the same. This is incorrect. Early stage detection is most likely responsible for an 81 percent five-year survival rate, whereas late stage detection is related to the 22 percent five-year survival rate. All of the other responses are correct. As of 1990 to 1995, the baseline was 35 percent of oral and pharyngeal cancers were detected during stage I, localized (early stage). The target is for 50 percent of these cancers to be detected early.

21-7.   (a) 13 percent. It is important to detect these types of cancers early because they can result in substantial illness and disfigurement, significant cost, and the loss of 8,000 lives annually. The target proportion is 20 percent of adults aged forty years and older reporting having had an oral and pharyngeal cancer examination within the past year.*

21-8.   (b) 50 percent. For the past thirty years there has been a dramatic decrease in dental caries due to fluoride exposure. Now most caries occur in molar teeth with pits and fissures, hence the need for increased application of sealants. As of 1994, the baseline percentage of those receiving molar teeth sealants was 23 percent for children eight years old, and 15 percent for adolescents fourteen years old.

21-9.   (c) 62 percent. Community water fluoridation is the adjustment of the natural fluoride concentration of a community's water supply to a level that is best for the prevention of dental decay. The target is 75 percent of the U.S. population being served by community water systems having optimally fluoridated water.

21-10.   (b) 44 percent. This is the percent of persons aged two years and older making a yearly dentist visit. The target is an increase to 56 percent. Regular dental visits provide an oppor-

---

*Ages adjusted to the year 2000 standard population.

tunity for the early diagnosis, prevention, and treatment of oral health diseases and other morbid conditions as well as for ensuring good self-care practices.

21-11. (b) 25 percent. As of 1997, only 19 percent of all nursing home residents received dental services. More data need to be collected on the status of this health concern. Apparently, the oral health needs of this population are unmet due to a number of factors, such as the residents having a number of other chronic diseases that might interfere with oral health practices. It is important that this population receive regular dental care because they might be taking medications that compromise their oral health.

21-12. (d) All of the above are correct. Coverage for pediatric dental services is covered by Medicaid and state children's health insurance programs, but still, lower income children have poor oral health and receive fewer services than those from higher incomes. As of 1996, only 20 percent of children and adolescents under age nineteen years at or below 200 percent of the federal poverty level received any preventive dental service. The target is for 57 percent of this population to receive such services.

21-13. (c) Many school-based health centers include an oral health component. This is incorrect. Although school-based health centers have been increasing in numbers nationwide, a low number of them provide preventive oral health services.

21-14. (b) 34 percent. The target is 75 percent of local jurisdictions and health centers having oral health components that typically provide services to socioeconomically disadvantaged persons.

21-15. (c) Pertaining to the head and face. As of 1997, twenty-three states and the District of Columbia had systems for recording and referring children with craniofacial anomalies, such as cleft lips and palates. The target is for all states and the District of Columbia to institute such systems.

21-16. (a) 0 percent. The target is for all states and the District of Columbia to have surveillance systems. These systems help to assess oral health needs and determine trends in oral diseases. This is the basis for program implementation and evaluation.

21-17.   (d) All of the above are correct. In 1999, only twenty-nine states had full-time state dental directors; fourteen states had part-time directors; and eight states had no director. At the local level, about two-thirds of health departments have a dental program.

Focus Area 22

22-1.   (b) 40 percent. For most, the best opportunity to be physically active is during leisure time. The target is to reduce this percentage to 20 percent of adults aged eighteen years and older who engage in no leisure time physical activity.

22-2.   (c) Activities that use large muscle groups and are at least equivalent to brisk walking. Examples are swimming, cycling, dancing, gardening and yardwork, and various domestic and occupational activities. Preferably, moderate physical activity should last at least thirty minutes a day, but the equivalent is intermittent physical activity in three ten-minute sessions daily. The baseline in 1997 was 15 percent of adults aged eighteen years and older engaged in moderate physical activity for at least thirty minutes five or more days per week, and the target is to increase to 30 percent.

22-3.   (b) 30 percent. Whereas moderate physical activity reaps benefits such as caloric expenditure, improved cardiovascular efficiency, muscular strength gains, and better flexibility, even greater health benefits can be gained through vigorous physical activity. Engaging in moderate physical activity for at least thirty minutes per day will help ensure that sufficient calories are burned to provide health benefits. As of 1997, 23 percent of adults aged eighteen years and older engaged in vigorous physical activity three or more days per week for twenty or more minutes per occasion.

22-4.   (d) 82 percent. Muscular strength and endurance activities would be weight training and resistance activities (e.g., using elastic bands or dumbbells). The baseline was 18 percent of adults aged eighteen years and older who performed physical activities that enhance and maintain strength and endurance two or more days per week, and the target is an increase to 30 percent.

22-5. (d) All of the above are correct. At first, flexibility might appear to be a minor component of physical fitness. However, the consequence of rigid joints affects all aspects of life, including walking, stooping, sitting, avoiding falls, and driving a vehicle. The 1998 baseline was 30 percent of adults aged eighteen years and older did stretching exercises in the past two weeks, and the target is to increase to 43 percent.

22-6. (c) Many children are physically active and their physical activity increases during adolescence. This is incorrect since many children are less physically active than recommended, and physical activity declines during adolescence. The 1999 baseline was 27 percent of students in grades nine through twelve engaged in moderate physical activity for at least thirty minutes on five or more of the previous seven days, and the target is to increase that number to 35 percent.

22-7. (d) 65 percent. The target is to increase to 85 percent of students in grades nine through twelve engaged in vigorous physical activity three or more days per week for twenty or more minutes per occasion.

22-8. (a) Middle, 17 percent; secondary, 2 percent. Middle comprises junior and generally represents grades six through nine, whereas secondary can be grades nine through twelve. The target is to increase to 25 percent of middle schools and 5 percent of secondary schools requiring daily physical education for students. This objective relates to a physical education requirement and not an elective.

22-9. (b) 29 percent. The target is for 50 percent of students in grades nine through twelve to participate in daily school physical education. Participating in school physical education ensures a minimum amount of physical activity and fosters learning experiences that develop into practices, which can be continued into adulthood.

22-10. (b) 38 percent. The target is for 50 percent of students in grades nine through twelve who are physically active in physical education class for more than twenty minutes, three to five days per week. This is a feasible target and should be pursued since it would provide a substantial portion of the recommended physical activity time for adolescents. This includes adaptive physical education for students with disabilities.

22-11. (c) 75 percent. As of 1999, the baseline was 57 percent of students in grades nine through twelve viewed television two or fewer hours per school day. In fact, about 25 percent of students spend at least four hours daily in front of the television.

22-12. (a) Participation in regular physical activity depends, in part, on the availability and proximity of community facilities and on environments conducive to physical activity. The other responses are incorrect. The greater the distance by driving, the less likely the facility will be used. Interestingly, people are more likely to use a facility if they can drive rather than walk or bike to it.

22-13. (c) 46 percent. The target is for 75 percent of work sites with fifty or more employees to offer physical activity and/or fitness programs at the work site or through their health plans. These programs can reach large numbers of persons and have demonstrated the ability to increase fitness levels, at least in the short term. There is also evidence of cost effectiveness.

22-14. (a) People prefer walking travel for over 75 percent of all trips less than one mile. This is incorrect because people prefer automobile travel to walking. Walking is a very popular form of physical activity in the U.S., yet people need the opportunity to walk safely. The declines in walking by persons of all ages have negative health implications.

22-15. (a) 0.6 percent. For adolescents biking to school two miles or less, it was 2.4 percent. The target for adults is an increase to 2.0 percent of trips, and for adolescents an increase to 5.0 percent of trips. Bearing in mind the need for safe conditions during travel, bicycling may be used by both children and adults for distances that may not be feasible, practical, or efficient to cover on foot.

Chapter 12

Trials

EPIDEMIOLOGICAL TRIALS

Trials are experimental studies on the effectiveness of interventions designed to treat or prevent disease. Sometimes a trial is called an intervention study because it is designed to test a hypothesized cause-effect relationship by modifying a causal factor in a group or population. A trial can be classified according to the level of prevention within which it operates. If primary prevention is the focus, then the study is considered a **prophylactic trial,** which targets subjects at low health risk. An **interventive trial,** by contrast, operates at the secondary level of prevention and targets subjects who are at high health risk. If treatment is the focus, a **therapeutic trial** is conducted since it operates at the tertiary level of prevention and targets persons who are cases of the disease (see Figure 12.1).

Trials are also distinguished by their subjects. A **clinical trial** considers individual persons among its subjects. Clinical trials are often designed to test new drugs, vaccines, and medical treatments. Accordingly, if the subject is a group of persons, it is deemed a community trial. **Community trials** are conducted to test the effectiveness of educational and clinical service programs in a defined population. The results of both clinical and community trials are applied to preventive health services (see Figure 12.2).

Trials	Levels of Prevention
Prophylactic	• Primary—low health risk
Interventive	• Secondary—high health risk
Therapeutic	• Tertiary—disease case

FIGURE 12.1. Trials and levels of prevention (*Source:* Adapted from Lilienfeld and Stolley, 1994, p. 157)

Trials	Subject	Examples
Clinical	Individual	New drugs and treatments
Community	Groups	Risk reduction programs

FIGURE 12.2. Trials and subjects (*Source:* Adapted from Lilienfeld and Stolley, 1994, p. 157)

Similar to analytic studies, trials can be used to determine causal relationships and their results can directly infer causality. That is because the research design within an epidemiological trial is more rigorous than within an analytic study. It controls for the unwanted influences of variables other than the intervention—be it a kind of treatment or program. Subjects are usually randomly selected from a population and then randomly assigned to either a treatment or control group. Many times a comparison group is used in lieu of a control. Unlike analytic studies, the intent of a trial is to determine if an intervention can effect change in a person, group, or population. Hence, the focus of the study is on change brought about by an intervention rather than determining the cause of disease.

Steps for conducting a clinical trial have been presented by Lilienfeld and Stolley (1994, p. 160):

- Develop study's rationale and background
- Generate study's objectives
- Present a concise statement regarding study's design
- Set criteria for subject selection and assignment
- Outline procedure for the treatment and within this define the methods (clinical, etc.)
- Assure data integrity
- Determine how outcomes will be measured
- Prepare for side effects in subjects
- Decide how to address problem cases
- Secure human subject review approval
- Arrange periodic review of the trial's progress
- Set up means of analyzing data and interpreting findings
- Establish means of communicating results to all interested professionals

---

The Tamoxifen Clinical Trial

Since 1994, an interventive clinical trial has been under way involving 11,000 U.S. and Canadian women taking either **tamoxifen,** an anti-estrogen drug for treating and preventing breast malignancy, or a placebo daily. The trial is set to conclude in 2003. Researchers hypothesized that when two groups are compared in 1999 and later years, the number of breast cancer cases will have been reduced by one-third in the tamoxifen treatment group. By 1999, the observed incidence of breast cancer cases was 15 percent less than expected in the treatment group. The subjects in the treatment group are at high risk for breast cancer: family history of breast cancer, personal history of breast biopsies, and age.

The trial does pose ethical challenges regarding tamoxifen side effects. By taking the powerful anticancer drug, the experimental group has a threefold increased risk of developing uterine cancer and life-threatening blood clots. Still, thousands of female subjects agreed to participate, realizing the potential benefit to themselves and to others. To address the increased uterine cancer risk, subjects are given annual endometrial biopsies to check for precancerous cell changes. All participants receive biannual breast and pelvic exams, blood tests, and an annual mammogram.

Epidemiologists recruited cancer-free female subjects who had twice the breast cancer risk compared to the general population. In response, approximately 97 percent of the subjects are white, middle-class, and well-educated—the same demographic profile that tends to volunteer for most clinical trials. One difference is that about one-third of the subjects have had hysterectomies, thus placing them at low risk for uterine cancer. Roughly 40 percent are below the age of fifty, and it has been easiest for the centers to attract pre-menopausal women with a strong family history of the disease (Herman, 1994; Landis, Murray, and Bolden, 2000).

This relates to Healthy People 2010 Objective 23-17: *Increase in the proportion of federal, tribal, state, and local public health agencies that conduct or collaborate on population-based prevention research* (Healthy People 2010, 2000, 23-20). (See Chapter 12 activities for more information.)

Problem-Solving Steps Within a Clinical Trial

As seen in previous chapters, there are generic problem-solving steps to conducting an investigation as well as a study. These steps can also be applied in an epidemiological trial:

1. *Determine the problem.* In response to the need to test a treatment or program, subjects are usually randomly selected from the population until a predetermined sample size has been met. The sample size is selected to ensure that the study has adequate

statistical power—that is, relationships between independent and dependent variables deemed statistically significant by researchers have a high probability of being actual relationships, rather than attributing the significance to chance occurrence. Subjects are usually randomly assigned to either the treatment/program group or control group.

2. *Study the problem.* Based on the results of analytic studies (e.g., case control and cohort), the researchers should have a pretty good idea as to the agents or risk factors of the disease. It is this relationship that will be intervened, meaning that the epidemiologists will want to introduce a treatment, an independent variable, that should nullify the influence of the agent or risk factor onto the dependent variable, the disease.

3. *Suggest a solution.* Epidemiologists generate a hypothesis, a logical expected influence of the introduced independent variable on the subjects, meaning that the treatment should reduce the incidence or prevalence of the dependant variable, the disease.

4. *Test the solution.* Epidemiologists implement the treatment and then collect and analyze pre- and postmeasurements of the dependent variable in either a quasi-experimental or experimental design. Quasiexperimental design means subject selection/assignment was nonrandom. Those not receiving the treatment are sometimes called the comparison group. The research lacks full control over the allocation and/or timing of the intervention. The experimental group does include subject randomness and utilizes a control group. Sometimes it is called a randomized controlled trial since individuals are randomly allocated; in some experiments (e.g., fluoridation of drinking water) whole communities have been (nonrandomly) allocated to experimental and control groups.

5. *Evaluate the solution.* Epidemiologists make a decision whether to accept the hypothesis. Essentially, they are deciding if the treatment works. Various techniques are used to reduce bias in the preceding steps. Besides randomization, **masking** may be necessary. Masking is the procedure intended to keep participants in a study from knowing some facts or observations that might bias or influence their actions or decisions regarding the study. That means the subjects and/or those conducting the

study do not know who received the treatment until the results are compiled. Of course, other techniques would need to be applied such as accuracy of measurement and consideration of other factors that might have inadvertently influenced the results of the study. Ethical concerns also need to be addressed, such as should a possibly beneficial treatment be withheld from a control (a patient in a clinical trial) in order to complete the study?

Clinical Trials for Exercise-Induced Asthma

Exercise-induced asthma (EIA) is a common condition impeding physical activity in persons of all ages. About 90 percent of people with chronic asthma display EIA. It is also likely to occur in persons with other allergies. Physicians advocate performing small-scale clinical trials to determine the appropriate treatment for individual patients. The physician gathers the patient's history to spot subtle EIA indicators, such as fatigue or poor athletic performance. A physical exam would rule out conditions that mimic EIA, such as respiratory distress. A pulmonary function test assesses the severity of the condition and establishes a baseline for treatment efficacy. The treatment could be better management of the exercise environment and warm-up routines. Several medications can help patients avoid symptoms and participate fully in activities. To determine the right regimen, a safe level of medication would be administered before exercise to see if EIA symptoms diminish during the workout. If the treatment has some effect, then the regimen would be increased accordingly. This research design is simple and practical and can be implemented during clinical practice. It does not determine if the patient has chronic asthma of which exercise is the antagonist or whether the person has solitary EIA. This is important because treatment is different for chronic asthma exacerbated by exercise versus solitary EIA. That is why the physician is careful in prescribing medications and relies heavily on before-and-after pulmonary function tests and on monitoring medical symptoms. Clinical trials of a greater scale (large number of patients) could be used for diagnostics and for determining the better clinical treatment (Lacroix, 1999).

This relates to Healthy People 2010 Objective 24-4: *Reduction in activity limitations among persons with asthma* (Healthy People 2010, 2000, 24-17). (See Chapter 12 activities for more information.)

Clinical Decision Making

Clinical decision making is the guiding principle in the treatment of disease and other morbid conditions. The clinician orders screenings, diagnostic tests, and procedures, ascertains a diagnosis, and then recommends appropriate clinical care. The decision making is based on necessary and essential choices. To implement this principle, clinicians are encouraged to frame a question and to create a decision tree. The decision tree is a valuable concept and involves assigning probabilities and utilities to the possible outcomes as well as performing a follow-up sensitivity analysis.

The following example best illustrates decision tree use. Epidemiologists wanted to answer the question, "Is walking during labor an effective treatment for ensuring less complicated labor/delivery and other maternal/fetal outcomes?" They conducted a clinical trial. The results indicated that walking during labor is no more effective than usual care for pregnant women during labor. This would be the basis of clinical decision making by obstetrical health care workers. The professional would likely inform pregnant women that walking was not necessary to ensure uncomplicated labor, delivery, and outcomes (Bloom et al., 1998). In fact, walking does not appear to worsen or lessen labor complications. Therefore, some of the outcomes would *not* be further considered in the clinical decision (e.g., by walking the labor conditions get worse, or by not walking the labor conditions get worse) (see Figure 12.3).

In another example, a clinical trial was staged to determine the more effective treatment for low back pain among three options: a physical therapy prescription, a chiropractic manipulation, or a patient education booklet (see Figure 12.4). Although there were some improvements in patients receiving either of the two therapies com-

Decision Tree

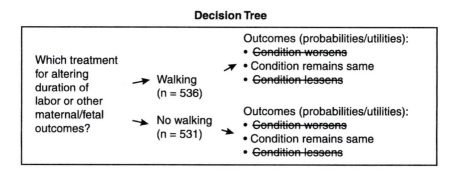

FIGURE 12.3. Decision tree applied to walking treatment during maternal labor (*Source:* Adapted from Timmreck, 1998, p. 362)

Decision Tree

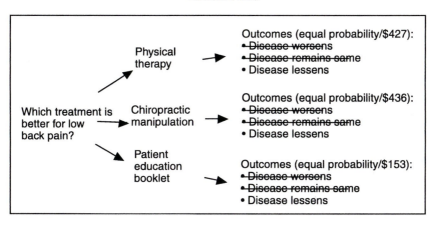

FIGURE 12.4. Decision tree applied to best treatment for low back pain (*Source:* Adapted from Timmreck, 1998, p. 362)

pared to the booklet, for the most part there were no statistically significant differences over time. The three kinds of treatment in this clinical trial had comparable effects on the patients. Therefore, the possible outcomes of the disease/condition getting worse or remaining the same are no longer considered (crossed out) in the decision, but rather each treatment seems to help lessen the condition somewhat. One overriding aspect of the treatment utility was patient satisfaction, of which a greater percentage of persons receiving therapies rated the care good to excellent. Another aspect of treatment utility was cost of treatment, of which the patient education was least expensive (Cherkin et al., 1998).

An important consideration during clinical decision making is minimizing error. For example, during a clinical trial of an experimental medication, the objective is to determine if the treatment is effective in reducing the clinical phase of a disease. During the trial, there are two determinations that can be made about the treatment: either it is effective or it is ineffective. For each of the two determinations there are two possible realities: the determination was correct, or the determination was incorrect. So there are actually four possible outcomes to a trial that must be considered during clinical decision making (see Figure 12.5). A clinician can determine whether a medicine is effective and can be either correct or incorrect in this decision. Likewise, a clinician can determine that a medicine is ineffective and can be either correct or incorrect in this decision.

Given the four possible outcomes, it stands to reason that a clinician wants to be correct in his or her decision making. Technically, the clinician wants to minimize the occurrence of error. The implications of this are vast. A clinician wants to avoid saying a medication is effective when in fact it is not—a false positive or Type I error. A clinician also wants to avoid saying that a medication is ineffective when in fact it is effective—a false negative or Type II error. A well-designed trial minimizes the likelihood of committing Type I or II errors by utilizing a proper subject sample size and strengthening the trial's measurement efforts to discern minimum treatment effectiveness.

Problem Solving Within a Community Trial

The community trial considers groups or communities as the subjects. Sometimes called a lifestyle intervention trial or field trial, entire communities are assigned to either treatment or control (or comparison) groups. There are a few reasons for such an epidemiological study. Perhaps the researchers find it difficult to select and assign individual subjects randomly. For instance, the researcher might not have access to individual students and instead has access to individual classes within a school building. Perhaps the factor under study, be it an agent or a risk, is not readily detectable, meaning that high-

Four Outcomes in a Clinical Trial		
Treatment effective:	Correct	Incorrect Type I error
Treatment ineffective:	Correct Type II error	Incorrect

FIGURE 12.5. Trial outcomes and possible errors (*Source:* Lilienfeld and Stolley, 1994, p. 161)

risk persons are difficult to identify. The epidemiologists would have to use more of a broad-brush approach to selecting subjects by recruiting groups rather than individual persons as subjects. Another compelling reason for a community trial is the opportunity to study a larger subject entity, which allows researchers to better generalize results to the overall population.

The stages within a community trial have been proposed by Lilienfeld and Stolley (1994, p. 181):

- Develop a protocol
- Select and recruit groups or communities to receive treatment or act as control (comparison)
- Establish baseline and community level surveillance systems
- Select and apply the treatment
- Oversee trial progress and monitor data collection analysis and interpretation
- Evaluate results

It would be repetitious to go through the problem-solving steps in a community trial, given how a clinical trial is performed. Rather, let's focus on the distinguishing features of the community trial. Simply put, the independent variable, such as a health education program, has to be uniformly applied to the treatment community and withheld from the comparison group. The treatment can be introduced as a mass media, extensive health education/services provision, or as enacted policy for citizen compliance. Of course, the hypothesis represents whether the introduced program or policy has an impact on the community receiving it. Dependent measures at pre- and postprogram stages are usually prevalence rates of disease or risk factors. The results of trials are applied to preventive health services.

A good example of a community trial is the Stanford Three Community Study during the 1970s. It was conducted as a prophylactic interventive trial to reduce risk factors to cardiovascular disease. One community was assigned a mass media health education campaign (e.g., health announcements on the six o'clock news) while another community received the same telecasts as well as invitations to participate in health education class sessions. A third community acted as a control. The most impressive finding was that there was a significant drop in the prevalence of tobacco smoking in the community that had the media health education classes, and about a third of citizens who stopped smoking stayed smoke-free a year after the study (Farquhar, 1978).

Another example of a community trial involved the introduction of fluoride into the municipal water supply of Kingston, New York, while the neighboring city, Newburgh, with its separate water supply, acted as a control. By the 1930s, it became known that fluoridated water was associated with decreased dental caries, especially in children and young adolescents. So by a flip of a coin, the Kingston water supply was selected to be fluoridated at a rate (or level) of one part per million. Over a ten-year period children were measured for decayed, missing, or filled teeth (DMF). The differences were statistically significant in that the Kingston children had a lower DMF index compared to the Newburgh youth (Lilienfeld and Stolley, 1994, pp. 5-7).

SUMMARY

The focus of an epidemiological trial can be prophylactic, interventive, or therapeutic. That is, a trial can test prevention efforts for persons at low or high risk for a disease, and it can test treatments for cases of disease. A trial can be clinical, in that it can be designed for individual persons acting as subjects. Accordingly, the trial can be a community trial wherein groups of persons act as the subjects. Trials are used to determine causal relationships between independent and dependent variables. The research design can be described according to the five problem-solving steps. Also, clinical decision making and its relationships to trials were discussed in so far as the clinician wants to be correct when determining the likely outcome of a particular prevention or treatment effort.

REVIEW QUESTIONS

1. What is an epidemiological trial and how is it similar to and different from an analytic study?
2. Do you know the definitions of terms in bold print throughout this chapter?
3. How can an epidemiological trial be classified?

4. If given an example, could you describe the problem-solving steps in a clinical trial? A community trial?
5. What is clinical decision making? What is its relationship to clinical trials? If given a description of a clinical trial, could you draw a decision tree and explain a clinician's decision-making options?
6. Can you distinguish between Type I and Type II errors and explain why a clinician wants to minimize committing either of these errors?
7. Do you know the answers to the following chapter activity questions based on objectives from Healthy People 2010 focus areas 23 and 24?

WEB SITE RESOURCES

Albert B. Sabin Vaccine Institute
<http://www.sabin.org/>

Center for AIDS Prevention Studies
<http://www.caps.ucsf.edu/>

The Cleveland Clinic, Clinical Trials
<http://www.clevelandclinic.org/>

Emory University, Clinical Cancer Trials
<http://www.winshipcancerinstitute/research/clinical_trials.htm>

National Cancer Institute, Cancer Trials
<http://cancer.gov/clinical_trials>

National Institutes of Health, Clinical Center
<http://www.cc.nih.gov/>

REFERENCES

Bloom, S.L., McIntire, D.D., Kelly, M.A., Beimer, H.L., Burpo, R.H., Garcia, M.A., and Leveno, K.J. (1998). Lack of effect of walking on labor and delivery. *New England Journal of Medicine* 339(2): 76-79.
Cherkin, D.C., Deyo, R.A., Battie, M., Street, J., and Barlow, W. (1998). A comparison of physical therapy, chiropractic manipulation, and provision of an educa-

tional booklet for the treatment of patients with low back pain. *New England Journal of Medicine* 339(15): 1021-1029.

Farquhar, J.W. (1978). The community-based model for cardiovascular health. *Lancet* 1: 1192-1195.

Healthy People 2010 (2000). *Healthy People 2010: Objectives for improving health.* Washington, DC: Office of Disease Prevention and Health Promotion, U.S. Department of Health and Human Services.

Herman, R. (1994). Tamoxifen on trial. *Washington Post* August 23, Health: 8-11.

Lacroix, V.J. (1999). Therapeutic trial for treating exercise-induced asthma. *The Physician and Sportsmedicine* 27(12): 1-6.

Landis, S.H., Murray, T., and Bolden, S. (2000). Cancer Statistics, 2000. *Cancer Journal for Clinicians* 50(1): 2398-2424.

Lilienfeld, D.E. and Stolley, P.D. (1994). *Foundations of epidemiology* (Second edition). New York: Oxford Press.

Timmreck, T.C. (1998). *An introduction to epidemiology,* (Second edition). Boston, MA: Jones and Bartlett Publishers.

Purpose: (1) to acquaint the reader with Healthy People 2010 targets for improvement and (2) present examples of epidemiology as the underlying science to health promotion and disease prevention.

Directions: Check out your knowledge of these Healthy People 2010 focus areas by taking the following tests (answers follow in a separate section).

FOCUS AREA 23:
PUBLIC HEALTH INFRASTRUCTURE

This focus area's goal is to ensure that federal, tribal, state, and local health agencies have the infrastructure to provide essential public health services effectively.

Data and Information Systems

23-1. *Increase in the proportion of tribal, state, and local public health agencies that provide Internet and e-mail access for at least 75 percent of their employees and that teach employees to use the Internet and other electronic information systems to apply data and information to public health practice (developmental).* As of 1999, what proportion of health departments had staff members who could search for and access public information on the Internet?
   a. 23 percent
   b. 43 percent
   c. 63 percent
   d. 83 percent

23-2. *Increase in the proportion of federal, tribal, state, and local health agencies that have made information available to the* public in the past year on the Leading Health Indicators, Health Status Indicators, and Priority Data Needs (developmental). Related to this objective, what are Leading Health Indicators?

a. A set of ten key determinants that influence health and can serve as a barometer for evaluating the health of the nation
b. Eighteen measures of health status defined in 1991 that represent a broad overview of a community's health and that can be used by various levels of government
c. Sixteen measures of status and risk behaviors of public health significance that were not included in the 1991 list of Health Status Indicators because of insufficient data at all levels of government
d. Twenty-eight focus areas of health promotion and disease prevention initiative for the nation

23-3.   *Increase in the proportion of all major national, state, and local health data systems that use geocoding to promote nationwide use of geographic information systems (GIS) at all levels.* Related to this objective, what is geocoding?

a. Connecting and interacting with learners through distributed learning resources that are separated by place and time
b. The process of address matching and assignment of a street address to a corresponding latitude and longitude
c. A health improvement plan comprised of action steps for providers of essential public health services in addressing problems and gaps that have been identified in a needs assessment
d. Research to identify effective public health prevention practices for particular populations

23-4.   *Increase in the proportion of population-based Healthy People 2010 objectives for which national data are available for all population groups identified for the objective.* What proportion of population-based objectives have available national databases?

a. 11 percent
b. 31 percent
c. 51 percent
d. 71 percent

23-5. *Increase in the proportion of Leading Health Indicators, Health Status Indicators, and Priority Data Needs for which data—especially for select populations—are available at the tribal, state, and local levels (developmental).* Considering each state has its own Healthy People plan, on the average what percentage of states' objectives had baseline data?
    a. 16 percent
    b. 36 percent
    c. 56 percent
    d. 76 percent

23-6. *Increase in the proportion of Healthy People 2010 objectives that are tracked regularly at the national level.* What is the targeted proportion of objectives that will be tracked regularly at the national level?
    a. 25 percent
    b. 50 percent
    c. 75 percent
    d. 100 percent

23-7. *Increase in the proportion of Healthy People 2010 objectives for which national data are released within one year of the end of data collection.* What is the targeted proportion of objectives whose national data are released within the year of collection?
    a. 25 percent
    b. 50 percent
    c. 75 percent
    d. 100 percent

Workforce

23-8. *Increase in the proportion of federal, tribal, state, and local agencies that incorporate specific competencies in the essential public health services into personnel systems (developmental).* Related to this objective, what is a competency essential to public health services?
    a. Knowing how to use information technology effectively for networking, communication, and access to information

    b. Being culturally and linguistically competent to understand the needs of and deliver services to select populations and to have sensitivity to diverse populations

    c. Having specialized knowledge in one or more areas of biostatistics, environmental and occupational health, social and behavioral aspects of health and disease, and preventive and clinical medicine

    d. All of the above

23-9. *Increase in the proportion of schools for public health workers that integrate into their curricula specific content to develop competency in the essential public health services (developmental).* Related to this objective, within which university schools are the graduate programs in public health?

    a. Nursing

    b. Environmental health

    c. Medicine, dentistry, and veterinary medicine

    d. All of the above

23-10. *Increase in the proportion of federal, tribal, state, and local public health agencies that provide continuing education to develop competency in essential public health services for their employees (developmental).* Related to this objective, which of the following is correct?

    a. There is an ongoing need to train and educate people employed in public health as new areas, problems, threats, and potential disasters emerge.

    b. Federal, tribal, state, and local public health agencies do not necessarily have to provide the education, but they need to ensure its availability to employees.

    c. Employees in organizations that are not formally part of the public health system but deliver health services also should have continuing education.

    d. All of the above are correct.

Public Health Organizations

23-11. *Increase in the proportion of state and local public health agencies that meet national performance standards for essential public health services (developmental).* Related to this objective, all of the following are correct except:

a. The measurement of performance is new to most health departments.
b. Comprehensive, systematic performance evaluation is not being done.
c. Standard performance indicators and systematic comparisons are useful in setting benchmarks for improvement.
d. National performance standards could be used to improve quality, increase accountability for dollars invested, and create credibility with internal and external constituents.

23-12. *Increase in the proportion of tribes, states, and the District of Columbia that have a health improvement plan and increase the proportion of local jurisdictions that have a health improvement plan linked with their state plan.* As of 1997, what proportion of states have a health improvement plan?
a. 18 percent
b. 38 percent
c. 58 percent
d. 78 percent

23-13. *Increase in the proportion of tribal, state, and local health agencies that provide or assure comprehensive laboratory services to support essential public health services (developmental).* Which would be such a service?
a. Laboratory quality assessment and improvement
b. Outbreak investigation
c. Laboratory-based surveillance
d. All of the above

23-14. *Increase in the proportion of tribal, state, and local public health agencies that provide or assure comprehensive epidemiology services to support essential public health services (developmental).* Related to this objective, what is epidemiology?
a. A formal process—which is the first step in a community health improvement process—of identifying problems and assessing the community's capacity to address health and social service needs
b. Research to identify effective public health prevention practices for particular populations

c. Branch of medical science dealing with the distribution and determinants of health-related events in specified populations and the application of this study to the control of health problems

d. The systematic application of information and computer science and technology to public health practice, research, and learning

23-15. *Increase in the proportion of federal, tribal, state, and local jurisdictions that review and evaluate the extent to which their statutes, ordinances, and bylaws assure the delivery of essential public health services (developmental).* Related to this objective, state and local health departments are usually authorized to enforce laws that:

a. Control diseases or classes of diseases

b. Limit certain kinds of businesses such as restaurants and health facilities

c. Monitor the treatment of waste materials such as sewage and garbage

d. All of the above

Resources

23-16. *Increase in the proportion of federal, tribal, state, and local public health agencies that gather accurate data on public health expenditures, categorized by essential public health service (developmental).* Related to this objective, which of the following is correct?

a. Financial resources fuel the public health infrastructure.

b. Understanding the nation's investment in public health and the origin and destination of these financial resources is critical.

c. To allocate resources appropriately and to ensure efficient performance, expenditures must be documented and explained.

d. All of the above are correct.

Prevention Research

23-17. *Increase in the proportion of federal, tribal, state, and local public health agencies that conduct or collaborate on population-based prevention research (developmental).* Related to this objective, which of the following is correct?
   a. Public health research is both funded and conducted by federal, state, and local public health agencies, academic institutions, private industry, and philanthropic institutions.
   b. Opportunities and incentives should be provided to attract new researchers and to encourage collaboration among federal agencies, states, local communities, and academic institutions.
   c. Collaboration between federal, state, and local constituents should result in a research agenda for the nation's public health infrastructure.
   d. All of the above are correct.

FOCUS AREA 24: RESPIRATORY DISEASES

This focus area's goal is to promote respiratory health through better prevention, detection, treatment, and education efforts.

Asthma

24-1. *Reduction in asthma deaths.* Related to this objective, which of the following is correct?
   a. The number of deaths annually from asthma is high compared to other chronic diseases.
   b. Death from asthma is two to six times more likely to occur among African Americans and Hispanics than among whites.
   c. The death rate for children and young adults had decreased by 50 percent in recent years.
   d. All of the above are correct.

24-2.   *Reduction in hospitalizations for asthma.* Related to this objective, effective asthma management is comprised of:
a. Controlling exposure to factors that trigger asthma-episodes
b. Adequately managing asthma with medicine
c. Monitoring the disease by using objective measures of lung function
d. All of the above

24-3.   *Reduction in hospital emergency department visits for asthma.* Which age group has the highest rate of asthma-related visits to the hospital emergency department?
a. Children under age five years
b. Children and adults aged five to sixty-four years
c. Adults aged sixty-five years and older
d. All age groups have same rate

24-4.   *Reduction in activity limitations among persons with asthma.* As of 1994-1996, what percentage of persons having asthma experienced activity limitations due to this condition?
a. 20 percent
b. 40 percent
c. 60 percent
d. 80 percent

24-5.   *Reduction in the number of school or work days missed by persons with asthma due to asthma (developmental).* Related to this objective, school and work absenteeism represent an indirect cost of asthma. Another example would be:
a. Caregiver costs
b. Travel and waiting time
c. Early retirement due to disability
d. All of the above

24-6.   *Increase in the proportion of persons with asthma who receive formal patient education, including information about community and self-help resources, as an essential part of the management of their condition.* What is the targeted proportion of persons with asthma receiving patient education?
a. 10 percent
b. 30 percent
c. 50 percent
d. 70 percent

24-7.   *Increase in the proportion of persons with asthma who receive appropriate asthma care according to the National Asthma Education and Prevention Program (NAEPP) guidelines (developmental).* Which is a guideline for receiving appropriate asthma care?
   a. Persons with asthma receiving written asthma management plans from their health care provider
   b. Persons with asthma with prescribed inhalers receiving instruction on how to use them properly
   c. Persons with asthma receiving education about recognizing early signs and symptoms of asthma episodes and how to respond appropriately
   d. All of the above

24-8.   *Establishment of, in at least twenty-five states, a surveillance system for tracking asthma death, illness, disability, impact of occupational and environmental factors on asthma, access to medical care, and asthma management (developmental).* Related to this objective, efforts directed at improving the environmental management of asthma include:
   a. Reducing exposure to allergens and irritants
   b. Reducing exposure to environmental tobacco smoke
   c. Reducing exposure to outdoor air pollution from ozone, sulfur dioxide, and particulate diesel matter
   d. All of the above

Chronic Obstructive Pulmonary Disease

24-9.   *Reduction in the proportion of adults whose activity is limited due to chronic lung and breathing problems.* As of 1997, what proportion of adults have respiratory problems that limit their activity?
   a. 2.2 percent
   b. 22.2 percent
   c. 42.2 percent
   d. 62.2 percent

24-10. *Reduction in deaths from chronic obstructive pulmonary disease (COPD) among adults.* How much of a reduction is targeted in deaths from COPD?
a. 25 percent
b. 50 percent
c. 75 percent
d. 100 percent

Obstructive Sleep Apnea

24-11. *Increase in the proportion of persons with symptoms of obstructive sleep apnea whose condition is medically managed (developmental).* Related to this objective, what is obstructive sleep apnea?
a. Abnormal permanent enlargement of the airspaces in the lungs accompanied by coughing and difficulty breathing
b. Shortness of breath
c. A condition characterized by snoring, partial or complete cessation of breathing during sleep, reductions in blood oxygen levels, severe sleep disruptions, and excessive daytime sleepiness
d. A lung disease characterized by airflow obstruction due to chronic bronchitis and emphysema

24-12. *Reduction in the proportion of vehicular crashes caused by persons with excessive sleepiness (developmental).* Related to this objective, what is the probability of a person with excessive sleepiness being involved in multiple vehicular crashes?
a. Two times more likely
b. Seven times more likely
c. Twelve times more likely
d. Seventeen times more likely

TEST ANSWERS

Focus Area 23

23-1. (d) 83 percent. Although this proportion is capable of using the Internet for work-related responsibilities, a smaller percentage actually have access.

23-2. (a) A set of ten key determinants that influence health and can serve as a barometer for evaluating the health of the nation. Leading health indicators include individual behaviors, the social and physical environment, and community health programs, and address areas that most influence the health of individuals, communities, and the nation. Health Status Indicators are the eighteen measures of health status defined in 1991 that represent a broad overview of a community's health that can be used by various levels of government. Priority Data Needs are the sixteen measures of health status and risk behaviors of public health significance that were not included in the 1991 list of Health Status Indicators because of insufficient data at all levels of government. Healthy People 2010 includes twenty-eight focus areas of health promotion and disease prevention initiative for the nation.

23-3. (b) The process of address matching and assignment of a street address to a corresponding latitude and longitude. Distance learning is connecting and interacting with learners through distributed learning resources that are separated by place and time. A health improvement plan comprises action steps for providers of essential public health services in addressing problems and gaps that have been identified in a needs assessment. Population-based prevention research is research to identify effective public health prevention practices for particular populations.

23-4. (a) 11 percent. More national data systems are needed to determine baseline and target rates and percentages that comprise many of the Healthy People 2010 objectives. These data can help determine if there are disparities between select groups within the population and if the nation is successful in bridging these gaps by year 2010.

23-5.   (d) 76 percent. Just like the national plan for Healthy People, each objective should have a baseline database. For the states, three-quarters of their objectives (operationalized to their respective populations) had baseline data.

23-6.   (d) 100 percent. Tracking should take place once every three years and only 66 percent of the Healthy People 2000 objectives met this criterion.* That is why it has been increased to 100 percent.

23-7.   (d) 100 percent. For Healthy People 2000 objectives, only 36 percent of the objectives met this criterion. Timeliness of data releases will be facilitated through greater use of electronic data systems.

23-8.   (d) All of the above. All of these competencies are essential in addition to having a basic knowledge of public health.

23-9.   (d) All of the above. A graduate program in public health is any academic postbachelor's degree program that specifically trains public health workers. Besides separate schools of public health, this discipline is also found in other university schools.

23-10. (d) All of the above are correct. An example of a possible area in which public health workers need continuing education and training is the threat of bioterrorism or the increased impact of any natural or technological disaster.

23-11. (a) The measurement of performance is new to most health departments. Measuring performance is not new, but comprehensive, systemic performance evaluation is. National organizations, such as the Joint Commission on Accreditation of Healthcare Organizations and the National Commission on Quality Assurance, have models for performance standards that can be used by the states and local jurisdictions.

23-12. (d) 78 percent. The target is for 100 percent of states and local public health organizations having a health plan articulated with local jurisdictions.

23-13. (d) All of the above. In addition, comprehensive laboratory services would involve emergency preparedness and response, population screening, and technology transfer. A national

*Healthy People 2000 information from the National Center for Health Statistics (2000). *Healthy People 2000 Review.* Bethesda, MD: Institutes of Health, U.S. Public Health Service.

laboratory network would benefit public health by helping assure safe water, food, and air, and by supporting programs such as newborn screening and lead-poisoning prevention.

23-14. (c) Epidemiology is a branch of medical science dealing with the distribution and determinants of health-related events in specified populations and the application of this study to the control of health problems. Needs assessment is the first step in a community health improvement process. Population-based prevention research identifies effective public health prevention practices for particular populations. Public health informatics is the systematic application of information, computer science, and technology to public health practice, research, and learning.

23-15. (d) All of the above. A review of state public health statutes shows significant variations among accepted frameworks of the essential public health services—a matter that is being addressed by this objective.

23-16. (d) All of the above are correct. Documenting finances will allow communities to identify gaps in expenditures that they can help fill, in partnership with public health agencies. State and local leaders need to know where gaps exist and how funding is changing to ensure that public health agencies can protect the nation's health.

23-17. (d) All of the above are correct. The federal government has a strong commitment to health research, as evidenced by the billions of dollars allocated to the National Institutes of Health, the Centers for Disease Control and Prevention, the Agency for Healthcare Research and Quality, the Health Resources and Services Administration, and other U.S. public health service agencies. State governments, private foundations, and private industry also are strong supporters of health research.

Focus Area 24

24-1. (b) Death from asthma is two to six times more likely to occur among African Americans and Hispanics than among whites. The other responses are incorrect. The number of annual deaths from asthma is low compared to other chronic diseases. The death rate for children and young adults has doubled in recent years.

24-2.   (d) All of the above. In addition, another component of effective asthma management is educating asthma patients to become partners in their own care.

24-3.   (a) Children under age five years. As of 1995-1997, the age group had a baseline rate of 150 per 10,000 hospital visits. The target is to reduce to 80 per 10,000 hospital visits.

24-4.   (a) 20 percent. The target is 10 percent persons with asthma experiencing activity limitations.*

24-5.   (d) All of the above. In addition, premature death accounts for about 50 percent of the total costs of asthma.

24-6.   (b) 30 percent. As of 1998, 8.4 percent of persons with asthma received formal patient education. Patients receiving asthma education in terms of self-management skills are better able to manage and control their disease than those not receiving this education.

24-7.   (d) All of the above. In addition, other guidelines involve persons with asthma who receive medications, need follow-up care, and require assistance in managing exposure to environmental risk factors.

24-8.   (d) All of the above. Working with local community groups to mobilize community resources for a comprehensive, culturally and linguistically competent approach to controlling asthma among high-risk populations is a priority. The states will need to track occupational and environmental factors that cause or trigger asthma episodes. Efforts will also have to be directed toward improving the environmental management of asthma.

24-9.   (a) 2.2 percent. This was the baseline for adults aged forty-five years and older experiencing activity limitations due to chronic lung and breathing problems. The target is to reduce to 1.5 percent.

24-10. (b) 50 percent. As of 1998 the baseline was 119.4 deaths from COPD per 100,000 persons aged forty-five years and older, and the target is a reduction to sixty deaths per 100,000 adults.

---

*Ages adjusted to the year 2000 standard population.

24-11. (c) Obstructive sleep apnea is characterized by snoring, partial or complete cessation of breathing during sleep, reductions in blood oxygen levels, severe sleep disruptions, and excessive daytime sleepiness. OSA is a chronic breathing problem with serious effects on individual health and productivity, including an inheritable risk of sudden infant deaths, behavior and learning disturbances, injury from accidents, and reduced quality of life. Emphysema is enlargement of the airspaces making breathing difficult. Shortness of breath is also known as dyspnea. Chronic obstructive pulmonary disease is a lung disease characterized by airflow obstruction due to chronic bronchitis and emphysema.

24-12. (b) Seven times more likely. Persons who have obstructive sleep apnea experience excessive sleepiness. In turn, excessive sleepiness increases the risk of multiple vehicular crashes sevenfold.

Chapter 13

Epidemiology and Programs

WHAT IS A PROGRAM?

A **program** is an organized response to undesirable health and disease conditions and situations. It is composed of three processes: planning, implementing, and evaluating. **Program planning** involves assessing the needs of a target group, persons to whom the program is directed. With needs identified, the program should be composed of goals and objectives, statements of the desired state of the target group, and steps toward that state. Thereafter, the intervention would be designed, which incorporates theory, activity, and necessary resources. **Program implementation** involves initiating and maintaining the intervention activity. This usually requires controlling the amount of activity and degree of participation until safe, efficient, and effective service delivery can be assured. During implementation, staff input is invited and participant feedback is encouraged regarding the quality of service delivery. This information can also be used as part of program evaluation. **Program evaluation** involves efforts at improving as well as proving the efficacy of the program. Evaluative efforts take place before, during, and after implementation. Through evaluation questions are being answered, such as how well the program was implemented, and whether the program achieved short-term and long-term success. To answer these questions, data are collected, analyzed, and reported.

Illustrative of our definitions of programs, Healthy People 2010 (2000, p. 1) is a nationwide program responding to undesirable health and disease conditions of Americans. Priority data needs have been identified and act as the basis in the establishment of the following leading health indicators used to measure the health of the nation over the next ten years:

- Physical activity
- Overweight and obesity
- Tobacco use
- Substance abuse
- Mental health
- Injury and violence
- Environmental quality
- Immunization
- Responsible sexual behavior
- Access to health care

Healthy People 2010 rests on two goals: (1) increasing the quality and years of healthy life, and (2) eliminating health disparities among different segments of the population. To reach these goals, 467 objectives, illustrative of program implementation efforts, act as targets within twenty-eight focus areas by design. Health promotion and disease prevention activity are directed at reaching these objectives by 2010. These activities will be undertaken at all levels in governmental agencies and among private nonprofit and for-profit organizations. Regular reviews, or program evaluations, of action and progress on the Healthy People 2010 objectives will be held throughout the 2000s based on DATA 2010, a data tracking system operated by the National Center for Health Statistics, Centers for Disease Control and Prevention (Healthy People 2010, 2000).

Healthy People 2010 is a macro health promotion and disease prevention program, which means it is designed for the general community (McKenzie and Smeltzer, 2001). Underlying its planning, implementation, and evaluation are the work and findings of epidemiologists. Surveillance helps to establish needs and evaluate if goals and objectives are reached. Health promotion and disease prevention activity is designed after successful efforts at investigating and studying diseases and other morbid conditions. Interventions specific to the twenty-eight focus areas have been researched and tested by epidemiologists (see Figure 13.1).

More and more communities are using community health planning processes to address the health and quality of living of their members. Examples of program planning modes include Assessment Protocol for Excellence in Public Health (APEX/PH), Healthy Cities, Healthy Communities, and Planned Approach to Community Health (PATCH)

Needs assessment	Goals and Objectives	Design	Implementation	Evaluation
Based on epidemiological surveillance systems of Healthy People 2010 Health Indicators	Based on Healthy People 2010 goals (2) and objectives (447)	Based on epidemiological investigations and studies, and Healthy People 2010 focus areas (28)	Based on health promotion and disease prevention activity by professionals, organizations, and coalitions	Based on interim review and achieving Healthy People 2010 goals and objectives

FIGURE 13.1. Health promotion and disease prevention programming

(Katz and Kreuter, 1997). For instance, the PATCH model is based on community organization principles such as coalition building. With local support, participation, and leadership, community members rely on local health data to determine their health problems, set goals and objectives, carry out interventions, and evaluate results. A team approach is used during which the people of the community work together with technical assistance from local and state health departments as well as the CDC. A good example of this collaborative model in action is the Commonwealth of Virginia's Turning Point Project. It consists of rethinking future roles and responsibilities for public health, improving knowledge and appreciation for community health, placing community health leaders and partners in a position to support information-based decision making, and insuring the commonwealth has a skilled workforce to perform core community health functions (VDH, 2000).

HIV Education for Teachers

A grant-funded project by the Virginia Department of Education was implemented through the state with the purpose of preparing school teachers and personnel to better meet the educational needs of their students regarding HIV. For two days, educational professionals attended lectures, listened to speakers, and participated in a variety of learning activities. The objectives of the training program were to increase participants' knowledge about HIV disease in school students, explore issues and examine attitudes toward HIV, and develop strategies for bringing sound HIV education into their schools. A measurement of HIV knowledge and attitudes was administered, demonstrating that participants had gains in knowledge and improvements in attitudes toward HIV disease in the school population (Miller and Hagaman, 1992).

This relates to Healthy People 2010 Objective 25-8: *Reduction in HIV infections in adolescent and young adult females aged 13 to 24 years that are associated with heterosexual contact* (Healthy People 2010, 2000, 25-23). (See Chapter 13 activities for more information.)

PREVENTION LEVELS DURING PROGRAMMING

Program planning, implementing, and evaluating should be seen as one continual process that can operate at various prevention levels. Data from health assessments and screenings such as health risk appraisals can be used to place persons in health risk categories. A person is considered at low health risk if his or her appraised age does not exceed chronological age. Moderate health risk is reached when his or her appraised age exceeds chronological age. High health risk is noted when the difference between appraised and chronological age is five or more years (Miller et al., 1990).

It is important to know these risk categories because they represent opportunities for disease prevention at the three prevention levels. A person at low heath risk is the most appropriate target for **primary level prevention** efforts, which include those that can prevent a health problem from occurring. **Secondary level prevention** focuses on persons at moderate health risk and takes places during the early stages of a health problem. It is important to note that many health screenings are designed to detect early stage health problems. **Tertiary level prevention** is directed at high health risk persons in late stages of a health problem. Cases of disease receive treatment and rehabilitation. During recovery, they are assisted in relapse prevention. These prevention levels represent strategies for changing health behaviors and improving health status.

Levels of prevention are also used to categorize health promotion and disease prevention activity. Examples of primary prevention include educating persons about the agents and risks of disease and other conditions, such as educating about how overnutrition contributes to the risk of hypertension. Other primary prevention activities include health care services, medical tests, counseling, health education, and other actions designed to prevent the onset of a targeted condition. Routine immunization of healthy individuals is another example of primary prevention.

Secondary prevention activities include screenings to detect risk factors to disease, for example, blood pressure screening for hypertension. Secondary prevention measures also include health care services designed to identify or treat individuals who have a disease or risk factors but who are not yet experiencing symptoms of the disease. Once a disease case has been diagnosed, tertiary prevention is applied through health care, which can include possible medication and lifestyle management counseling.

Tertiary prevention can include preventive health care measures or services that are part of treatment and management plans of persons with clinical illnesses. Examples of tertiary prevention include cholesterol reduction for patients with coronary heart disease and insulin therapy to prevent complications of diabetes (Pozzilli, 1996).

HEALTHY PEOPLE 2010 AND PREVENTION

As previously described, Healthy People 2010 has twenty-eight focus areas containing numerous objectives that pertain to primary, secondary, and tertiary prevention programming. The following examples come from all three areas of prevention programming.

Primary Prevention

7-5.   Increase the proportion of work sites that offer a comprehensive employee health promotion program to their employees (Healthy People 2010, 2000, 5-18).

9-11.   Increase the proportion of young adults who have received formal instruction before turning age eighteen years on reproductive health issues, including all of the following topics: birth control methods, safer sex to prevent HIV, prevention of sexually transmitted diseases, and abstinence (Healthy People 2010, 2000, 9-26).

16-7.   (Developmental) Increase the proportion of pregnant women who attend a series of prepared childbirth classes (Healthy People 2010, 2000, 16-28).

Secondary Prevention

3-10.   Increase the proportion of physicians and dentists who counsel their at-risk patients about tobacco use cessation, physical activity, and cancer screening (Healthy People 2010, 2000, 3-22).

12-11. Increase the proportion of adults with high blood pressure who are taking action (for example, losing weight, increasing physical activity, or reducing sodium intake) to help control their blood pressure (Healthy People 2010, 2000, 12-22).

28-11. (Developmental) Increase the proportion of newborns who are screened for hearing loss by age one month, have audiologic evaluation by age three months, and are enrolled in appropriate intervention services by age six months (Healthy People 2010, 2000, 28-14).

Tertiary Prevention

2-8. (Developmental) Increase the proportion of persons with arthritis who have had effective, evidence-based arthritis education as an integral part of the management of their condition (Healthy People 2010, 2000, 2-16).

4-3. Increase the proportion of treated chronic kidney failure patients who have received counseling on nutrition, treatment choices, and cardiovascular care twelve months before the start of renal replacement therapy (Healthy People 2010, 2000, 4-13).

5-1. Increase the proportion of persons with diabetes who receive formal diabetes education (Healthy People 2010, 2000, 5-12).

Each focus area in the Healthy People 2010 program contains a section on opportunities for achieving the objectives. The primary means of accomplishment is through programming at the three levels of prevention. Here are some selected examples:

- Educational and behavioral interventions can relieve symptoms and reduce disability. For example, arthritis self-help programming has been shown to reduce pain up to 20 percent beyond what was achieved through conventional medical care. It counters myths about arthritis and emphasizes applying available interventions that can help reduce the impact of this health problem (Lorig, Lubeck, and Kraines, 1985).
- Epidemiological evidence suggests that several types of cancer can be prevented through a healthy lifestyle and that the prospects for surviving cancer continue to improve (Greenwald, Kramer, and Weed, 1995). Various types of resources must be applied such as providing culturally and linguistically appropriate information on prevention, early detection, and treatment to the public and to health care professionals. There also has to be mechanisms or systems for providing people with access to state-of-the-art preventive services and treatment.
- As useful information is gathered by environmental epidemiologists on individual health risks due to environmental factors, new programs are under way to improve the management of en-

vironmental hazard exposure. One such effort is increasing public awareness of environmental health issues through Web sites operated by the National Institutes of Health and the EPA (NLOM, 2001).

- Since 1972, the National High Blood Pressure Education Program began public outreach and education efforts to reduce incidence of high blood pressure. Combined with state and local level initiatives, such as the American Heart Association, there has been a dramatic increase in the population's control of hypertension through lifestyle changes and antihypertensive medications. Whereas 16 percent of hypertensive persons were exhibiting control of their condition, the proportion has increased to 65 percent. Impressively, 90 percent of all adults have their blood pressure checked every two years, and the average blood pressure level per capita has fallen 10-12 mm/Hg since the 1970s (NCHS, 1998; Roccella and Horan, 1998).

- Programming to reduce HIV transmission will continue to focus on the disproportionate impact of HIV/AIDS among certain racial and ethnic groups as well as particularly high-risk and hard-to-reach persons such as injection drug users, homeless persons, runaway youth, mentally ill, and incarcerated persons. However, there is a growing emphasis on increasing the number of people who learn their HIV status in order to detect HIV infection when the potential for transmission is greatest and the need for prevention, care, and treatment, including HAART, is greatest. **HAART** is highly active antiretroviral therapy comprised of protease inhibitors and reverse transcriptase inhibitors whose purpose is to reduce HIV load infection to undetectable levels (UN, 1998).

- Many potentially effective culturally and linguistically competent intervention strategies for violence prevention exist, such as parent training, mentoring, home visitation, and education. Evaluation of ongoing programs is a major component to help identify effective approaches for violence prevention. The public health approach to violence prevention is multidisciplinary, encouraging experts from scientific disciplines, organizations, and communities to work together to find solutions to violence in the United States (NCIPC, 1999).

Project LIFE Targets Substance-Involved Youth

A U.S. Department of Education grant-funded project was implemented in rural school districts throughout upstate New York. Teachers, school personnel, and community agency representatives were invited to participate in an intensive five-day training program that addressed substance-involved youth. The program was initiated in response to the alarming numbers of school-age youth who are already substance involved. A variety of learning experiences was designed for the participants that encouraged knowledge and attitude growth opportunities. The participants also worked on action plans for their school districts. Examples were instituting no-tolerance policies in the school district, instructing colleagues on how to spot substance involvement, and becoming competent and confident in constructively confronting substance-abusing youth. Measurements of attitudes toward drug abuse indicated that over the span of the five-day workshop, the participants had significant gains in positive attitudes toward discouraging youth substance involvement (Metz and Miller, 1993, pp. 22-30).

This relates to Healthy People 2010 Objective 26-10: *Reduction in past-month use of illicit substances.* (Healthy People 2010, 2000, 26-25). (See Chapter 13 activities for more information.)

SUMMARY

This chapter examined programs, what comprises them, as well as various types and applications. Healthy People 2010 is an example of a nationwide program. Each program process, which includes planning, implementation, and evaluation, is based on epidemiolgical surveillance, investigation, and research. A program can operate at primary, secondary, and tertiary levels of prevention, based on the health risk of the target group. Refer to this chapter for examples of program applications based on Healthy People 2010 objectives and opportunities for improvement.

REVIEW QUESTIONS

1. What is a program? Can you identify and describe the three program processes? How is Healthy People 2010 a nationwide program? Can you explain how the Healthy People 2010 program processes are based on epidemiological surveillance, investigations, and studies?

2. How is health risk related to levels of prevention? What are the three risk categories and how is each determined? What are the three levels of prevention? Which risk category relates to which prevention level?
3. Can you explain what a primary prevention program is? Secondary prevention program? Tertiary prevention program? Can you provide examples?
4. Are you familiar with Healthy People 2010 objectives that relate to programming? Can you identify examples?
5. Do you know the answers to the following chapter activity questions based on objectives from Healthy People 2010 focus areas 25 and 26?

WEB SITE RESOURCES

Arizona Tobacco Use Prevention Plan
<http://www.tepp.org>

CDC National Prevention Information Network
<http://www.cdcnpin.org>

CDC's State Data on Health Status Indicators and Priority Data Needs
<http://www.cdc.gov/nchs>

National Committee for Quality Assurance
<http://www.NCQA.org/>

National Institute on Deafness and Other Communication Disorders, WISE EARS!
<http://www.nidcd.nih.gov/>

REFERENCES

Greenwald, P., Kramer, B., and Weed, D.L. (Eds.) (1995). *Cancer prevention and control.* New York: Marcel Dekker.

Healthy People 2010 (2000). *Healthy People 2010: Objectives for improving health*. Washington, DC: Office of Health Promotion and Disease Prevention, U.S. Department of Health and Human Services.

Katz, M.F. and Kreuter, M.W. (1997). Community assessment and empowerment. In F.D. Scutchfield and C.W. Keck (Eds.), *Principles of public health practice* (pp. 147-156). Albany, NY: Delmar Publishers.

Kost, K., Landry, D., and Darroch, J. (1998). The effects of pregnancy planning status on birth outcomes and infant care. *Family Planning Perspectives* 30(5): 223-230.

Lorig, K., Lubeck, D., and Kraines, R. (1985). Outcomes of self-help education for patients with arthritis. *Arthritis Rheumatism* 28(6): 680-685.

McKenzie, J.F. and Smeltzer, J.K. (2001). *Planning, implementing, and evaluating health promotion programs,* (Third edition). Boston: Allyn and Bacon.

Metz, G.J. and Miller, R.E. (1993). Drug attitudinal change in rural school personnel. *Wellness Perspectives* 10: 22-30.

Miller, R.E., Golaszewski, T.G., Pfieffer, G., and Edington, D.W. (1990). Significance of the lifestyle system to employee wellness and assistance. *Health Values* 14(1): 41-49.

Miller, R.E. and Hagaman, E. (1992). Comprehensive Health Education Teacher-Training Center. Richmond, VA: Commonwealth of Virginia, Department of Education.

NCHS (1998). *Health, United States, 1998*. Hyattsville, MD: National Center for Health Statistics.

NCIPC (1999). *Best practices for preventing violence by children and adolescents: A source book*. Atlanta, GA: National Center for Injury Prevention and Control, Centers for Disease Control and Prevention.

NLOM (2001). Toxnet7 and Internet Grateful Med. Bethesda, MD: National Library of Medicine.

Pozzilli, P. (1996). Prevention of insulin-dependent diabetes. *Diabetes Metabolism Review* 12: 27-136.

Roccella, E.J. and Horan, M.J. (1998). The National High Blood Pressure Education Program: Measuring progress and assessing its impact. *Health Psychology* 7: 237-303.

UN (1998). The UNAIDS Report. Joint United Nations Programme on HIV/AIDS. Geneva, Switzerland.

VDH (2000). Turning Point. Richmond, VA: Virginia Department of Health. Accessed online: <http://www.vdh.state.va.us/tpoint/index.htm>.

Purpose: (1) to acquaint the reader with Healthy People 2010 targets for improvement and (2) present examples of epidemiology as the underlying science to health promotion and disease prevention.

Directions: Check out your knowledge of these Healthy People 2010 focus area by taking the following tests (answers follow in a separate section).

FOCUS AREA 25:
SEXUALLY TRANSMITTED DISEASES

This focus area's goal is to promote responsible sexual behaviors, strengthen community capacity, and increase access to quality services to prevent sexually transmitted diseases (STDs) and their complications.

Bacterial STD Illness and Disability

25-1.   *Reduction in the proportion of adolescents and young adults with* Chlamydia trachomatis *infections.* Related to this objective, which kind of disease is this?
a. Bacterial sexually transmitted disease
b. Viral sexually transmitted disease
c. Protozoan sexually transmitted disease
d. Metazoan sexually transmitted disease

25-2.   *Reduction in gonorrhea.* Related to this objective, all of the following are correct except:
a. African Americans (non-Hispanic blacks) accounted for about 77 percent of the total number of reported cases of gonorrhea.

   b. Infertility and ectopic pregnancy resulting from unrecognized or undiagnosed chlamydia or gonorrhea.
   c. Gonorrhea ranks in the top ten of infectious diseases reported to the states by local health departments.
   d. Adults over twenty-four years old have the highest rates of gonorrhea infection.

25-3. *Elimination of sustained domestic transmission of primary and secondary syphilis.* Related to this objective, which of the following is correct?
   a. Syphilis is easy to detect and cure, given adequate access to and use of care.
   b. Nationally, syphilis is at the highest rate ever recorded.
   c. It is highly prevalent and has spread to a high number of geographic areas.
   d. All of the above are correct.

Viral STD Illness and Disability

25-4. *Reduction in the proportion of adults with genital herpes infection.* As of 1988-1994, what proportion of adults had genital herpes?
   a. 17 percent
   b. 37 percent
   c. 57 percent
   d. 77 percent

25-5. *Reduction in the proportion of persons with human papillomavirus (HPV) infection (developmental).* Related to this objective, all of the following are correct except:
   a. Epidemiologists have established the central role of HPV in the pathogenesis of cervical cancer.
   b. Reducing the number of new HPV cases will not help to minimize the overall number of cases of cervical cancer in females aged fifteen to forty-four years.
   c. About 20 million persons in United States have HPV infection.
   d. About 5.5 million new HPV infections occur each year.

STD Complications Affecting Females

25-6.   *Reduction in the proportion of females who have ever required treatment for pelvic inflammatory disease (PID).* What is the targeted proportion of females requiring PID treatment?
a. 5 percent
b. 25 percent
c. 45 percent
d. 65 percent

25-7.   *Reduction in the proportion of childless females with fertility problems who have had a sexually transmitted disease or who have required treatment for pelvic inflammatory disease (PID).* How much of reduction is targeted in childless females with fertility problems either having a STD or treatment for PID?
a. 24 percent reduction
b. 44 percent reduction
c. 64 percent reduction
d. 84 percent reduction

25-8.   *Reduction in HIV infections in adolescent and young adult females aged thirteen to twenty-four years that are associated with heterosexual contact (developmental).* Related to this objective, which of the following is correct?
a. Young heterosexual women, especially minority women, are increasingly acquiring HIV infection and developing AIDS.
b. As of 1998, 41 percent of reported AIDS cases in persons aged 13 to 24 years occurred in young women.
c. The spread of HIV infection in the United States through heterosexual transmission is similar to other STD epidemics.
d. All of the above are correct.

STD Complications Affecting the Fetus and Newborn

25-9.   *Reduction in congenital syphilis.* Related to this objective, what is congenital syphilis?
a. A condition causing permanent damage to the female reproductive tract which can lead to ectopic pregnancy, infertility, or chronic pelvic pain

b. The standard medical definition of infertility
c. A condition in a fetus or newborn caused by infection with the syphilis bacteria from an untreated mother
d. A serious health problem that occurs following an acute bacterial or viral STD

25-10. *Reduction in neonatal consequences from maternal sexually transmitted diseases, including chlamydial pneumonia, gonococcal and chlamydial ophthalmia neonatorum, laryngeal papillomatosis (from human papillomavirus infection), neonatal herpes, and preterm birth and low birth weight associated with bacterial vaginosis.* Which of these STDs is responsible for newborn eye infections and loss of sight?
a. Gonorrhea
b. Chlamydia
c. HPV
d. Both a and b

Personal Behaviors

25-11. *Increase in the proportion of adolescents who abstain from sexual intercourse or use condoms if sexually active.* As of 1999, what was the proportion of adolescents either abstaining or using condoms?
a. 25 percent
b. 45 percent
c. 65 percent
d. 85 percent

25-12. *Increase in the number of positive messages related to responsible sexual behavior during weekday and nightly prime-time television programming (developmental).* Which of the following would be such a positive message?
a. Abstinence
b. Delaying sexual intercourse
c. Using effective methods to prevent STDs and pregnancy
d. All of the above

Community Protection Infrastructure

25-13. *Increase in the proportion of tribal, state, and local sexually transmitted disease programs that routinely offer hepatitis B vaccines to all STD clients.* As of 1998, what proportion of states routinely offered hepatitis B vaccine to all STD clients?
a. 5 percent
b. 25 percent
c. 45 percent
d. 65 percent

25-14. *Increase in the proportion of youth detention facilities and adult city or county jails that screen for common bacterial sexually transmitted diseases within twenty-four hours of admission and treat STDs (when necessary) before persons are released (developmental).* Related to this objective, a group that is disproportionately affected by STDs is:
a. Sex workers (people who exchange sex for money, drugs, or other goods)
b. Adolescents
c. Persons in detention
d. All of the above

25-15. *Increase in the proportion of local health departments that have contracts with managed care providers for the treatment of nonplan partners of patients with bacterial sexually transmitted diseases (gonorrhea, syphilis, and chlamydia) (developmental).* Related to this objective, since most STD care in the United States is delivered in the private sector, who should work together to overcome barriers to rapid and effective treatment of the nonplan sex partners of health plan members?
a. Private health care providers
b. Managed care organizations
c. Public health departments
d. All of the above

Personal Health Services

25-16. *Increase in the proportion of sexually active females aged twenty-five years and under who are screened annually for genital chlamydia infections (developmental).* Related to this objective, which of the following is correct?
   a. Most STDs produce clear symptoms or signs which are hard to disregard.
   b. STD-infected persons often seek medical care.
   c. As many as 15 percent of women with chlamydia have no symptoms.
   d. Routine screening for asymptomatic chlamydia during pelvic examination is recommended for all sexually active females, especially those at high risk.

25-17. *Increase in the proportion of pregnant females screened for sexually transmitted diseases (including HIV infection and bacterial vaginosis) during prenatal health care visits, according to recognized standards (developmental).* Related to this objective, which of the following is correct?
   a. Evidence is insufficient to make a recommendation concerning routine screening of pregnant females for STDs.
   b. The benefits of early intervention in HIV-asymptomatic pregnant women are known.
   c. Similar benefits have been demonstrated in detecting and treating asymptomatic chlamydia infection in pregnancy.
   d. All of the above are correct.

25-18. *Increase in the proportion of primary care providers who treat patients with sexually transmitted diseases and who manage cases according to recognized standards.* As of 1998, what proportion of primary care providers treat STDs according to recognized standards?
   a. 30 percent
   b. 50 percent
   c. 70 percent
   d. 90 percent

25-19. *Increase in the proportion of sexually transmitted disease clinic patients who are being treated for bacterial STDs (chlamydia, gonorrhea, and syphilis) and who are offered provider referral services for their sex partners (developmental)*. Related to this objective, all of the following are correct except:

a. With partner treatment, the initially infected person benefits from a reduced risk of reinfection from an untreated partner.
b. With partner treatment, the partner avoids acute infection and its potential complications.
c. With partner treatment, future sex partners are at greater risk of being infected by the bacterial STDs.
d. With partner treatment, the community benefits because the chain of transmission has been broken.

FOCUS AREA 26: SUBSTANCE ABUSE

This focus area's goal is to reduce substance abuse to protect the health, safety, and quality of life for all, especially children.

Adverse Consequences of Substance Use and Abuse

26-1. *Reduction in deaths and injuries caused by alcohol- and drug-related motor vehicle crashes.* How much of a reduction is targeted in injuries by alcohol-related motor vehicle crashes?
a. 22 percent reduction
b. 42 percent reduction
c. 62 percent reduction
d. 82 percent reduction

26-2. *Reduction in cirrhosis deaths.* Related to this objective, all of the following are correct except:
a. Sustained heavy alcohol consumption is the leading cause of cirrhosis.
b. Cirrhosis is one of the top ten leading causes of death in the United States.
c. Cirrhosis occurs when healthy liver tissue is replaced with scarred tissue until the liver is unable to function effectively.
d. There has been an increase in cirrhosis deaths for the past three decades.

26-3.   *Reduction in drug-induced deaths.* Related to this objective, what is a cause of drug-induced death?
a. Drug psychosis
b. Drug dependence
c. Suicide
d. All of the above

26-4.   *Reduction in drug-related hospital emergency department visits.* How much of a reduction is targeted in these kinds of emergency department visits?
a. 15 percent reduction
b. 35 percent reduction
c. 55 percent reduction
d. 75 percent reduction

26-5.   *Reduction in alcohol-related hospital emergency department visits (developmental).* As of 1996, what percent of emergency department visits were alcohol related?
a. 2.4 percent
b. 22.4 percent
c. 42.4 percent
d. 62.4 percent

26-6.   *Reduction in the proportion of adolescents who report that they rode, during the previous thirty days, with a driver who had been drinking alcohol.* As of 1999, what proportion of adolescents rode in the past month with a driver who was under the influence?
a. 13 percent
b. 33 percent
c. 53 percent
d. 73 percent

26-7.   *Reduction in intentional injuries resulting from alcohol- and illicit drug-related violence (developmental).* Related to the objective, all of the following are correct except:
a. A majority of homicide offenders were drinking when they committed the offense.
b. Drugs as well as alcohol are factors in a significant number of firearm-related deaths.

    c. Juvenile and adult arrestees testing positive for drugs had been arrested frequently for violent offenses.

    d. A small percent of victims who experienced violence by an intimate partner reported that alcohol had been involved.

26-8. *Reduction in the cost of lost productivity in the workplace due to alcohol and drug use (developmental).* Related to this objective, as of 1995, the majority of alcohol-related productivity losses were attributed to:

    a. Alcohol-related illness

    b. Alcohol-related crime

    c. Alcohol-related violence on the job

    d. Alcohol-related consumption on the job

Substance Use and Abuse

26-9. *Increase in the age and proportion of adolescents who remain alcohol and drug free.* What is the average age for first use of alcohol or marijuana?

    a. Eleven

    b. Thirteen

    c. Fifteen

    d. Seventeen

26-10. *Reduction in past-month use of illicit substances.* As of 1998, what proportion of adolescents aged twelve to seventeen were alcohol/drug free during the past thirty days?

    a. 39 percent

    b. 59 percent

    c. 79 percent

    d. 99 percent

26-11. *Reduction in the proportion of persons engaging in binge drinking of alcoholic beverages.* What is the targeted proportion of college students involved in binge drinking within past two weeks?

    a. 20 percent

    b. 40 percent

    c. 60 percent

    d. 80 percent

26-12. *Reduction in average annual alcohol consumption.* What is the targeted annual alcohol consumption?
a. 1 gallon
b. 2 gallons
c. 3 gallons
d. 4 gallons

26-13. *Reduction in the proportion of adults who exceed guidelines for low-risk drinking.* A person might be at risk for alcohol-related problems if he or she consumes more than:
a. One drink per occasion for either gender
b. Two drinks per occasion for either gender
c. Two drinks per occasion for females and three drinks for males
d. Three drinks per occasion for females and four drinks for males

26-14. *Reduction in steroid use among adolescents.* Related to this objective, a behavioral health problem associated with steroid use is:
a. Suicide
b. Other substance abuse
b. Homicide
d. All of the above

26-15. *Reduction in the proportion of adolescents who use inhalants.* As of 1998, what proportion of adolescents used inhalants in the past year?
a. 2.9 percent
b. 12.9 percent
c. 22.9 percent
d. 32.9 percent

Risk of Substance Use and Abuse

26-16. *Increase in the proportion of adolescents who disapprove of substance abuse.* As of 1998, what proportion of eighth graders reported disapproval of having one or two alcoholic drinks nearly every day?
a. 37 percent
b. 57 percent

c. 77 percent
d. 97 percent

26-17. *Increase in the proportion of adolescents who perceive great risk associated with substance abuse.* What is the targeted proportion of adolescents who report perceived risks associated with substance abuse?
a. 20 percent
b. 40 percent
c. 60 percent
d. 80 percent

Treatment for Substance Abuse

26-18. *Reduction in the treatment gap for illicit drugs in the general population (developmental).* What is the "treatment gap"?
a. Average consumption of illicit drugs per capita of the population
b. The difference between the number of persons who need treatment for the use of illicit drugs and the number of persons who are receiving treatment in a given year
c. As perception of harmfulness decreases, use tends to increase
d. The difference between licit and illicit drugs

26-19. *Increase in the proportion of inmates receiving substance abuse treatment in correctional institutions (developmental).* Related to this objective, which of the following is correct?
a. There has been a large increase in the number of individuals incarcerated for drug-related offenses (e.g., possession).
b. Criminal offenders frequently have high occurrences of a substance abuse history.
c. Criminal offenders not receiving needed drug treatment have a greater likelihood of committing a criminal offense.
d. All of the above are correct.

26-20. *Increase in the number of admissions to substance abuse treatment for injection drug use.* How much of an increase is targeted in admitting injection drug users to treatment?
a. 19 percent
b. 39 percent

    c. 59 percent
    d. 79 percent

26-21. *Reduction in the treatment gap for alcohol problems (developmental).* Related to this objective, all of the following are correct except:
    a. Alcohol problems can be described by their duration (acute, intermittent, chronic) and severity (mild, moderate, substantial, severe).
    b. Availability of resources and access to clinically appropriate and effective treatment for alcohol problems are limited.
    c. The size of the treatment gap is well defined in terms of treatment capacities and utilization in local jurisdictions.
    d. Increasing the availability of treatment for alcohol problems is critical because of the pervasive impact these problems have on all aspects of society.

State and Local Efforts

26-22. *Increase in the proportion of persons who are referred for follow-up care for alcohol problems, drug problems, or suicide attempts after diagnosis or treatment for one of these conditions in a hospital emergency department (developmental).* Related to this objective, emergency departments should be prepared to assess and refer patients with the following behavioral risk factor(s):
    a. Hazardous patterns of alcohol consumption
    b. Use of illicit drugs
    c. Predisposition to suicidal thoughts or actions
    d. All of the above

26-23. *Increase in the number of communities using partnerships or coalition models to conduct comprehensive substance abuse prevention efforts (developmental).* Related to this objective, improving the environment means:
    a. Changing local ordinances and policies
    b. Coordinating local prevention services
    c. Increasing resident participation
    d. All of the above

26-24. *Extend administrative license revocation laws, or programs of equal effectiveness, for persons who drive under the influence of intoxicants.* As of 1998, how many states had administrative license revocation laws for persons who drive under the influence of intoxicants?
a. Twenty-one states
b. Thirty-one states
c. Forty-one states
d. Fifty-one states

26-25. *Extend legal requirements for maximum blood alcohol concentration levels of 0.08 percent for motor vehicle drivers aged twenty-one years and older.* As of 1998, how many states had these legal requirements?
a. Sixteen states
b. Twenty-six states
c. Thirty-six states
d. Forty-six states

TEST ANSWERS

Focus Area 25

25-1.   (a) Bacterial sexually transmitted disease. Like gonorrhea and syphilis, chlamydia is a curable sexually transmitted disease. In 1997, 12.1 percent of females and 15.7 percent of males aged fifteen to twenty-four years attending STD clinics had chlamydia. The target is a reduction in this age group to 3 percent.

25-2.   (d) Adults over twenty-four years old have the highest rates of gonorrhea infection. This is incorrect. As of 1997, females aged fifteen to nineteen years and males aged twenty to twenty-four years had the highest reported rates of both gonorrhea and chlamydia. The target is to reduce the rate of gonorrhea to nineteen new cases per 100,000 population.

25-3.   (a) Syphilis is easy to detect and cure, given adequate access to and use of care. The other two responses are incorrect. Nationally, syphilis is at its lowest recorded rate and it is limited to a small number of geographic areas. As of 1997, the baseline rate of primary and secondary syphilis was 3.2 cases per 100,000 population, and the target is a reduction to 0.2 cases per 100,000 population.

25-4.   (a) 17 percent. This was the baseline for adults aged twenty to twenty-nine years with genital herpes infection as measured by herpes simplex virus type 2 antibody. The targeted proportion is 14 percent of adults. One way to reach this target is through safer sexual practices.

25-5.   (b) Reducing the number of new HPV cases will not help to minimize the overall number of cases of cervical cancer in females aged fifteen to forty-four years. This is incorrect. Reducing the number of new HPV cases can help to minimize the overall number of cases of high-risk subtypes associated with cervical cancer in females aged fifteen to forty-four years.

25-6.   (a) 5 percent. As of 1995, the baseline was 8 percent of females aged fifteen to forty-four years required treatment for PID. PID is a most serious threat to women's reproductive health. Gonorrhea and chlamydia infection most likely cause

PID when the bacteria ascend into the uterus, fallopian tubes, and then into the pelvic cavity.

25-7. (b) 44 percent reduction. As of 1995, the baseline was 27 percent of childless females aged fifteen to forty-four years with fertility problems had a history of STDs or PID treatment. The target is 15 percent (a reduction of 44 percent). The significance of this objective is that many females who are interested in becoming pregnant do not know that past STD infection or PID treatment may have compromised their fertility. They need to be tested and evaluated.

25-8. (d) All of the above are correct. More than 80 percent of AIDS cases reported in females thirteen to twenty-four years occurred in certain racial and ethnic groups, mostly African Americans or Hispanics.

25-9. (c) A condition in a fetus or newborn caused by infection with the syphilis bacteria from an untreated mother. Infected newborns show a wide spectrum of clinical signs, and only severe cases are clinically apparent at birth. Severe illness or death can result after birth if the newborn is not treated. Regarding the other responses, pelvic inflammatory disease is a condition that causes permanent damage to the female reproductive tract and can lead to ectopic pregnancy, infertility, or chronic pelvic pain. A fertility problem is the standard medical definition of infertility. STD complication refers to a serious health problem that occurs following an acute bacterial or viral STD.

25-10. (d) Both a and b. Infections in a fetus or newborn also include conditions such as congenital syphilis, neonatal herpes, HIV infection, and pneumonia.

25-11. (d) 85 percent. This was the baseline for adolescents in grades nine through twelve. Fifty percent had never experienced sexual intercourse; 14 percent had but not in the past 3 months; and 21 percent were sexually active and used a condom at last intercourse. The target is an increase to 95 percent of adolescents either abstaining or using condoms.

25-12. (d) All of the above. Television messages hold the potential to promote responsible sexual behaviors such as those identified in these positive messages.

25-13. (a) 5 percent. This was the baseline for state and local STD programs offering hepatitis B vaccines to clients in accordance with CDC guidelines. The target is 90 percent. High rates of acute hepatitis B continue to occur in young adult risk groups, particularly persons with a history of another sexually transmitted disease and persons with multiple sex partners.

25-14. (d) All of the above. Another group would be migrant workers. STDs disproportionately affect disenfranchised persons and persons who are in social networks in which high-risk sexual behavior is common and either access to care or health-seeking behavior is compromised. Without publicly supported STD services, many people in these categories would lack access to STD care.

25-15. (d) All of the above. Active partner notification and partner treatment generally have been the responsibility of personnel in public STD clinics. Currently, the trend is to share this responsibility with the private sector.

25-16. (d) Routine screening for asymptomatic chlamydia during pelvic examination is recommended for all sexually active females, especially those at high risk. The other responses are incorrect. The majority of STDs either do not produce any symptoms or signs, or they produce symptoms so mild that they are often disregarded. This results in a low index of suspicion by infected persons who often do not seek necessary medical care. Many resulting in a low index of suspicion by infected persons who should but often do not seek medical care. As many as 85 percent of women with chlamydia have no symptoms.

25-17. (d) All of the above are correct. STDs in pregnant women can cause serious health problems and threaten the living status of the fetus or newborn. These infections can also complicate the pregnancy by causing spontaneous abortion, stillbirth, premature rupture of the membranes, or preterm delivery.

25-18. (c) 70 percent. The target is for 90 percent of primary care providers to follow CDC STD Treatment Guidelines.

25-19. (c) With partner treatment, future sex partners are at greater risk of being infected by the bacterial STDs. This is incorrect. With partner treatment, future sex partners will be protected

from the risk of STD infection. Identifying and treating partners of persons with curable STDs to break the chain of transmission in a sexual network always have been integral to organized control programs. Early antimicrobial prophylaxis
of the exposed partner reduces the likelihood of transmission
and thwarts infection.

Focus Area 26

26-1. (b) 42 percent reduction. As of 1998, the baseline rate was
113 alcohol-related injuries per 100,000 population and the
target is 65 such injuries per 100,000. Related to this, the
baseline rate for alcohol-related motor vehicle crash deaths
was 5.9 per 100,000 and the target is 4 per 100,000. Baseline
and target rates for drug-related injuries and deaths are developmental.

26-2. (d) There has been an increase in cirrhosis deaths for the past
three decades. This is incorrect. There has been a decline since
1973 due to availability of alcoholism treatment, greater consumer awareness, and the imposition of higher state excise tax
rates on distilled spirits. Yet cirrhosis is a leading killer. As of
1998, the baseline rate was 9.5 cirrhosis deaths per 100,000
population and the target is 3.0 deaths per 100,000 population.*

26-3. (d) All of the above. Additional causes are intentional and accidental poisonings. Declining initiation, number of cases,
and intensity of drug abuse should be reflected in fewer drug-
induced deaths. However, the prevention of suicide, accidental poisoning, and fatal interaction among medications contributes to changes in the statistics measured in this objective.
As of 1998, the baseline rate was 6.3 drug-induced deaths per
100,000 population. The target is one death per 100,000 population.

26-4. (b) 35 percent reduction. As of 1998, the baseline was
542,544 hospital emergency department visits were drug-
related. The target is a reduction to 350,000 visits per year. A
drug-related episode results from the nonmedical use of a

---

*Age adjusted to the year 2000 standard population.

drug including the unprescribed use of prescription drugs, use of drugs contrary to approved labeling, and use of illicit drugs.

26-5.   (a) 2.4 percent. That amounts to 2.2 million emergency department visits. Alcohol consumption is associated with a wide range of events that can result in emergency department visits such as motor vehicle crashes, violence, and alcohol poisoning.

26-6.   (b) 33 percent. The target is to reduce to 30 percent of students in grades nine through twelve reportedly riding during the previous thirty days with a driver who had been drinking alcohol. Since motor vehicles crashes are a leading explanation for adolescent deaths, the risky behavior of riding with another adolescent driver who has been drinking contributes significantly to the likelihood of a fatal alcohol-related crash.

26-7.   (d) A small percent of victims who experienced violence by an intimate partner reported that alcohol had been involved. This is incorrect since two-thirds of these victims reported alcohol had been involved. In addition, among spousal victims, three out of four incidents involved an offender who was drinking. Thirty-one percent of strangers who were victimized believed that the offender was using alcohol.

26-8.   (a) Alcohol-related illness. These costs, measured as impaired earnings among those with a history of alcohol dependence, may result from increased unemployment, poor job performance, and limited career advancement.

26-9.   (b) Thirteen. Actually, the average age for first alcohol use was 13.1, and for first marijuana use was 13.7. The targets are 16.1 for alcohol and 17.4 for marijuana. Being able to resist the influence to start alcohol and drug use during youth is an important capability that will be later employed during adulthood, long after family constraints and other support mechanisms are less available.

26-10. (c) 79 percent. The target is for 89 percent of adolescents aged twelve to seventeen years reporting no alcohol or illicit drug use in the past thirty days. Although the invlovement in drugs/alcohol of persons aged eighteen and older in the past thirty-days has remained relatively unchanged over the past few years, younger adolescents have been increasing their involvement.

26-11. (a) 20 percent. As of 1998, 39 percent of college students admitted to engaging in binge drinking during the past two weeks. The target is to reduce this number by 49 percent.

26-12. (b) Two gallons. This is a reduction of 9 percent. As of 1997, the baseline was 2.18 gallons of ethanol consumed per person aged fourteen years and older. These estimates are based on population figures as they relate to information on beverage sales, tax receipt data, or both. The data come primarily from states, with some data provided by beverage industry sources.

26-13. (d) Three drinks per occasion for females and four drinks for males. In addition, risk drinking is seven or more drinks weekly for females, and fourteen or more weekly for males.

26-14. (d) All of the above. There are also physical health problems associated with steroid use such as liver damage and heart attacks.

26-15. (a) 2.9 percent. The target is to reduce this proportion to less than 1 percent of adolescents aged twelve to seventeen years who used inhalants in the past year. Examples of inhalants are amyl nitrate, nitrous oxide, and toluene (glue).

26-16. (c) 77 percent. Accordingly, 75 percent of tenth graders and 69 percent of twelfth graders registered the same disapproval. The target is for at least 83 percent of students in these grade levels to disapprove daily alcohol use.

26-17. (d) 80 percent. Examples would be perceiving the risk of consuming five or more alcoholic drinks at a single occasion once or twice a week, smoking marijuana once per month, and using cocaine once per month.

26-18. (b) The difference between the number of persons who need treatment for the use of illicit drugs and the number of persons who are receiving treatment in a given year. This objective is in place because accepted estimates of the number of persons who need treatment and the number who receive treatment are not available.

26-19. (d) All of the above. Drug dependence is a chronic, relapsing disorder with addicted persons frequently engaging in self-destructive and criminal behavior. Treatment can help end dependence on addictive drugs and reduce the consequences of addictive drug use on society.

26-20. (a) 19 percent. As of 1997, there were 167,960 admissions for injection drug use and the target is to increase to 200,000 admissions.

26-21. (c) The size of the treatment gap is well defined in terms of treatment capacities and utilization in local jurisdictions. Actually, the size of the gap is not well defined. Wide variability exists among jurisdictions in areas such as total treatment capacity and in how that capacity is distributed among settings and modalities.

26-22. (d) All of the above. The effectiveness of emergency departments, interventions for these risk factors is determined by how well the affected patients are evaluated and treated, and by the extent of communication and coordination with other settings and organizations in the community.

26-23. (d) All of the above. Another technique would be communicating with the local media on how it portrays local communities. A comprehensive community program is crucial to effective substance abuse prevention. These programs address issues related to their environments, not just their at-risk populations.

26-24. (c) Forty-one states. Actually, it was forty-one states plus the District of Columbia. The target is for all states to have this kind of law.

26-25. (a) Sixteen states. The target is for all states and the District of Columbia to have legal requirements for maximum blood alcohol concentration levels of 0.08 percent for motor vehicle drivers aged twenty-one years and older.

Chapter 14

Future Epidemiology

THE FIRST AND SECOND ERAS

Recall that Chapter 2 covered historical perspectives of epidemiology. The time period before the mid-nineteenth century can be considered the first era of epidemiology. It was largely a time of replacing mystical and natural notions about disease with epidemiological reasoning. As the nineteenth century approached, several persons were responsible for establishing the scientific notion of disease. Rather than inferring cause from the coincidence of two events, the epidemiological reasoner observed closely and took into account all possible factors in the physical, social, and biological environments that might influence disease events.

During the mid-1800s, epidemiologists such as Snow, Koch, Pasteur, and others laid the groundwork to what is called the second era of epidemiology. Through their work, the occurrence and distribution of diseases such as cholera, anthrax, and malaria were better understood. Diagnostic techniques were invented to determine the cause of infectious diseases, and epidemiologists were able to establish protocols for conducting investigations into outbreaks. Epidemiologists such as Graunt and Shattuck were proponents of surveillance systems so that communities could monitor the incidence and prevalence of disease and death. During the twentieth century, the Centers for Disease Control and Prevention supported a multitude of retrospective, prevalence, and prospective studies to better understand what causes infectious and noninfectious diseases and other health-affecting conditions. The improvement of inoculation programs significantly reduced many pathogenic and virulent diseases such as polio, rubella, pertussis, hepatitis, and others. These studies also established the relationship between risk factors and leading causes of death, such as coronary heart disease, malignant neoplasm (cancer), chronic obstructive lung disease (e.g., emphysema), and others. But as the twentieth century waned, epidemiological focus shifted. Although epidemiologists continue to practice surveillance, investigations, and studies, the kinds of diseases and other health-affecting conditions have changed.

THE THIRD ERA

Beginning in the late twentieth century, a third era of epidemiology has evolved. Epidemiologists established an agenda of action that pertains to the following diseases and conditions:

- Reemerging infectious diseases
- Continuing relationships between environmental toxins and health
- Behavioral and social agents to disease and other health affecting conditions
- Genetic agents to disease (Stone et al., 1996)

Reemerging Infectious Diseases

Recently several infectious diseases have reemerged as national and international public health alerts. As some examples, bubonic and pneumonic plague were once considered under control, but outbreaks continue in currently developing countries. Nationally and internationally, the sexually transmitted disease chlamydia is only recently being comprehensively screened and included in surveillance systems. There have been recent outbreaks of encephalitis and other arboviral diseases such as West Nile virus in the United States. Lyme disease continues to increase in incidence, especially in the northeastern region of the nation. The incidence of toxic shock syndrome and related syndromes alarmed the public in the 1970s—sporadic outbreaks of this streptococcal infection continue today. There is even a strain that "eats flesh." Herpes, a viral sexually transmitted disease, still persists in the U.S. population. Antibiotic-resistant tuberculosis bacteria explain the increased incidence of tuberculosis nationally and internationally. Viral diseases, such as Marburg fever and dengue fever, as well as the protozoan disease malaria, were believed contained in tropical areas of the globe until international travel facilitated **autolochronous transmission.** This transmission takes place when an infected source host visits a place free of the disease and inadvertently allows an indigenous vector to transmit the disease to new hosts in that place. Although human cases of rabies, a highly virulent viral disease, have been controlled, there are increasing numbers of domestic pets contracting this disease from wildlife. Internationally, there have been devastating outbreaks of other highly virulent viral diseases such as ebola and lassa. There have been impressive advances in the prevention and treatment of HIV disease and other bloodborne pathogens such as hepatitis B, but epidemiologists now realize that there is more than one strain of each of these viruses. The commonly experienced human papaloma virus, which causes genital warts, is now considered a biological agent to cervical cancer. Unknown to epidemiologists until the latter 1900s, virulent hemorrhagic diseases such as legionellosis and hanta have broken out in the nation. There are probably more *E. coli* bacteria in one person's gut than the population count of the U.S. population, but when this pathogenic bacterial disease is introduced as a foodborne disease, severe illness and possible death occur (Karlen, 1996).

As mentioned above, there are a growing number of bacteria resistant to antibiotics. The increased use of antibiotics has contributed to this trend. There is alarm because several bacterial infections might become untreatable as a result. For example, the pneumococcal bacterium implicit in meningitis is now resistant to all antibiotics save vancomycin. The Centers for Disease Control and Prevention in conjunction with the American Academy of Pediatricians have developed recommendations for the careful use of antibiotics. The guidelines apply to diagnoses of **otitis media,** middle ear infection; **rhinitis** and **sinusitis,** common cold and sinus infections respectively; **pharyngitis,** sore throat; cough illness; and **bronchitis,** lower respiratory tract infection. Health care practitioners are guided in clinical decision making—when antibiotic treatment is appropriate and when it should be refrained. Anticipating patient and parent demand for the obligatory prescription, the guidelines offer explanations that can be shared by the health care practitioner regarding his or her clinical decision making (CDC, 2000).

The preceding was not meant as alarmism but merely as a reminder that the national and international communities must maintain an agenda of infectious disease control. One such example is CDC's strategy for the twenty-first century that targets the disparity in vaccination rates among preschool children of certain racial and ethnic populations. Efforts are under way to increase vaccination coverage for children living in poverty. Whereas vaccines and treatments can successfully address the process of many of these diseases, there is no substitution for hand washing, proper food preparation, safer sex, and other prudent methods of standard infection control. Large numbers of undervaccinated children reside in urban areas representing a population at risk for outbreaks of disease. Many adults remain at risk for vaccine-preventable diseases. Although more adults sixty-five years and older in nonwhite populations are taking advantage of pneumococcal and influenza vaccines, the coverage in African-American and Hispanic communities is far below the general population (CDC, 1999).

ENVIRONMENTAL TOXINS

It is hard to imagine what little attention was given to chemical and physical environmental agents to disease prior to the 1970s. Today there is an intense effort to study this relationship. Perhaps the pioneer in this effort was Rachel Carson, who during the 1960s alerted the public of the deleterious effects of **environmental estrogens** (DDT, PCBs, and others) on the food chain, specifically the reproductive capabilities of wildlife, especially birds, linked to continual exposure to DDT-laden insecticides. Epidemiologists and environmental health specialists are particularly concerned about these environmental estrogens and their suspected contributory role in cancer formation. Environmental estrogens (EEs) are found in nature or synthetically made and mimic the actions of estrogen in the body. The Environmental Protection Agency, which maintains its priority list of toxins threatening personal and public health, monitors proper storage and disposal of EEs and other hazardous substances.

Toxicity of Secondhand Smoke

It is hard to imagine, but there are over 4,000 chemicals in tobacco smoke and forty-three of them are carcinogenic. It is estimated that 3,000 nonsmokers die annually from lung cancer because of their exposure to secondhand smoke. Between 150,000 to 300,000 infants and children under age eighteen months experience lower respiratory tract infections, asthma, and other respiratory conditions triggered or worsened by tobacco smoke. Epidemiologists have also determined that secondhand smoke exposure causes heart disease among adults. Secondhand smoke is so pervasive that about 88 percent of U.S. persons over age four have detectable amounts of serum cotinine, a biological marker for exposure to secondhand smoke. Both home and workplace environments have contributed to the widespread exposure to secondhand smoke (Pirkle, Flegal, and Bernet, 1996).

This relates to Healthy People 2010 Objective 27-13: *Establishment of laws on smoke-free indoor air that prohibit smoking or limit it to separately ventilated areas in public places and work sites* (Healthy People 2010, 2000, 27-27). (See Chapter 14 activities for more information.)

Physical agents such as solid waste and energy sources (e.g., radioactive material) have been regulated through environment-related legislation. Still, these agents will continue to represent a source of disease, a potentially deadly legacy handed down to future generations. Great effort and money are dedicated to the proper disposal or storage of these known agents of disease. Epidemiologists will have to continue investigations and studies regarding the long-term exposure to presently produced and poorly stored agents of disease.

Behavioral and Social Agents of Disease

The abstract nature of behavioral and social agents of disease has challenged the traditionally minded epidemiologist. Whereas cardiovascular disease risk factors such as elevated cholesterol and blood pressure are biomedically measurable, some researchers are stymied when explaining the role of stress or physical inactivity in heart disease. To address this matter, the prospective medicine movement began in the mid-twentieth century. Its chief accomplishment was the invention of the health risk appraisal, which was discussed in Chapter 7. Even so, epidemiologists admit that about 20 percent of the predictive value of behavioral agents to disease has been established through retrospective and prospective diseases, meaning that common sense is used when stating that exercising reduces the risk of several diseases. Evidence to support these claims is still being compiled. The reason for this is because physical inactivity appears to be more of a moderating rather direct agent to disease. That is, physically inactive persons tend to accumulate other risk factors and their combined effect increases the risk of early morbidity and mortality.

Epidemiologists have also looked at other behavioral agents that can explain the leading causes of death. For all age groups, unintentional injuries represent one of the leading causes of death. These behavioral agents are given the designation **human factors** or **misactions.** Behavioral health conditions such as anxiety and mood disorders might not explain early morbidity, except perhaps in incidence of suicide, but these morbid conditions still have recognizable behavioral agents such as stress, unresolved conflict, and early life trauma. So, despite the conceptual aspects of behavioral agents, epidemiologists have been able and will continue to demonstrate the benefits of healthy and safe behaviors.

An expanding front for epidemiological action has been the relationship of social agents to disease and other morbid conditions. Traditionally minded epidemiologists scratch their heads and question if epidemiological concepts and principles can be applied to social agents of depressed socioeconomic conditions, psychosocial influences from media or peers, discrimination, severe civil unrest, and war. More contemporary-minded epidemiologists have set out to show that social agents such as gang behavior, domestic violence, and suicide can be investigated and controlled to reduce the likelihood of intentional injuries and death.

Heredity and Other Factors That Influence Vision and Hearing

Among the five senses, people depend on vision and hearing to provide the primary cues for conducting the basic activities of daily life. At the most basic level, vision and hearing permit people to navigate and to stay oriented within their environment. These senses provide the portals for language, whether spoken, signed, or read. They are critical to most work and recreation and allow people to interact more fully. For these reasons, vision and hearing are defining elements of a person's quality of life. Either, or both, of these senses may be diminished or lost because of heredity, aging, injury, or disease. Such loss may occur gradually, over the course of a lifetime, or traumatically in an instant.

(continued)

(continued)

Conditions of vision or hearing loss that are linked with chronic and disabling diseases pose additional challenges for patients and their families. From the public health perspective, the prevention of either the initial impairment or additional impairment from these environmentally orienting and socially connecting senses requires significant resources. Prevention of vision or hearing loss or their resulting disabling conditions through the development of improved disease prevention, detection, or treatment methods or more effective rehabilitative strategies must remain a priority (Freid, Makuc, and Rooks, 1998).

This relates to Healthy People 2010 Objective 28-2: *Increase in the proportion of preschool children aged five years and under who receive vision screening (developmental);* and 28-11: *Increase in the proportion of newborns who are screened for hearing loss by age one month, have audiologic evaluation by age three months, and are enrolled in appropriate intervention services by age six months* (Healthy People 2010, 2000, 27-27, 28-14). (See Chapter 14 activities for more information.)

Genetic Agents of Disease

A new frontier for epidemiologists is further understanding the role of genetic agents in the disease process. Presently, the Human Genome Project has completed mapping the genes of the human body. The next step will be to make connections between genetic material and protein synthesis. The efforts at mapping genetic material will lead to futuristic developments in medicine that are difficult to imagine. Ostensibly, epidemiologists will gain insight into the direct role of genes and genomes in disease causation. For instance, it is now known that about 5 percent of all breast cancer cases are due to a defective gene. Likewise, 10 percent of osteoporosis cases, primarily in males, are linked directly to the presence of a particular gene. But how will the public handle the indirect role of these genetic agents along with the increasing realization of genetic predisposition to disease? Just as there are health risk appraisals, future epidemiologists will likely develop genetic risk appraisals of disease. These researchers will be squarely in the middle of a looming ethical concern. Will society responsibly address and treat diseases and conditions that might be "out of our hands"? Epidemiologists will have to face issues of privacy and confidentiality while conducting their work, especially if their work deals with human genetic makeup (Gordis, 1996).

THE FUTURE

Throughout this text, epidemiology's relationship with health promotion and disease prevention has been explored. Epidemiology is the underlying science to health promotion and disease prevention. Through surveillance, investigations, and studies, epidemiology acts as the foundation to the Healthy People 2010 National Initiative, and its twenty-eight focus areas that have been presented as chapter activities. These focus areas with their respective Healthy People 2010 objectives represent the future of epidemiology and how it will be realized through health promotion and disease prevention activity.

SUMMARY

Epidemiological action in our society can be viewed in three eras. Whereas past eras gradually replaced early notions of disease with epidemiological reasoning, the current era is faced with challenges of reemerging infectious diseases, environmental toxins and health, behavioral/social agents to disease, and newly discovered genetic agents to disease. Since epidemiology is the underlying science to health promotion and disease prevention activity, Healthy People 2010 represents the future of epidemiology.

REVIEW QUESTIONS

1. Can you distinguish the first, second, and third eras of epidemiology?
2. Do you know the definitions of terms in bold print throughout this chapter?
3. Can you identify reemerging infectious diseases?
4. What is the public health concern regarding environmental estrogens and other toxic substances?
5. Can you think of examples of how epidemiologists are trying to explain the relationship of behavioral/social agents to disease?
6. What is an ethical concern associated with the discovery of genetic agents to disease?

7. Do you know the answers to the following chapter activity questions based on objectives from Healthy People 2010 focus areas 27 and 28?

WEB SITE RESOURCES

CDC's Adult Immunization Action Plan
<http://www.cdc.gov/od/nvpo/adult.htm>

CDC's Plan for Preventing Emerging Infectious Diseases
<http://www.cdc.gov/ncidod/emergplan>

Program for Monitoring Emerging Diseases (ProMed)
<http://www.fas.org/promed/>

World Wide Virtual Library of Epidemiology
<http://www.epibiostat.ucsf.edu/epidem/epidem.html>

REFERENCES

CDC (1999). Preventing Emerging Infectious Diseases Threat: A Strategy for the 21st Century. Atlanta, GA: Centers for Disease Control and Prevention.

CDC (2000). Careful antibiotics use. Recommendations by the CDC/AAP to promote judicious antibiotics use. Atlanta, GA: Centers for Disease Control and Prevention.

Freid, V.M., Makuc, D.M., and Rooks, R.N. (1998). Ambulatory health care visits by children: Principal diagnosis and place of visit. *Vital and Health Statistics* 13(137): 17, 1-23

Gordis, L. (1996). *Epidemiology*. Philadelphia, PA: W.B. Saunders.

Karlen, A. (1996). *Men and microbes*. New York: G.P. Putnam and Sons.

Pirkel, J.L., Flegal, K.M., and Bernet, J.T. (1996). Exposure of the U.S. population to environmental tobacco smoke. *Journal of the American Medical Association* 275: 1233-1240.

Stone, D.B., Armstrong, W.R., Macrina, D.M., and Pankau, J.W. (1996). *Introduction to epidemiology*. Madison, WI: Brown and Benchmark.

Purpose: (1) to acquaint the reader with Healthy People 2010 targets for improvement and (2) present examples of epidemiology as the underlying science to health promotion and disease prevention.

Directions: Check out your knowledge of these Healthy People 2010 focus areas by taking the following tests (answers follow in a separate section).

FOCUS AREA 27: TOBACCO USE

This focus area's goal is to reduce illness, disability, and death related to tobacco use and exposure to secondhand smoke.

Tobacco Use in Population Groups

27-1.   *Reduction in tobacco use by adults.* As of 1998, what proportion of adults smoked cigarettes?
   a. 14 percent
   b. 24 percent
   c. 34 percent
   d. 44 percent

27-2.   *Reduction in tobacco use by adolescents.* What is the targeted percent of adolescents using tobacco products within the past month?
   a. 11 percent
   b. 21 percent
   c. 31 percent
   d. 41 percent

27-3.   *Reduction in the initiation of tobacco use among children and adolescents (developmental).* All of the following are correct except:

    a. A majority of tobacco use initiates in adolescence.

    b. Adolescent tobacco use is more experimentation and initiation when compared to adult tobacco use.

    c. Adolescent cigarette smoking is a notifiable condition, meaning providers are required to report cases to local health departments.

    d. Measuring tobacco use in adolescents involves spit tobacco and cigars in addition to cigarettes.

27-4.   *Increase in the average age of first use of tobacco products by adolescents and young adults.* As of 1997, what was the average age for adolescents (ages twelve to seventeen) to start using tobacco products?

    a. Ten

    b. Twelve

    c. Fourteen

    d. Sixteen

Cessation and Treatment

27-5.   *Increase in smoking cessation attempts by adult smokers.* What is the targeted percentage of adult smokers attempting to quit smoking?

    a. 35 percent

    b. 55 percent

    c. 75 percent

    d. 95 percent

27-6.   *Increase in smoking cessation during pregnancy.* What is the targeted percent of pregnant women who stop smoking during pregnancy?

    a. 10 percent

    b. 30 percent

    c. 50 percent

    d. 70 percent

27-7.   *Increase in tobacco use cessation attempts by adolescent smokers.* As of 1999, what percent of adolescents who smoke daily tried quitting their habit?

    a. 16 percent

    b. 36 percent

c. 56 percent
d. 76 percent

27-8. *Increase in insurance coverage of evidence-based treatment for nicotine dependency.* As of 1997-1998, what percentage of health maintenance organizations offered some kind of coverage for nicotine dependency treatment?
   a. 15 percent
   b. 35 percent
   c. 55 percent
   d. 75 percent

Exposure to Secondhand Smoke

27-9. *Reduction in the proportion of children who are regularly exposed to tobacco smoke at home.* As of 1994, what proportion of children were exposed to secondhand smoke at home?
   a. 7 percent
   b. 27 percent
   c. 47 percent
   d. 67 percent

27-10. *Reduction in the proportion of nonsmokers exposed to environmental tobacco smoke.* Between 1988 and 1994, what was the proportion of nonsmokers exposed to secondhand smoke?
   a. 25 percent
   b. 45 percent
   c. 65 percent
   d. 85 percent

27-11. *Increase in smoke-free and tobacco-free environments in schools, including all school facilities, property, vehicles, and school events.* What is the targeted percent of schools being tobacco/smoke-free?
   a. 25 percent
   b. 50 percent
   c. 75 percent
   d. 100 percent

27-12. *Increase in the proportion of work sites with formal smoking policies that prohibit smoking or limit it to separately venti-*

lated areas. As of 1998-1999, what proportion of work sites had such policies?
a. 19 percent
b. 39 percent
c. 59 percent
d. 79 percent

27-13. *Establishment of laws on smoke-free indoor air that prohibit smoking or limit it to separately ventilated areas in public places and work sites.* What is the targeted number of states having such laws?
a. Twenty-one states
b. Thirty-one states
c. Forty-one states
d. Fifty plus the District of Columbia

Social and Environmental Changes

27-14. *Reduction in the illegal sales rate to minors through enforcement of laws prohibiting the sale of tobacco products to minors.* As of 1998, what number of states had 5 percent or less sales rate to minors?
a. No states
b. Ten states
c. Twenty states
d. Thirty states

27-15. *Increase the number of states and the District of Columbia that suspend or revoke state retail licenses for violations of laws prohibiting the sale of tobacco to minors.* As of 1998, what number of states could suspend or revoke sales licenses due to these violations?
a. Four states
b. Fourteen states
c. Twenty-four states
d. Thirty-four states

27-16. *Elimination of tobacco advertising and promotions that influence adolescents and young adults.* Related to this objective, limiting the appeal of tobacco products to young people involves:

a. Restricting tobacco advertising
b. Restricting tobacco promotions
c. Countering the ability of tobacco advertising to reach large segments of the population quickly and efficiently
d. All of the above

27-17. *Increase in adolescents' disapproval of smoking.* As of 1998, what percent of eighth graders disapproved of smoking?
a. 20 percent
b. 40 percent
c. 60 percent
d. 80 percent

27-18. *Increase in the number of tribes, territories, states, and the District of Columbia with comprehensive, evidence-based tobacco control programs (developmental).* Related to this objective, which of the following is correct?
a. Evidence indicates that comprehensive tobacco control programs are effective.
b. Investments in such programs to date have been seriously limited.
c. The ability to sustain reductions in per capita consumption due to excise tax increases is greater when the tax increase is combined with a comprehensive tobacco control program.
d. All of the above are correct.

27-19. *Elimination of laws that preempt stronger tobacco control laws.* As of 1998, how many states had preemptive tobacco control laws in the areas of clean indoor air, minors' access laws, or marketing?
a. No states
b. Ten states
c. Twenty states
d. Thirty states

27-20. *Reduction in the toxicity of tobacco products by establishing a regulatory structure to monitor toxicity (developmental).* Related to this objective, which of the following is correct?
a. There have been recent efforts at reducing the harm in tobacco through alternative forms of nicotine delivery.

  b. Although efforts focus on making tobacco products safer, there is really no such thing as a "safe cigarette."
  c. Proposed hard reduction strategies would be reducing tar/ nicotine levels, tobacco-specific nitrosamines, and specific additives.
  d. All of the above are correct.

27-21. *Increase in the average federal and state tax on tobacco products.* What is the targeted average federal/state tax on tobacco products?
  a. $.50
  b. $1.00
  c. $1.50
  d. $2.00

FOCUS AREA 28: VISION AND HEARING

This focus area's goal is to improve the visual and hearing health of the nation through prevention, early detection, treatment, and rehabilitation.

Vision

28-1. *Increase in the proportion of persons who have a dilated eye examination at appropriate intervals (developmental).* Related to this objective, which of the following is correct?
  a. Many eye diseases and disorders have no symptoms or early warning signs.
  b. Dilated eye examinations should be performed at appropriate intervals to detect changes in the retina or optic nerve or both.
  c. Eye care professionals can view the back of the eye for subtle changes and, if necessary, initiate treatment at the right time.
  d. All of the above are correct.

28-2. *Increase in the proportion of preschool children aged five years and under who receive vision screening (developmental).* Related to this objective, all of the following are correct except:

a. Many vision problems begin well before children reach school.

b. Every effort must be made to ensure that children receive a screening examination from their health care provider before age five.

c. Early recognition of disease results in more effective treatment that can be sightsaving or even lifesaving.

d. Myopia, or nearsightedness, is found in 20 percent of children entering school.

28-3. *Reduction in uncorrected visual impairment due to refractive errors (developmental).* Which is a visual device that can used to correct refractive errors?

a. Magnifying spectacles

b. Hand-held magnifiers

c. Stand magnifiers

d. All of the above

28-4. *Reduction in blindness and visual impairment in children and adolescents aged seventeen years and under.* How much of a reduction is targeted in blindness and visual impairment in this age group?

a. 20 percent reduction

b. 40 percent reduction

c. 60 percent reduction

d. 80 percent reduction

28-5. *Reduction in visual impairment due to diabetic retinopathy (developmental).* Related to this objective, what is diabetic retinopathy?

a. Cloudiness of the lens that may prevent a clear image from forming on the retina

b. Complication of diabetes that damages the retina

c. Deterioration of the macula that results in a loss of sharp central vision

d. Developmental abnormality of the central nervous system that causes impaired vision in one or both eyes

28-6. *Reduction in visual impairment due to glaucoma (developmental).* All of the following are correct except:

a. Glaucoma is a leading cause of visual impairment.

b. If left untreated glaucoma causes progressive optic nerve damage that leads to blindness.

c. Glaucoma is the number one cause of blindness in whites compared to other racial groups in the U.S. population.

d. Although treatments are available, at least half of people with glaucoma are not receiving treatment because they are unaware of their condition.

28-7. *Reduction in visual impairment due to cataract (developmental).* Related to this objective, which of the following is correct?

a. Cataract is a leading cause of visual impairment in the U.S. population.

b. People with diabetes also are more likely to have cataracts.

c. Cataract is a cloudiness of the lens that may prevent a clear image from forming on the retina.

d. All of the above are correct.

28-8. *Reduction in occupational eye injury (developmental).* Related to this objective, which could be an adaptive device used by visually impaired or blind persons on the job?

a. Large-print reading materials (books, newspapers)

b. Check writing guides

c. High-contrast watch dials

d. All of the above

28-9. *Increase in the use of appropriate personal protective eyewear in recreational activities and hazardous situations around the home (developmental).* Related to this objective, which of the following is correct?

a. Almost all eye injuries can be prevented.

b. Many sports and recreation activities, including baseball, basketball, tennis, racquetball, and hockey, carry some risk of eye injury.

c. Activities at home, such as cooking and yard work, also present eye injury risk.

d. All of the above are correct.

28-10. *Increase in vision rehabilitation (developmental).* Related to this objective, which of the following is correct?

a. Rehabilitation addresses the needs in daily living skills that are directly related to vision.
b. A visual aid could be an optical or nonoptical device that helps people with low vision make use of their remaining sight.
c. Both visual and adaptive devices can be used by persons with visual impairments.
d. All of the above are correct.

Hearing

28-11. *Increase in the proportion of newborns who are screened for hearing loss by age one month, have audiologic evaluation by age three months, and are enrolled in appropriate intervention services by age six months (developmental).* Related to this objective, hearing loss may be caused by:
a. Genetic factors
b. Noise or trauma
c. Sensitivity to certain drugs or medications
d. All of the above

28-12. *Reduction in otitis media in children and adolescents.* How much of a reduction is targeted in inner ear infection in younger persons?
a. 15 percent reduction
b. 25 percent reduction
c. 45 percent reduction
d. 65 percent reduction

28-13. *Increase in access by persons who have hearing impairments to hearing rehabilitation services and adaptive devices, including hearing aids, cochlear implants, or tactile or other assistive or augmentative devices (developmental).* Related to this objective, early detection and rehabilitation of hearing problems is crucial because:
a. Untreated cases may progress to total hearing loss
b. Hearing loss in children is often sufficient to prevent the spontaneous development of spoken language

      c. Minimal hearing loss also is an important factor in school success and psychosocial development

      d. All of the above

28-14. *Increase in the proportion of persons who have had a hearing examination on schedule (developmental).* In adults between the ages of nineteen and fifty years old, hearing examination for impairment and disability should occur:

      a. Every year

      b. Every five years

      c. Every ten years

      d. Only when there is reason to suspect hearing is being impaired

28-15. *Increase in the number of persons who are referred by their primary care physician for hearing evaluation and treatment (developmental).* Related to this objective, what is involved in an audiologic evaluation?

      a. Tests of conduction

      b. Tests of speech perception and speech discrimination

      c. Case history of hearing health

      d. All of the above

28-16. *Increase in the use of appropriate ear protection devices, equipment, and practices (developmental).* Related to this objective, hearing conservation involves:

      a. Engineering controls

      b. Noise monitoring and measuring

      c. Employee notification

      d. All of the above

28-17. *Reduction in noise-induced hearing loss in children and adolescents ages seventeen years and under (developmental).* Related to this objective, which of the following is correct about noise-induced hearing loss?

      a. Noise-induced hearing loss is caused only by one-time exposure to loud noise.

      b. All noise-induced hearing loss is immediate and permanent.

    c. Noise-induced hearing loss may be accompanied by tinnitus, which is a ringing, buzzing, or roaring in the ears or head.

    d. Tinnitus takes place only at the time of first injury to the inner ear.

28-18. *Reduction in adult hearing loss in the noise-exposed public (developmental).* Related to this objective, which is a significant factor in the prevention of noise-induced hearing loss?

    a. Knowledge of potentially dangerous noise

    b. Fitting and use of hearing protection

    c. Careful product selection

    d. All of the above

TEST ANSWERS

Focus Area 27

27-1. (b) 24 percent. The target is 12 percent of adults eighteen years and older smoking cigarettes. At little over 2 percent of adults are involved in spit tobacco and cigar use and the target is to reduce to 1 percent.*

27-2. (b) 21 percent. Tobacco products involve cigarettes, smokeless tobacco, and cigars. The 1999 baseline was 40 percent of adolescents having used such a product within the past month.

27-3. (c) Adolescent cigarette smoking is a notifiable condition, meaning providers are required to report cases to local health departments. This is incorrect because adult cigarette smoking is what gets reported to health departments. For the first time in notifiable disease surveillance, a behavior—cigarette smoking—is considered a condition that needs to be reported.

27-4. (b) Twelve. The target is to increase the average age of tobacco use initiation to fourteen. Since most tobacco use initiation occurs in adolescence, direct measures of tobacco use in adolescence are important health indicators.

27-5. (c) 75 percent. The baseline in 1998 was 41 percent of adult smokers aged eighteen years and older who stopped smoking for one day or longer because they were trying to quit.

27-6. (b) 30 percent. As of 1998, the baseline was 14 percent of females aged eighteen to forty-nine years stopped smoking during the first trimester of their pregnancy. Smoking during pregnancy is implicated in spontaneous abortions, low birth weight, and sudden infant death syndrome.

27-7. (d) 76 percent. The target is for 84 percent of everyday smokers in grades nine through twelve to attempt to quit smoking. About half of cigarette smoking adolescents believe they will stop within five years, however, only about 25 percent of them actually achieve this goal.

27-8. (d) 75 percent. The target is 100 percent of HMOs either partially or fully covering one or more smoking cessation inter-

*Ages adjusted to the year 2000 standard population.

ventions (e.g., self-help materials, smoking cessation classes, pharmaceutical treatments, etc.).

27-9.   (b) 27 percent. 27 percent of children aged six years and under lived in a household where someone smoked inside the house at least four days per week. The target is to reduce this to 10 percent.

27-10. (c) 65 percent. 65 percent of nonsmokers aged four years and older had a serum cotinine level above 0.10 ng/mL. This is significant because about 37 percent of adult nontobacco users were aware enough of their exposure to report having been exposed to secondhand smoke either at home or at work. The target is a reduction to 45 percent exposure to secondhand smoke.

27-11. (d) 100 percent. The baseline in 1994 was 37 percent of middle, junior high, and senior high schools were smoke free and tobacco free.

27-12. (d) 79 percent. The target is for 100 percent of work sites with fifty or more employees having formal smoking policies that prohibited or limited smoking to separately ventilated areas.

27-13. (d) Fifty plus the District of Columbia. As of 1998, states with laws prohibiting smoking established these areas: private workplaces, 1; public workplaces, 13; restaurants, 3; public transportation, 16; day care centers, 22; and retail stores, 4.

27-14. (a) No states. The target is for all states including the District of Columbia to have tobacco sales rates to minors at no more than 5 percent.

27-15. (d) Thirty-four states with some form of retail licensure could suspend or revoke the license for violation of minors access laws. The target is for all states including the District of Columbia.

27-16. (d) All of the above. Because of their appeal, the mass media can serve as a powerful tool for tobacco control. Television and radio stations, magazines, and other media can deliver information and educational messages directly to targeted audiences, build public support for tobacco control programs and policies, reinforce social norms supporting the nonuse of tobacco, and counteract messages and images of tobacco marketing and public relations campaigns.

27-17. (d) 80 percent. The target is 90 percent of eighth graders, tenth graders, and twelfth graders disapproving of smoking a pack of cigarettes a day.

27-18. (d) All of the above are correct. Tobacco control programs comprise school-based curriculum, community-based activities, and mass media interventions.

27-19. (d) Thirty states. The target is to have zero states with these kinds of preemptive laws. A preemptive state tobacco control law prevents local jurisdictions from enacting restrictions that are more restrictive than or vary from state law.

27-20. (d) All of the above are correct. Issues raised by products or technologies that purport to reduce risk require the establishment of an appropriate scientific and regulatory framework within the federal government. Much work needs to be done before scientific and regulatory agencies are in a position to evaluate the issues raised by these technologies and to inform the public about risks.

27-21. (d) $2.00. As of 1998, the average federal/state tax on cigarettes was $.63.

Focus Area 28

28-1. (d) All of the above are correct. Periodic dilated eye examinations can detect diseases such as diabetic retinopathy and age-related macular degeneration.

28-2. (d) Myopia, or nearsightedness, is found in 2 percent of children entering school and about 15 percent of those entering high school. In children, visual impairment is associated with developmental delays and the need for special educational, vocational, and social services, often into adulthood.

28-3. (d) All of the above. Visual devices use lenses or combinations of lenses to provide magnification. Besides the ones listed as correct responses, there are stand magnifiers, computer monitors with large type, and closed-circuit televisions.

28-4. (a) 20 percent reduction. As of 1997, the baseline rate was twenty-five per 1,000 children and adolescents aged seventeen years and under were blind or visually impaired. The target is a reduction to twenty per 1,000.

28-5. (b) Complication of diabetes that damages the retina. People with diabetes are at risk of developing this disease, which is a major cause of visual impairment and blindness.

28-6. (c) Glaucoma is the number one cause of blindness in whites compared to other racial groups in the U.S. population. This is incorrect because it is African Americans who have higher rates of blindness related to glaucoma. This is true in both U.S. and Caribbean populations.

28-7. (d) All of the above are correct. Cataracts' effect on vision can be accommodated through visual devices.

28-8. (d) All of the above, such as talking computers, are auditory aids.

28-9. (d) All of the above are correct. In addition, it is worth noting that some injuries may go unnoticed because only one eye is involved.

28-10. (d) All of the above are correct. In addition, it is worth noting that legal blindness determines eligibility for benefits from the federal government, however, it has little or no value for rehabilitation purposes.

28-11. (d) All of the above. In addition, other causes of hearing loss, especially in young persons, are viral or bacterial infections.

28-12. (a) 15 percent reduction. As of 1997, the baseline rate was 344.7 per 1,000 doctor office visits for otitis media in the under-eighteen-year-old age group. The target is to reduce that number to 294 visits per 1,000. Otitis media is commonly called ear infection—an inflammation of the middle ear caused by viral or bacterial infection. It accounts for 24.5 million doctor office visits and is the most frequent reason for children's emergency department visits.

28-13. (d) All of the above. During rehabilitation, assistive technology can facilitate a hearing-impaired person's ability to have an equal opportunity in schools, in workplaces, and in society.

28-14. (c) Every ten years. For persons in this age group, hearing screening should take place every decade. However, persons after age fifty should have more frequent monitoring.

28-15. (d) All of the above. Audiologic evaluation comprises tests and procedures that measure the ability to hear. The evaluation identifies type and degree of hearing loss and includes recommendations about appropriate assistive devices.

28-16. (d) All of the above. In addition, an occupational hearing conservation program provides audiometric testing and evaluation, health education, and follow-up that includes hearing protection and fitting and/or audiologic/otologic evaluation.

28-17. (c) Noise-induced hearing loss may be accompanied by tinnitus, which is a ringing, buzzing, or roaring in the ears or head. This is correct; the other responses are incorrect. Noise-induced hearing loss can be caused by repeated exposure to sounds at various levels over an extended period of time as well as by one-time exposure. Most cases of noise-induced hearing loss develop gradually over time rather than immediately and permanently. Likewise, tinnitus, which usually accompanies noise-induced hearing loss, accompanies this condition over years of development.

28-18. (d) All of the above. In addition, audiologic/otologic evaluation is important in the prevention of noise-induced hearing loss.

Glossary

absolute risk: The number of cases of disease occurring in a given time period (N) divided by the population exposed to the risk, and the quantity multiplied by 100. *See* GENERIC RATE FORMULA.

active immunity: Attained either from exposure to a highly immunogenic agent or being inoculated against the agent.

activities of daily living: An indicator of recovery from disease in which the host resumes independent functioning in basic living areas, such as dressing, feeding, toileting, etc., with special equipment if needed.

actuarial data: Life table information used to determine life expectancy.

adoption studies: A version of twin studies in which twin siblings were separated and raised in different home life situations.

agent: A necessary factor for the occurrence of disease or other health-affecting condition.

age-specific death rates: The numerator (N) contains death counts, and the denominator denotes the population of a specified age group. Quotient is multiplied by a power of ten. *See* GENERIC RATE FORMULA.

alcohol-related fatal crash: When either a deceased driver of an automobile or nonoccupant (e.g., pedestrian) had a blood alcohol concentration of greater than or equal to 0.01 g/dL in a police-reported traffic accident.

allergy: A hypersensitive immune defense to an antigen, in this case, known as an allergen.

amniotic fluid: The water medium within the amniotic sac that houses the unborn.

analytic studies: Focus on the risk factors and the cause of disease and behaviors affecting health status.

anaphylaxis: A severe allergic reaction.

angioplasty: Widening of an artery via inserted balloons.

anthrax: A bacterial infection characterized by a boillike lesions and swelling of the lymph glands close to the lesion.

antibiotic: A substance (e.g., penicillin) from bacteria, fungi, and other organisms that destroys or inhibits bacterial growth.

antibodies: White blood cells and other proteins that counteract an antigen.

antigen: A biological agent whose presence will likely stimulate the immune defense system to produce antibodies.

antisepsis: The destruction of disease-causing microorganisms to prevent infection.

arthritis (and other rheumatic conditions): An inflammatory and possibly degenerative disease of the joints, muscles, fascia, tendons, bursa, ligaments, and other connective tissues of the body.

artifactual difference: The faulty measurement of a disease.

asbestosis: A fibrous lung disease caused by prolonged inhalation of asbestos fibers.

asthma: A common noninfectious, chronic disease with symptoms of breathing difficulty caused by temporary constriction of the bronchi, the airways connecting the trachea to the lungs.

astrology: The study of celestial bodies, their activity, and their presumed influence on natural events and human affairs.

at risk: Being at greater risk of developing a disease or other health-affecting condition.

attack (or case) rate: The most specific kind of morbidity rate in which only persons exposed to an identified agent or factor can be included in the denominator. *See* GENERIC RATE FORMULA.

attributal risk: Portion of disease occurrence that appears to be explained by exposure to a factor.

audiometric significant shift: When a person loses ability to distinguish pitch—the highness or loudness of sound produced by frequency of waves.

autolochronous transmission: When an infected source host visits a place free of the disease and inadvertently allows an indigenous vector to transmit the disease to new hosts in that place.

bacteria: Microscopic parasites that lack nuclear membranes but can live in or outside of the cells of their hosts.

Baillou, Guillaume de: A French physician of the sixteenth and seventeenth centuries recognized as the parent of traditional epidemiology because he applied Hippocratic principles, or the natural notion, to disease causation.

B cells: Lymphocytes produced in bone marrow.

behavioral agents: Unhealthy life practices that lead to some infectious and many noninfectious diseases.

Behavioral Risk Factor Surveillance System (BRFSS): A state-level telephone survey used to monitor the prevalence of major behavioral agents in the adult population.

bias: Error caused by systematically favoring some study findings over others.

biological agents: Microorganisms such as bacteria, viruses, rickettesia, protozoa, and metazoa.

biological environment: Living things in our surroundings.

biological pollutants: Pathogenic microbes: bacteria, viruses, protozoa and metazoa; overgrowth of aquatic plants such as algae.

biomonitoring data: Information furnished by measurements of toxic substances in the human body.

biopsy: The excising of body tissue for the purpose of diagnostics.

biostatistics: The application of statistics to biological or medical problems.

bloodborne pathogens: Disease agents requiring blood or body fluid for transmission.

body mass index (BMI): Weight (in kilograms) divided by the square of height (in meters); or weight (in pounds) divided by the square of height (in inches) multiplied by 704.5. Because it is readily calculated, BMI is the measurement of choice as an indicator of healthy weight, overweightness, and obesity.

booster shot: An additional inoculation to ensure active immunity in a host.

bronchitis: An inflammation of the lower respiratory tract due to biological or chemical agent.

bubonic plague: A bacterial disease transmitted from rodents to human hosts through a flea vector, which if left untreated, has a case fatality of 60 to 90 percent.

cancer: Diseases characterized by abnormal and out-of-control cell division that can invade surrounding tissue and spread through the circulatory systems to other body parts. *See* MALIGNANT NEOPLASM—rapid multiplication of underdeveloped cells.

carbon monoxide (CO): A colorless, odorless gas produced as a result of incomplete burning of carbon-containing fuels that reduces the blood's ability to carry oxygen.

carcinogen: A cancer-causing agent.

cardiovascular disease (CVD): A collection of disorders of the heart tissue/valves or the blood vessels vasculating the organ.

carpal tunnel syndrome: A repetitive motion disorder in the wrist causing inflammation, swelling, tenderness, and numbness in the extremity.

carrier: An infected host who is progressing through the disease process, but many times does not display signs or symptoms, and who is capable of transferring the biological agent to other hosts.

case control studies: Analytic and retrospective in nature, incidence studies that utilize two groups.

case fatality rate: Persons who die from a disease or condition (N) divided by those who were diagnosed with the disease (population); the quotient is multiplied by 100. *See* GENERIC RATE FORMULA.

case studies: Examination, verification, and classification of disease cases during an outbreak.

cases (in a case control study): Persons with the disease.

Centers for Disease Prevention and Control (CDC): A U.S. Public Health Services agency comprised of centers dealing with epidemiology, international health, laboratory improvement, prevention services, environmental health, occupational health, infectious diseases, and professional development.

chain of infection: The mechanism of an infectious agent spreading from its source and entering new hosts.

chemical agents: Pollutants as well as toxic substances.

chi square test: A nonparametric inferential statistical analysis.

chlamydia: A sexually transmitted bacterial disease that primarily infests the urogenital tract.

chlorofluorocarbons (CFCs): Simple, gaseous compounds used in refrigerants, aerosols, and insulators that are suspected in the destruction of the ozone layer in the Earth's upper atmosphere, which is said to allow more ultraviolet radiation from the sun, which damages plants and greatly increases people's risk of skin cancer.

cholecystectomy: Gallbladder removal.

cholera: A water- or foodborne bacterial disease causing severe diarrhea, dehydration, vomiting, and cramps.

cholesterol: A blood lipoprotein necessary for hormonal production, cell integrity, and other functions of the body.

chronic back condition: Low back pain and other conditions affecting only the back.

chronic obstructive pulmonary diseases: Emphysema, asthma, and chronic bronchitis. These diseases cause airways to become partly blocked or narrower, making it difficult for air to move through them.

cirrhosis: A severe liver disease that occurs when scar and fibrous tissue replace liver cells.

clinical stage: When pathological changes become clearly apparent and diagnosable.

clinical trial: An experimental study in which the subjects are individual persons.

clustering: When any number of rare or special diseases cases occur and are distributed due to the interaction of person, place, or time characteristics.

cochlea: An organ in the inner ear.

cohort: A group comprised of same-aged persons with varying degrees of risk exposure.

cohort study: A prospective study in which a group of persons without the disease are assessed periodically for long periods of time to see if there is a factor exposure-disease incidence relationship.

common source epidemic: When each case was exposed to the same source host or environment.

communicability: The ability of an agent to be transmitted from host to host.

community trial: An experimental study in which the subjects are groups of persons.

concept: A general idea obtained or deduced from specific phenomena or happenings.

concurrent prospective study: A cohort study that starts in the present and proceeds into the future.

congenital diseases: Disorders present at birth.

congenital rubella syndrome: Includes deafness, cataracts, heart defects, and mental retardation occurring in babies born to mothers who contracted rubella during pregnancy.

contagion: The spread of disease through direct or indirect contact.

controls (in a case control study): Persons without the disease.

convalesces: Recovering from disease.

cross-contamination: Indirect transmission of a biological agent to a host via one fomite to another.

crossover effect: Observed when a characteristically high rate of mortality in a group decreases as the persons progress through a disease life cycle while other groups experience increases in mortality rates.

cross-sectional sampling: When the proportions of person characteristics in the sample are similar to those of the population.

crude rate: The general mortality rate of the population.

cumulative incidence: New cases of disease occurring in a period of time in which everyone in the population was susceptible to the disease.

cyclical variation: Case distribution according to sociocultural designations of the year, such as when children attend school.

cytopatholoy: The study of diseased cells.

death certificate: A vital statistic surveillance instrument for gathering data on mortality.

demography: The statistical study of human populations.

demonic belief (in disease): Disease explanation due to mystical and spiritual influences.

dependent variable (DV): A condition or factor dependent on an independent variable (IV).

descriptive statistic: A numerical value resulting from a calculation that represents a person, place, or time characteristic.

descriptive studies: Focus on the distribution of disease and other health-affecting conditions.

diabetes: An endocrine disorder which disrupts insulin production or absorption in the body.

diphtheria: A severe bacterial infection of the upper respiratory tract.

direct method (of rate adjustment): Uses age-specific cases within the local population multiplied by the age-specific case rates of the standardized population, with the products totaled and entered into the GENERIC RATE FORMULA.

direct transmission: When the agent is passed from a source host to another host, or from a source environment to another host.

disability: A general term used to represent the interactions between individuals with a health condition and barriers in their environment.

disease: A pathological condition of an organism resulting from various causes, characterized by clinical signs and/or symptoms of illness.

disease prevention programming: An array of health services and settings for the prevention, diagnosis, treatment, management, and rehabilitation of disease, injury, and disability centered on the continuum of care.

disease process: Pathological progress by way of successive stages starting with susceptibility, moving to exposure, clinical observation, and ultimately to a stage of full, partial, or no recovery.

disease-specific death rates (or cause of): Disease-specific death cases are placed in the numerator (N), divided by the population at midpoint of a reporting year, whose quotient is multiplied by a power of 10. *See* GENERIC RATE FORMULA.

distress: A health-affecting condition of mental discomfort.

Doll, Richard and Hill, Austin: Conducted studies during the mid-1900s that established the causal relationship between cigarette smoking and lung cancer.

droplet nuclei: Dried or congealed nasal/throat discharges that act as reservoirs for biological agents.

dysentery: A bacterial or protozoan-caused disease of the intestines resulting in inflammation, painful and bloody diarrhea, and dehydration.

dysplasia: Abnormal cell growth that can be a precursor to cancer.

ecological fallacy: Presuming physical environmental characteristics are the direct explanation of disease, when it could likely be sociocultural environmental influence.

ecology: The study of the interrelationships of organisms and their environment.

ecosystems: Living things that interact as functional units.

emphysema: Occurs from a breakdown of the lung alveoli resulting in significantly diminished breathing capacity.

endemic: The usual incidence and prevalence of disease or other behaviors affecting health status.

enterotoxin: The poisonous products from bacteria infesting the gastrointestinal tract.

environment: The physical, biological, and psychosocial conditions surrounding an organism affecting its growth, development, and survival.

environmental epidemiology: The study of physical, biological, and chemical factors in the external environment that may or may not affect human health. Can include examining specific populations or communities exposed to different ambient environments to clarify the relationship between physical, biological, or chemical factors and human health.

environmental estrogens: Found in nature or synthetically made (e.g., DDT or polychlorinated biphenyls (PCBs)) and mimic the actions of estrogen in the body.

environmental health: A related discipline to epidemiology since it also concerns itself with the occurrence, distribution, cause and control, treatment, and prevention of disease and other health-affecting conditions from an environmental perspective.

epidemic: A greater than expected or sudden increase in disease occurrence. *See* OUTBREAK.

epidemic curve: A charting along a time line of case appearance during an epidemic.

epidemiological reasoning: The close observation and accounting of all possible factors in the physical, social, and biological environments that might influence a disease event.

epidemiological triad: A principle comprising the concepts of agent, host, environment, and time to explain disease occurrence.

epidemiology: The study of the occurrence and distribution, cause and control, and prevention and treatment of diseases and other health-affecting conditions.

ergonomics: An applied science of workplace design that maximizes productivity and minimizes worker fatigue and injury.

Escherichia coli: Naturally found bacteria and an integral part of the normal gastrointestinal inner environment. Sewage-contaminated water, milk, or food (e.g., undercooked beef) can transmit them.

etiology: Cause of disease.

eutrophicates: Water pollutants such as phosphates and nitrates in fertilizers.

experimental studies (trial): Determine the effectiveness of interventions meant to treat or prevent disease. The subjects are randomly selected and assigned to treatment and control groups.

exposure: When the host lays open to the agent.

factual difference: When the trend in disease cases, such as regional differences, is truly due to place factors.

fatality rate: The death rate in a designated series of persons exposed to or affected by a simultaneous event like a disaster.

fecal coliform: A bacterium that subsists in human or animal waste and causes gastrointestinal disease.

firearm-related injury: A penetrating injury from a weapon using a powder charge to fire a bullet or other projectile.

fomite: An inanimate vehicle during disease transmission, such as clothing or a drinking glass.

foodborne disease: Relies on food as a vehicle of transmission.

food contamination (or intoxication): When a host consumes a toxic substance and then proceeds through a disease process as a result of the exposure.

food cycle: The production, processing, and preparation of food.

food infection: When a host consumes a microorganism carried by food and then proceeds through a disease process as a result of the agent incubating and growing in number inside the host.

food poisoning: When a host consumes a microorganism carried by food and then proceeds through a disease process as a result of the toxins or poisons produced by the agent.

formal diabetes education: Self-management training that includes a process of initial individual patient assessment; instruction provided or supervised by a qualified health professional; evaluation of accumulation by the diabetic patient of appropriate knowledge, skills, and attitudes; and ongoing reassessment and training.

Fracastoro, Girolamo: The parent of germ theory. Proposed germ explanation of disease three centuries before its scientific demonstration.

Galen: The parent of anatomy. Perfected the skills of bodily dissection and surgery.

gastroenteritis: The inflammation of the gastrointestinal tract, with symptoms such as nausea, vomiting, and anorexia, and can be accompanied by fever, abdominal discomfort, and diarrhea.

generic rate formula: A basic formula used to calculate and illustrate various epidemiological findings. The formula considers the number of cases or events (N) divided by a measure of the population and the quotient is multiplied by some power of ten. $\left(\frac{(N)}{\text{population}} \right) 10^{(n)}$

genetic agents: Chemical instructions within genetic material that inadvertently cause or contribute to disease or other morbid conditions.

genetic shifting: The ability of an agent to develop subtypes or strains at irregular intervals.

giardiasis: A protozoan-caused infectious disease whose mode of transmission is intestinal discharge and consumption of contaminated food and water (fomites). Signs and symptoms are gastrointestinal problems.

Goldberger, Joseph: Conducted his work on pellagra, a disease from the deficiency of niacin.

gonorrhea: A sexually transmitted bacterial disease that primarily infests the urogenital tract.

Graunt, John: The parent of vital statistics. Studied patterns in municipal death rates.

HAART: Highly active antiretroviral therapy comprised of protease inhibitors and reverse transcriptase inhibitors whose purpose is to reduce HIV load infection to undetectable levels.

handicap: A disadvantage for a given individual, resulting from an impairment or a disability, that limits or prevents the fulfillment of a role that is normal, depending on age, sex, social, and cultural practice for that individual.

harmful contact incidents: Intentional or unintentional injuries.

Healey, Bernadette: The first female director of the National Institutes of Health during the 1980s and 1990s. She promoted greater female representation both as investigators and as subjects in analytical research.

health promotion and disease prevention (HP/DP): The aggregate of all purposeful activities designed to improve personal and public health.

health promotion programming: Any planned combination of educational, political, regulatory, and organizational supports for actions and living conditions conducive to the health of individuals, groups, or communities.

health status: A person's standing in terms of physical functioning, emotional well-being, daily life activity performance, and feelings of fulfillment, productivity, and social responsibility. It is considered the appraised age of an individual compared to his or her actual age.

Healthy People 2010: A national health promotion and disease prevention initiative that brings together national, state, and local government agencies; nonprofit, voluntary, and professional organizations; businesses; communities; and individuals to improve the health of all Americans, eliminate disparities in health, and improve years and quality of healthy life.

healthy worker effect: Employed persons have a higher health status than unemployed persons.

hemophilia: A blood-clotting disorder.

hepatitis B: A blood/body fluid-borne viral infection of the liver, also called serum hepatitis.

hepatitis C: A blood/body fluid-borne viral infection of the liver.

herd immunity: When a population is immune to a disease.

Highly Active Antiretroviral Therapy: *See* HAART.

Hippocrates: The parent of medicine. Established a rational approach to disease causation and treatment through direct and intense observation.

historical cohort study: Uses control subjects from whom data were collected at a time preceding that of the group being studied.

host: An organism on or within which another organism lives.

HP/DP: *See* HEALTH PROMOTION AND DISEASE PREVENTION.

human factors or **misactions:** Unsafe practices.

Human Genome Project: An international scientific program, with the intention of mapping all of the chemical instructions found in genes that control heredity in human beings.

humours: Fluids of the body as presumed by HIPPOCRATES: blood, phlegm (mucous), yellow bile (secretions), and black bile (excretions).

hydrophobia: Fear of water.

hypercholesteremia: An elevated cholesterol level of ≥ 220 mg/dL blood.

hypertension: High blood pressure.

hypothesis (about disease outbreak): A tentative and testable explanation about how an outbreak happened.

hysteria: A mental health disorder in which symptoms are displayed without an organic cause.

iatrogenic: A condition created by behavioral agents in the course of health care delivery.

immunity: Capability of withstanding or not responding to the presence of a biological agent.

immunogenicity: The ability of a biological agent to elicit an immune defense response including immunity.

impairment: Any loss or abnormality of psychological, physiological, or anatomical structure or function.

incidence: New cases or new events of a disease or other morbid condition.

incidence rate: Calculated using new cases of a disease versus the total number of exposed persons. *See* GENERIC RATE FORMULA.

incidence rate, period: Calculated using new cases of disease occurring during a specified length of time, usually a year or greater. *See* GENERIC RATE FORMULA.

incidence rate, point: Calculated using new cases of disease occurrences during a specified length of time, usually less than a year. *See* GENERIC RATE FORMULA.

incubation period: When a host's immune defense has been activated in response to growing numbers of agent prior to symptoms. Also called SUBCLINICAL PHASE.

independent variable (IV): Has an actual or assumed directional relationship with a DEPENDENT VARIABLE (DV) so that change in the IV influences change in the DV.

indirect method (of rate adjustment): Uses age-specific cases within the standardized population multiplied by the age-specific case rates of the local population with the products totaled and entered into the standardized mortality (morbidity) ratio.

indirect transmission: When an intermediary passes the agent from a source to a host.

infection control: Practiced at all disease process stages during which standard precautions (e.g., cleanliness, protection, immunization) are performed to prevent the spread of infectious diseases.

infection rate: An incidence rate in which the numerator (N) includes both new cases and inapparent infection cases, persons who start a disease process but do not display symptoms, divided by the total number of exposed individuals. *See* GENERIC RATE FORMULA.

infectious disease: A pathological condition resulting from infection by a microorganism or its products. *See also* SUBCLINICAL PHASE *and* INCUBATION PERIOD.

infectivity or **infectibility:** The ability of a biological agent to enter and multiply within a host.

influenza: A viral infection of the respiratory tract.

***International Classification of Diseases* (ICD-10):** A three-digit code system under the direction of the World Health Organization to classify diseases, injuries, and other causes of death.

interventive trial: Operates as the secondary level of prevention and targets subjects who are at high health risk.

in utero: Within the womb.

investigations: Professional responses to disease occurrence, especially sudden increases in occurrence known as outbreaks or epidemics, with the twofold purpose of controlling the event and preventing any further occurrence.

investigative method: Involves determining the needs of a disease control program, designing appropriate interventive and preventive health services, and responding to the usual or unusual presence of disease in a population.

jaundice: When bilirubin levels rise in the blood causing a yellowish tint to skin and eyes.

Kannel, William and Dawber, Thomas: Were on the first research team for the Framingham Heart Study with others.

kidney disease: Renal dysfunction that most likely manifests in successive, irreversible stages of chronic renal insufficiency, chronic renal failure, and end-stage renal disease.

Koch, Robert: The parent of bacteriology. German physician who isolated the bacteria responsible for tuberculosis, cholera, and anthrax.

Koch's Postulates of Disease: Fundamental principles for understanding infectious disease causation.

latency period: The subclinical phase of a noninfectious disease process. *See* SUBCLINICAL PHASE *and* NONINFECTIOUS DISEASE.

laudanum: An early anesthetic comprised of alcohol and opiates.

lead: A metallic element used in manufacturing processes that is known to pollute the environment through dust and fumes released by industrial plants.

leptospirosis: An acute febrile illness caused by a bacterium.

levels of prevention: Gradient stages of risk for disease.

life expectancy: The projected average number of years of living for a birth cohort (or group) given the mortality rates at that time.

life expectancy free from disability: An estimate of life expectancy adjusted for activity limitations.

life table: Depicts age-specific survivorship and is used to predict the percentage of persons likely to live long enough to comprise the next age group.

lifetime prevalence: As in prevalence rate calculations, this is a subset wherein the total of persons who have ever had a disease some time in their life are figured into the numerator while the total at-risk population count remains in the denominator.

Lind, James: A naval surgeon during the eighteenth century, considered the parent of naval hygiene in England.

Livingston, Ivor Lensworth: The first to compile a comprehensive review of epidemiological research on health problems, issues, and policies pertaining to African Americans.

local population: The population under observation.

logistics: The handling of details in a process or operation such as procurement, distribution, maintainence, and replacement of resources needed for implementation.

Lyme disease: This is caused by a bacterium with symptoms of headache, muscular aches and pains, and fatigue.

Lyssavirus: A highly virulent viral disease that is usually transmitted from animal to human host. *See* RABIES.

malaria: A protozoan infection of the circulatory system resulting in periodic attacks of chills and fever, anemia, and enlarged spleen, often with fatal complications.

malignant neoplasm: Rapid multiplication of underdeveloped cells. *See* CANCER.

masking: As in an epidemiological study where the subjects and/or those conducting the study do not know who receives the treatment until the results are compiled.

measles: An acute viral disease causing rash, fever, and general discomfort.

mental disorders: Health conditions characterized by alterations in thinking, mood, or behavior (or some combination thereof) that are all mediated by the brain and associated with distress, impaired functioning, or both.

mesothelioma: A rare cancer in the membrane lining of the lungs and abdominal organs.

metazoa: Microscopic multicellular parasites.

miasmas: Poisonous gasses assumed to emanate from swamps and putrid matter to cause disease.

misactions or **human factors:** Unsafe practices.

morbid conditions: Any departures, subjective or objective, from physical or mental well-being.

morbidity: Illness.

morbidity rates: Measure disease occurrence and are calculated for attack, incidence, and prevalence of disease within a population. Normally, rates are set against 100, 1,000 or 10,000. *See* GENERIC RATE FORMULA.

mortality: Death.

mortality rates: Measure death occurrence in a population and are calculated as crude, disease-specific, age-specific, maternal, and natal. Usually measured against 10,000 or 100,000. *See* GENERIC RATE FORMULA.

multiple sclerosis: A neurological disease in which nerve fiber covering is damaged from an unknown agent, marked by partial or complete paralysis and jerking muscle tremors.

mystical notion of disease: Spiritual or mystical explanations of morbidity and mortality.

natality rates: Death counts occurring at specific stages of fetal or early life development calculated in proportion to live births, with fetal deaths included in fetal and perinatal natality rates. Rate is normally set against 1,000. *See* GENERIC RATE FORMULA.

National Center for Health Statistics: Organization that maintains morbidity and mortality data systems and conducts periodic surveys of the general public.

National Institute of Occupational Safety and Health (NIOSH): Organization that establishes, through research, workplace health and safety standards.

natural notion of disease: Influence of naturally concurring events as explanations of illness and death.

necessary factor: A factor that must be present for morbidity, although its presence alone does not necessarily lead to disease.

nicotine: A psychotropic drug found in tobacco products that can stimulate both sympathetic and parasympathetic portions of the autonomic nervous system.

nitrogen oxide (NO): A compound resulting from combustion of fossil fuels; a form of air pollution.

nonattainment area: A place that exceeds EPA standards for levels of air pollutants.

nonconcurrent prospective study: A cohort study that uses data collected in the past to construct future possible outcomes regarding risk factor exposure of a given population.

noninfectious disease: A pathological condition resulting from exposure to risk factors or nonliving substances. *See* SUBCLINICAL PHASE *and* LATENCY PERIOD.

nonlean body mass: Adipose tissue.

nonpoint source: A dispersed source of exposure usually distant from the originating or point source.

Norwalk virus: Causes a highly contagious disease characterized by nausea, vomiting, and diarrhea.

nosocomial infections: Infectious diseases inadvertently spread by health care professionals in the process of providing care.

obesity: Condition in which a person weighs 20 percent or higher than recommended body weight.

occupational diseases: Diseases resulting from exposure to agents on the job.

Occupational Safety and Health Administration (OSHA): Organization founded within the U.S. Department of Labor to ensure healthy and safe working conditions.

odds ratio: Calculated from an epidemiological two-by-two table wherein persons without the disease have been controlled.

official health agencies: State health departments.

otitis media: Middle ear infection.

osteoporosis: A bone disease characterized by a reduction of bone mass and deterioration of the microarchitecture of bone leading to bone fragility.

outbreak: A sudden increase in disease occurrence. *See* EPIDEMIC.

ozone (O_3): Also known as ground-level ozone. A form of oxygen that is a highly reactive gas resulting from the chemical reaction of sunlight on hydrocarbons and nitrogen oxides emitted in fossil fuel combustion.

pandemic: A wide geographic distribution of an epidemic.

particulate matter (PM 10): A complex and varying mixture of substances that includes carbon-based particles, dust, and acid aerosols that are emitted primarily from transportation sources.

passive immunity: The borrowing of antibodies from another host or from a serological preparation.

Pasteur, Louis: A French chemist and microbiologist who is most well known for his contributions to immunizations. Also known as the parent of vaccines.

pasteurization: The process of ridding milk products and other liquids of unhealthy microorganisms through parital sterilization.

pathogenicity: The ability of a biological agent to produce signs and symptoms of disease.

pathological: An anatomical or functional manifestation of disease.

pellagra: A disease associated with a deficiency of niacin resulting in general weakness, lowered appetite, skin and mucous membrane inflammation, gastrointestinal problems, and emotional discomfort.

people with disabilities: Persons identified as having activity limitations or who use assistance in normal everyday activity.

periodicity: A time characteristic of disease distribution in which cases recur during intervals.

period incidence rate: Calculated using new cases of disease occurring during a specified length of time, usually a year or greater. *See also* INCIDENCE RATE *and* GENERIC RATE FORMULA.

person characteristics: Inherited qualities or personal activities that determine who is at risk for disease and other morbid conditions.

person, place, and time characteristics: Detailed levels or features of the sufficiency factors to disease.

pertussis: A severe bacterial infection of the upper respiratory tract, also known as whooping cough.

pfisteria: Protozoan infection of fish usually occurring in algae-rich, oxygen-depleted waters containing elevated levels of nitrogen and phosphorus.

pharyngitis: A sore throat caused by inflammation of the pharynx.

phenylketonuria: An amino acid enzyme deficiency disorder.

physical agents of disease: Natural or human-made features of the physical environment that also act as pollutants.

physical environment: Naturally or human-made structures and conditions of our surroundings.

place characteristics: Inherent in the three kinds of environments: physical, biological, and sociocultural.

point incidence rate: Incidence rate calculated using new cases of disease occurrences during a specified length of time, usually less than a year. *See* GENERIC RATE FORMULA.

point source: The originating site of exposure.

pollutants: Chemical agents that degrade environmental quality and threaten personal and public health.

postexposure prophylaxis: Inoculating a person to bring about passive immunity.

prevalence: The number of instances of a given disease or condition in a given population at a designated time.

prevalence rate: A morbidity rate calculated using existing cases of a disease. *See* GENERIC RATE FORMULA.

prevalence study: Begins while a disease is presently occurring.

primary prevention: Disease or morbid condition prevention program which targets subjects at low health risk.

principle: The relationship between two or more concepts that acts as a rule of understanding.

principle of causality: A rule of understanding the cause of infectious and noninfectious disease.

problem solving: A principle applied to epidemiological investigations and studies that consists of five steps: (1) determine the problem, (2) study the problem, (3) suggest solution, (4) test solution, and (5) evaluate solution.

program: An organized response to undesirable health and disease conditions and situations.

program evaluation: This involves efforts at improving as well as proving the efficacy of the program.

program implementation: Initiating and maintaining intervention activity.

program planning: Assessing needs of a target group, composing goals and objectives, and designing the intervention.

propagated epidemic: When each case of a disease or morbid condition was exposed to a different source host.

prophylactic trial: Operates at the primary prevention level and targets subjects at low health risk.

proportionate mortality: The number of deaths from a specific cause per 100 in a selected group of persons.

prospective study: Begins before the disease has occurred and follows a group of persons into the future assessing subjects of risk exposure and disease occurrence.

protective factor: Any factor (e.g., healthy life practice) that decreases the possibility of morbidity or death.

protozoa: Microscopic single-cell parasites.

public health agencies: Organizations with a mission of protecting and promoting the population's health and environment by assuring safe food and water, adequate sanitation, preventive health services delivery, and formulation of relevant legislation, all within the context of disease prevention and control.

puerperal fever: Also known as "childbed" fever; systematic bacterial infection of the body.

pyelonephritis: Kidney infection.

quality-adjusted life years: A measure of wellness in a person's estimated remaining years of life.

quarantine: A disease control strategy involving detaining and isolating known source hosts from potential hosts.

quasiexperimental design: Study design in which subject selection/assignment was nonrandom. Those not receiving the treatment are sometimes called the comparison group.

rabies: A highly virulent viral disease that is usually transmitted from animal to human host. *See LYSSAVIRUS.*

radon: A colorless, odorless gas that is a product of decaying uranium and occurs naturally in soil and rock. As radon gas breaks down it becomes a respiratory tract carcinogen.

Ramazzini, Bernardino: A seventeenth-century Italian physician, considered the parent of occupational medicine.

ratio: Calculated using the generic formula, measured against 100. Technically, persons representing the numerator should not be contained within the denominator. A ratio is generally used to calculate risk compared to a rate that is used to express disease occurrence. *See* GENERIC RATE FORMULA.

recovery: Process in which the host returns to a normal state of function.

relative risk: The incidence rate of disease in exposed persons divided by incidence rate of disease in nonexposed persons.

research design: A predetermined procedure and method that researchers utilize during a study.

reservoir: A medium for storage and growth of a biological agent (e.g., humans or animals, the physical environment).

retrospective study: A study that begins after a disease has occurred.

Reye syndrome: A rare brain condition that can follow some cases of chicken pox and other viral diseases, especially when younger patients are given aspirin.

rhinitis: The common cold.

rickettsia: A kind of bacteria once considered a mix of virus and bacteria whose infectivity, pathogenicity, and especially virulence usually require health care intervention (e.g., Lyme Disease).

risk: The possibility of a group of persons experiencing morbidity or mortality.

risk factor: Any factor to which persons are exposed to that increases the possibility of morbidity (illness) or mortality (death).

Rocky Mountain spotted fever: A tickborne rickettsial disease that causes fever, rash, and discomfort. Cases cluster along the East Coast and south central part of the United States.

Sabin, Albert: Discovered the oral polio vaccine.

Sager, Ruth: A twentieth-century geneticist who pioneered breast cancer research.

Salk, Jonas: Discovered the injected polio vaccine.

scarlet fever: A streptococcal infection that starts as a sore throat and can progress to rheumatic heart disease.

sciatica: A painful condition of the legs due to inflammation of the sciatic nerve from musculoskeletal stress.

scientific notion of disease: Biological, physical, and social environments are considered the likeliest causes for morbidity and mortality. This notion represents the start of epidemiological reasoning.

scurvy: Nutritional deficiency of citric acid (vitamin C).

secondary attack rate: An expression of incidence in which anyone exposed to the first case of a disease is included in the denominator of the rate calculation. *See* GENERIC RATE FORMULA.

secondary prevention: A disease or morbid condition prevention program which focuses on persons at high health risk.

secular trend: A long-term trend of disease or death rates of at least one year, though usually comprised of ten years.

Semmelweis, Ignaz Philipp: Known as the parent of infection control because of his work in antisepsis.

serologic laboratory test: A range of measurements of blood and plasma-related protein molecules indicative of immune defense activity.

Shattuck, Lemuel: A leader in community-based disease control and therefore deserving of the honor, parent of U.S. public health.

sickle-cell anemia: A genetic disorder that forms abnormal hemoglobin and limits the capacity of red blood cells to carry oxygen. Occurs more prevalently in the African-American and selected Mediterranian populations.

signs: Objective indicators of disease based on professional observation.

sinusitis: Inflammation of the sinus.

Snow, John: Known as the parent of modern epidemiology for investigating cholera outbreaks in nineteenth-century England.

social agents of disease: Human-made features of the social environment that are experienced by groups of persons.

sociocultural environment: Human-made conventions and constructs of our surroundings.

solid waste: Refuse from households, agriculture, and businesses.

spiritual health: One's state of health as affected by transcending material existence and interconnecting with others.

spiritual notion of disease: Mystical explanations of morbidity.

spontaneous generation: An early belief that unhealthy environmental conditions automatically created germs and vermin.

spot mapping: Physically marking the locations of disease cases according to geographic areas on a map.

spurious relationship: Unauthentic relationship of agent, risk factor, and disease with regard to disease causation.

standard population: Any population used during rate adjustments.

standardized mortality (or morbidity) ratio: Observed cases divided by estimated cases and multiplied by 100.

Stern, Elizabeth: Canadian-born researcher known for her work in cytopathology.

strain: A genetic variety.

St. Vitus' dance: Chorea characterized by a lack of coordination and spasmodic movement that develops after a staphylococcus bacterial infection.

study: Research on the distribution and cause of disease, as well as on interventions to prevent and treat disease and other morbid conditions.

subclinical phase: Pathological changes are taking place in a host while subtle signs and symptoms are indicated. *See* LATENCY PERIOD *and* INCUBATION PERIOD.

substance abuse: The inappropriate and/or excessive involvement with a psychoactive substance that results in personal, family, social, and work problems.

suicide: Intentional self-inflicted injury leading to death.

sufficiency factors: Combine with the necessary factor for disease occurrence.

sulfur dioxide: A sulfur-oxygen compound produced as a result of fossil fuel combustion; represents of form of air pollution.

surveillance: The monitoring of a population's illness and death through data collection, analysis, interpretation, and reporting.

susceptibility stage: When agent, host, and environment factors are conducive to disease occurrence.

Sydenham, Thomas: A seventeenth-century physician and sometimes called the English Hippocrates. He was an intense observer of illness by meticulously recording details of disease.

symptoms: Subjective interpretations of feeling ill.

synergy (in occupational disease): When one agent works in conjunction with another agent to cause disease.

syphilis: A bacterial sexually transmitted disease that enters the body through skin breaks and has a high pathogenicity and virulence.

tamoxifen: An antiestrogen drug used for treating and preventing malignancy.

tar: A known carcinogen found in tobacco products.

taxonomy of disease: An orderly classification of diseases into appropriate categories on the basis of relationships among them.

Tay-Sachs disease: A rare genetic disease causing neurological damage and death, primarily occurs in infants of eastern European Jewish descent.

T cells: Lymphocytes produced in the thymus gland.

tertiary prevention: A disease and morbid condition prevention program that focuses on treatment of current disease cases.

therapeutic trial: Operates at the tertiary level of prevention and targets subjects who are disease cases.

thermal water pollutant: Water used in a manufacturing or other process that has been heated and returned to its source before cooling.

time (factor): A continuum of past, present, and future events comprising a disease occurrence.

time characteristics: Incubation and/or latency time, length of disease process, time of occurrence, and trends and cycles.

tinnitus: Ringing or buzzing in ears.

toxic shock syndrome: A systemic bacterial infection caused by exposure to a *Staphylococcus aureus*-based toxin.

toxic substances: Chemical agents distinguished by their poisonous, corrosive, or flammable nature.

traumatic brain injury (TBI): A syndrome of signs and symptoms such as headaches, sleep disturbances, and inability to concentrate that are indicative of a range of neurological damage from mild (impaired written and verbal test-taking abilities) to severe (long-term disability and death).

trial: An experimental study on the effectiveness of an intervention with regard to treating or preventing disease.

tuberculosis: A severe bacterial infection of the respiratory tract that is generally fatal unless successfully treated.

two-by-two table: Table composed of four squares that is used to analyze the relationship between agent exposure and disease.

typhus: A severe rickettsial infection causing fever, malaise, and body aches.

vaccine: A means of eliciting active immunity through inoculation.

van Leewenhoek, Antonie: Considered the parent of microbiology, he invented the first microscope used to detect bacteria and protozoa.

varicella (chicken pox): A contagious viral disease common in children. Symptoms include fever and lethargy, which is followed by an itchy blisterlike rash on the body.

vector: An animate transmitter of an agent (e.g., arthropod, rodent).

vehicle: An inanimate object that transmits an agent. Sometimes called a FOMITE.

vermin: Rodent carriers of disease.

virulence: The ability of a biological agent to produce severe, possibly life-threatening signs and symptoms in a host.

viruses: Submicroscopic parasites that reproduce within the cells of their hosts, upon which they depend for vital life processes.

vital statistics: Collected, analyzed, and summarized data on major life events—births, deaths, marriages, and divorces.

World Health Organization (WHO): A United Nations agency located in Zurich, Switzerland, that conducts worldwide public health campaigns.

yaws: A bacterial (spirochete) infection indistinguishable from syphilis except for its typical mode of transmission—contaminated water.

years of healthy living: The extent and duration (in years) of a person's ability to perform activities of daily living.

years of life lived: The actual number of years (including partial year) a person lives and is the unit of measurement used in mortality rates.

years of potential life lost: Calculated at time of death by subtracting a person's actual age in years from his or her expected length of life in years.

yellow fever: A viral disease spread by a mosquito which causes fever, chills, muscle aches, and possible death.

zoonosis: A disease acquired by a human from any other vertebrate animal.

Index

Page numbers followed by the letter "f" indicate figures; those followed by the letter "t" indicate tables.

Order a copy of this book with this form or online at:
http://www.haworthpressinc.com/store/product.asp?sku=4633

EPIDEMIOLOGY FOR HEALTH PROMOTION AND DISEASE PREVENTION PROFESSIONALS

_____ in hardbound at $69.95 (ISBN: 0-7890-1598-6)

_____ in softbound at $44.95 (ISBN: 0-7890-1599-4)

COST OF BOOKS_____

OUTSIDE USA/CANADA/
MEXICO: ADD 20%____

POSTAGE & HANDLING_____
*(US: $4.00 for first book & $1.50
for each additional book)
Outside US: $5.00 for first book
& $2.00 for each additional book)*

SUBTOTAL_____

in Canada: add 7% GST____

STATE TAX____
*(NY, OH & MIN residents, please
add appropriate local sales tax)*

FINAL TOTAL____
*(If paying in Canadian funds,
convert using the current
exchange rate, UNESCO
coupons welcome.)*

☐ **BILL ME LATER:** ($5 service charge will be added)
(Bill-me option is good on US/Canada/Mexico orders only;
not good to jobbers, wholesalers, or subscription agencies.)

☐ Check here if billing address is different from
shipping address and attach purchase order and
billing address information.

☐ Signature_____

☐ **PAYMENT ENCLOSED: $**_____

☐ **PLEASE CHARGE TO MY CREDIT CARD.**

☐ Visa ☐ MasterCard ☐ AmEx ☐ Discover
☐ Diner's Club ☐ Eurocard ☐ JCB

Account # _____

Exp. Date_____

Signature_____

Prices in US dollars and subject to change without notice.

NAME_____

INSTITUTION_____

ADDRESS_____

CITY_____

STATE/ZIP_____

COUNTRY_____ COUNTY (NY residents only)_____

TEL_____ FAX_____

E-MAIL_____

May we use your e-mail address for confirmations and other types of information? ☐Yes ☐No
We appreciate receiving your e-mail address and fax number. Haworth would like to e-mail or fax special
discount offers to you, as a preferred customer. **We will never share, rent, or exchange your e-mail address
or fax number.** We regard such actions as an invasion of your privacy.

Order From Your Local Bookstore or Directly From
The Haworth Press, Inc.
10 Alice Street, Binghamton, New York 13904-1580 • USA
TELEPHONE: 1-800-HAWORTH (1-800-429-6784) / Outside US/Canada: (607) 722-5857
FAX: 1-800-895-0582 / Outside US/Canada: (607) 722-6362
E-mail: getinfo@haworthpressinc.com
PLEASE PHOTOCOPY THIS FORM FOR YOUR PERSONAL USE.
www.HaworthPress.com

BOF02